Partner... Parents and Teachers: ...ent

Parents and Teachers: Partners in Language Development

Audrey Ann Simmons-Martin, Ed.D.
Karen Glover Rossi, M.A.

Foreword by S. Richard Silverman, Ph.D.
Director Emeritus,
Central Institute for the Deaf

Alexander Graham Bell Association for the Deaf
3417 Volta Place, N.W. • Washington, D.C. 20007

Library of Congress Cataloging in Publication Data

Simmons-Martin, Audrey Ann and Rossi, Karen Glover
Parents and Teachers:
Partners in Language Development

Library of Congress catalog card number 90-081334
ISBN 0-88200-167-1
© 1990 Alexander Graham Bell Association for the Deaf
3417 Volta Place, N.W.
Washington, D.C. 20007

Printed in the United States of America
10 9 8 7 6 5 4 3 2 1

iv

Foreword

The pages that follow constitute a comprehensive in-depth tutorial for parent-teacher partnership in fostering language development in young hearing-impaired children.

It is an impressive piece of work which should prove valuable to parents, parent-teachers and pre-school teachers.

As we read we are struck by the admirable manner in which Audrey Simmons-Martin and Karen Rossi have fashioned a felicitous combination of developmental theory and the fruits of a rich and long experience on the firing line in practicing what they recommend.

Their experience is distilled into a crystal-clear rationale with numerous scenarios that outline the roles of parents and teachers. The problem of language acquisition in layman's terms is important reading. The attention to the child's perception of meaning is noteworthy. With that focus the reader is advanced from procedures for family-centered teaching to child-oriented procedures. We note not only that the authors have been moved to apply the results of the burgeoning investigative activity in language description and language learning, but they recognize here and there, perhaps unconsciously, the impact of increasing research, even far back into infancy, of early perception and cognition. In doing so they stress the importance of focusing on the parents. Only to the extent to which the parent is "engrossed" in the child's development will more benefit accrue to the linguistic and overall communicative behavior of the child. While the level of literacy of a parent may influence the benefit to be derived from this book, the authors caution teachers to take account of this in communicating background rationale and constructive implementation. The fundamental message is that the parent and, of course, the teacher should be at all times mindful of the child's capabilities and not to underestimate them. This mind-set is indispensable if the teacher-parent partnership is to exploit fully and optimally the sound premises, this practical guidance and the clearly stated procedures offered by Simmons-Martin and Rossi.

S. Richard Silverman, Ph.D.
Director Emeritus, Central Institute for the Deaf

Contents

Foreword v
Contents vii
Preface xi
Notes to Reader xiii
Acknowledgements xv
Part I - Rationale
Chapter 1   The Child 1
               Talking 3
               Language 5
               Learning Environment 6
               Implications 8
               The Home 8
               Summary 12
Chapter 2   The Parents 15
               Parent Types 17
               Fathers 19
               The "Super Mother's" Role 20
               Parents' Role in Language Acquisition . . . 23
               Parent Intervention 24
               Parents of Hearing-Impaired Children:
                 Specific Factors 25
               Phases of Reaction to Diagnosis 28
               The Family 31
               Summary 34
Chapter 3   The Child Has Much to Learn 37
               1. Prelude to Language 39
               2. Language at the Prelinguistic Level . . . 43
               3. Fundamentals of Language 45
               4. Actual Language Begins 48
               5. Language Becomes Sophisticated 52
Chapter 4   The Parent Has Much to Learn 55
               1. Nurture the Child 57
               2. Tune in to the Child 62
               3. Talk *to* the Child 70
               4. Talk *for* the Child 79
               5. Talk *with* the Child 90

Chapter 5   Hear Ye! Hear Ye! More to Do! 97
               Early Detection 97
               Hearing 98
               Hearing Speech 99
               Critical Period of Learning 100
               Acoustic Facts 101
               Hearing Is Learned Behavior 102
               The Ear 104
               Hearing Aids 107
               Parent Objectives for Auditory Training . . 108
               Speech Perception Through Lipreading . . . 113
               Summary 116
Chapter 6   The Teacher 117
               Task of the Professional 117
               Role of the Professional 119
               Personal Qualities of Interveners 120
               Teacher Preparation 121
               Planning and Teaching 123
               Individual Curriculum Development . . . 126
               Summary 131
Chapter 7   Then There Is Language 133
               Language 135
               Phonology 137
               Morphology 141
               Syntax 142
               Semantics 148
               Conclusion 155
               Code Learning 155
Chapter 8   Preschool 159
               Auditory-Global 161
               Strategies 163
               Activities 174
               Techniques 191
               Summary 196
References 197

Part II - Implementation
Introduction to Part II 201
Area A   Nurture the Child 203
Area B   Tune In to the Child 233

Area C   Talk *To* the Child 255
Area D   Talk *For* the Child 275
Area E   Talk *With* the Child 295
Area F   Hearing Aid Use 315
Area G   Structuring the Environment 327
Area H   Awareness of Sound 339
Area I   Awareness of Speech 347
Area J   Auditory Recognition 357
Area K   Structuring the Visual Environment 365
Area L   Parents' Speech Patterns 373
Recommended Readings 385

Preface

Language development begins with bonding at birth and continues through concept growth in the classroom. An explanation of this phenomena is the basis of this book. The text is grounded in developmental theory and oriented to the principle that competent children are reared by capable parents and encouraged by knowledgeable teachers.

The essence of every child's achievement is the ability to communicate. Developing competency in spoken communication is the authors' focus. Meaningful interaction with the child is the objective.

Language acquisition is a complex process, extremely sensitive to differences in the child's early experiences, parents' rearing patterns and teacher's perception of individual needs. It is that environment that the authors want to influence parents and teachers to develop.

It is a well-established fact that the time from birth to six is crucial for the mastering of the "mother tongue". Infancy is so important that the child's parents must be his teachers. Their teaching comes from their daily contacts and routines within the child's own environment. Through loving, caring, interacting, talking, responding, reinforcing, playing and modeling the parents teach their child in the early months and years to communicate.

The authors see the development as following definite growth patterns, albeit at different rates. The growth proceeds along a relatively smooth continuum. At the earliest stage the process is parent-centered but it advances to a child-centered program. The vehicle children use to achieve competency is *MEANING*. The child must perceive the meaning and from it learn the language that clothes it.

That all children have the necessary potential for acquiring language is the thrust of the book. As the skills are discussed, it is readily apparent that the authors believe that early and continuous use of amplification is necessary for the deaf child. Both hearing and vision are essential even though the child may have minimal sensory ability. Parents and teachers must train the sense modalities to take in the maximum of which the child is capable.

The threefold purposes of this book are: 1) To give parents knowledge about language; 2) to help the professionals who assist the parents; and 3) to help the teachers who work with the children as they acquire language.

We visualize the professionals as *partners* who guide and synchronize with the parents. Both members of the partnership, the family on one hand and the professional on the other, must see appropriate steps, have identical goals and perceive the means for achieving the goal. The child benefits from a harmonious partnership.

Given the rationale, theory and procedures delineated in *Parents and Teachers: Partners in Language Development*, the parents and the professionals can originate their own ideas which are conducive to their life and teaching style. The more engrossed they become, the greater and longer lasting are the child's gains.

Factors to be considered in determining the parents' ability to benefit from guidance are the ways they learn and the degree of their involvement. Nevertheless, parents with *help* can all become "super parents."

Notes to the Reader

In order to minimize the confusion with the personal pronouns he/she, him/her, and she/he/they in referring to the child and his parents, the authors have chosen to refer to the child as "he" or "him." The parent will be referred to as "the mother" or "parent," and by the feminine pronouns, "she" or "her." References to the teacher will also be in the feminine gender "she" or "her."

Since the procedures described in the text are applicable to children with or without a hearing loss, the degree of hearing is not critical. Therefore, we have used the terms "hearing-impaired" and "deaf" to refer to hearing losses across the spectrum, from mild to profound. This does not mean that we do not have a great respect for every decibel of hearing a child has, but the procedures would remain as described.

Acknowledgements

The first author, Audrey Ann Simmons-Martin, would personally like to thank the wonderful staff that worked with her throughout the years at Central Institute for the Deaf. Through their dedication and untiring efforts they contributed much to the knowledge in teaching deaf infants and children and their families. In particular, she would like to thank: Mary Lou Koelkebeck, Phyllis Britt, Phyllis Rudman, and Rosemarie Smith.

Dr. Martin would also like to thank her husband, James Anthony Martin, who has given his continuing assistance, encouragement, and understanding so generously.

Karen Rossi wishes to thank her husband, Charlie, and their three children, Jennifer, Nicole, and Brian, for their patience during the writing of this book. She also thanks her parents for a lifetime of encouragement.

The authors express appreciation to Sister Joyce Buckler, Ed.D. Principal of St. Joseph Institute for the Deaf, for her valuable editorial comments.

PART I
RATIONALE

Chapter 1

The Child

A rose is a rose, so they say. With no hesitation we paraphrase — "A child is a child is a child." Although each rose differs from other roses in color, size, strength, perfume and type, it is more like other roses than different. Similarly, each child, while unique, is at the same time very like other children. As a child, each individual will advance through the sequences of development all children will experience. No child proceeds in a hit-and-miss pattern, but progresses at a relatively smooth pace even though the timing may vary. The exact time the new growth or development takes place is not nearly as important as what the parents and the child do to achieve maximally at each of these stages.

All children follow the same sequences of development physically, socially, emotionally, and mentally. So it is with the hearing-impaired child. He, too, is a CHILD, who is like other children. He just happens not to hear as well.

Physically, the baby will raise his arms and legs before he raises his body to sit. He will roll from side to side before he stands. He will crawl on his hands and knees before he takes steps. He can walk around in a playpen before he anchors to furniture or people. He walks independently before he climbs; goes up steps before he jumps. Such is the pattern for all children with or without a hearing impairment.

Too, there are sequences in every child's social development. He watches the adult's face before he responds to smiles. He responds to smiles before voices. He accepts his parent or caregiver before he tolerates strangers. In fact, he is apt to cry when approached by a stranger too quickly or too closely. He learns to get attention by whining, cooing or some "verbal-like" effort. Eventually, he advances to verbal expression for his feelings of anger, joy, displeasure, and happiness.

Cognitive or mental development is more difficult to trace

1

because it depends upon so many variables — the child's curiosity, his sensorimotor experiences, and most critically language, the topic of this text. Importantly, these cognitive factors can be stimulated, encouraged and trained. Regrettably, children who do not receive the needed assistance in development proceed much more slowly along the expected continuum.

All the experiences a child has assist him in his cognitive development. He moves from exploring his smaller world, by following a moving object with his eyes, to handling the object and taking it apart, to sharing in the universal world of knowledge. This movement depends heavily upon what adults do *with* the child during these critical stages. Teaching him the labels for things and experiences becomes the tool with which the child stores information while new concepts are added. On the other hand, a child may spend his life just seeing the whole object never knowing that it has parts; that it can do things; that it can change. He needs to experience that the teddy bear has a nose, eyes, a mouth and ears and "lo and behold!" so does Mommy and so does he. A child observes the wholeness before he sees the details, but without attention, he may never know the various parts.

Fortunately, there are innumerable texts or manuals available to the reader on the topic of child growth and development. Therefore, this text shall not perseverate on this topic, but refer the reader to the materials listed later.

Along with child development materials, there has been a proliferation of parenting "primers" which are being bought and read in increasing numbers. Almost all parents have read at least one or more books plus the articles published on this subject in magazines, newspapers and pamphlets. The most well-known is, of course, *Baby and Child Care* (Spock 1976) which has sold over twenty-eight million copies. Over a half million have been sold of each of the other classics: *How to Parent* (Dodson 1970) and *Between Parent and Child* (Ginot 1965). Recently, there has been effort to show parents how to stimulate development. Foremost among these authors are White (1975), Church (1973) and Bettleheim (1987).

One of the problems with child-care materials, however, is the seeming disregard for individual differences in family circumstances. Most often the experts offer parents and teachers guidelines, rules, and blanket suggestions as if they are equally applicable and appropriate for every family. Experts seem to assume that there is an ideal kind of child and one set of rules to produce the achievement in every child in every family. One must not lose track of the fact that each child is unique and has his own timetable of development which must be aided by his environment. While the child will proceed through the expected developmental stages, he will nevertheless perform at his own rate. The absolutes are:

1. Children follow the same developmental stages whether they hear or not.

2. Every child is unique and follows the pattern of development on his own time schedule.

3. Children need stimulation from the environment to move successfully along the continuum.

4. No child can develop in a vacuum.

Talking

Of all the developmental skills a child masters, learning to talk is the most difficult and the most marvelous. Unlike learning to sit, to crawl, or to walk, a child cannot learn to talk without close parental bonding, multiple examples, and patient teaching from the adults who surround him. The same is even more true for a child with a hearing impairment.

Talking implies oral language. The word "oral" with all of its derivations, has many connotations in professional and nonprofessional circles. To avoid the problem in semantics, perhaps we should define what the authors mean by "oral," "oralism," "orally," etc. To the authors, it is a way of life, a philosophy, yet also a process. "Oralism" is not something given to a hearing-impaired child within the confines of a classroom. Unlike reading, math, social studies, or spelling, it is not something that can be tutored. It is not something that can be packaged into a period of the day, regardless of the length of time. Drills and exercises can sharpen some parts of the act, i.e., articulation and phrasing, but without all of the components, such activities do not help the child to become "oral."

"Oral" means to be able to *speak* the "mother tongue." This linguistic act is made up of the components of phonation, pronunciation, articulation, intonation, rhythm, vocabulary, grammar, word order, and sentences. More important than any of its parts, talk is made up of *ideas*, of *meanings*. It is the *thought* emanating from the *speaker's mind* being transmitted to the *mind of the listener*. The thought in the mind of the speaker may be a description, a label, predications, relationships, associations, solutions to problems, and the like. The content may be a single word or many sentences relating more ideas, but always it is *meaningful* both to the speaker and the listener. It is an exchange of ideas in real-life situations.

This exchange of ideas must be in the same *mode of communication*. Contrary to some current opinion, deaf children do not do better when learning signs and speech simultaneously. As reported by Westerhouse (1988), Geers and Moog found conclusive evidence to this effect after studying three hundred profoundly deaf children. Some of the one hundred fifty children from Total Communication programs were learning to sign but were not learning to talk as well as those in oral programs. Furthermore, they were not learning to sign English at any higher level than the one hundred fifty orally educated children learning to speak English. They stated emphatically that "there was no evidence that showed a profoundly deaf child could be taught to sign and speak and do both well." (Westerhouse, 1988, p. 1)

The task of speech is to communicate and/or exchange ideas with parents, siblings, teachers, neighbors, and friends. The communicator needs to understand the messages spoken to him and then in turn respond by sending his own message. Communication involves turn-taking which parents do very early in the cooing play with infants. Baby says, "Gee, gee, gee" and the adult responds, "Gee, gee, yes, I hear you saying, 'Gee, gee'." Communication involves relating one idea to another which parents do when they say sentences about the child's toys, food, clothes and the many other objects and activities in his immediate environment. For example, the parent sees the child looking at his toy car and she says, "That's your car. It's your little red car. Can you make it go?" It is, of course, the content of communication which is important, *not* the specific language.

Too often, teachers talk about receptive language and then list words. Next, they discuss expressive language and list more words. To be sure, receptive language is an auditory (and visual) event while expressive language is the spoken form; however, the *message* is what is being exchanged, not lists of words. The *form* of the language used to express ideas or receive ideas is identical to that used to receive ideas. Receptive and expressive language are not two distinct entities but rather the spoken and listening events in transmitting thoughts and ideas.

Language

It is imperative that one is aware of the fact that the transmission of messages is the most abstract activity in which a child can be involved. Application of Einstein's theory pales in comparison to the successful use of language to decode the ideas of others and encode the meanings we wish to express.

How is language abstract? Take the word "big" for example. What mental image does this concept project? There are numerous words which can be used with "big;" however, the term can be applied only after being processed through the listener's complete network of concepts. These three simple letters represent a concept of bigness which varies according to the noun it modifies. An elephant is big, but a roach can also be big. Some babies are big; so are some adults. Some cookies are big, though few cakes really are. So the abstraction of the meaning of "big" is a generalized characteristic of "bigness" rather than its relation of one item to another.

The mental picture varies even more for such concrete words as "shoe." "Shoe" represents the object worn by a child, but it can also be worn by an adult and yes, even horses. It can be hightop, laced, slipped on, with or without heels. The word "shoe," then, represents something all of the objects have in common. The child's task is to abstract out of all these experiences that *shoes are worn on feet.*

What does a child abstract from the word, "ball" — its shape? a baseball? a football? a golf ball? a beachball? Does he abstract its function — to play with? to hit? to roll? to bounce? "Ball" is an abstraction and the meaning is signaled by words such as: throw, bounce, spin, toss, catch, hit, or pitch. These are needed in order for the child to decode the message: "The catcher missed the low ball."

Thus, we could go on and on about the abstractness of meaning of the symbols, i.e., *"Push"* is different from *"Pull"* because of the *action* represented. To do something *in an hour* is quite different from the concept of doing something *on the hour*. Concepts are the essence of language. It is impossible to delineate the concepts a child will encounter. The number is infinite. Try listing them for just fifteen minutes of a conversational day! What is of utmost importance is that adults are aware of the complexity of concepts a child is expected to develop.

Learning Environment

How does a child learn the concepts necessary to decode the language he receives and encodes for expressing himself? He learns them by being involved. He learns by handling things, seeing what happens to them, playing with them, having fun with them while, at the same time, the *concepts are being labeled.*

It is in the home that the child takes his first step. This event needs to be accompanied by language. He tumbles. This needs to be verbalized. He becomes physically involved with his toys, his body (especially his feet and fingers), his mother's pots and pans, his food and all of the milieu that surrounds him. He is curious. Exploring his environment needs to be encouraged. A safe home allows the freedom necessary to explore. It is at home that:

He tastes things — "bitter," sweet," sour."

He feels things — "soft," "hard," "rough."

He sees things — "big," "tiny," "small."

He meets friends and relatives — "Aunt Jane," "Uncle Joe."

He encounters pets — "puppy," "kitty," "gerbil."

He plays with toys and people.

He identifies and expresses his feelings and emotions.

By constant repetition, a child can learn combinations of things which he will eventually pair or categorize. He sees that "shoe and sock," "coat and hat," "cup and saucer," are usually paired. Someone puts the bananas, apples and oranges in the same bowl. Someday, if the family refers to them verbally, he will learn that those are categorized as "fruit," whereas carrots, celery, and potatoes are "vegetables." When asked if he wants a drink, he will eventually learn that milk, orange juice, soda and even Daddy's coffee are in the same category.

Certainly, he can learn that things are "all gone," or "almost ready" as he experiences situations many times a day. Other cognitive experiences abound in the home — "hot," "melt," "freeze." Things "dissolve," "absorb," "float," etc. As a child's whole person experiences his daily world, all of these concepts need to be labeled for storage. Retrieval of the concepts and the associated language will be made by the child in not too many years.

In the home, the child — *all of him* — experiences first hand things that lead to his physical, emotional, sensory, cognitive, and linguistic development. Fortunately, these experiences occur over and over. If language is associated with them, the learning situation is ideal. *First-hand experiences with much repetition is a given rule in the process of learning.*

Basic to this development and learning is the parents' or caregivers' style of "teaching." This governs language development. Under no circumstances do the experts in language development (the psycholinguists) think of that "teaching" as something done with certain materials at given times in a day. At no time do they even consider that the process of learning to speak the "mother tongue" can be accomplished between the hours of eight o'clock and three o'clock; five days a week; or for thirty-two weeks per year, or for that matter in an academic setting. Psycholinguists are unanimous in their thinking that real language learning goes on hour in and hour out *from the instant of birth — in the home.*

It is not by accident that the term "mother tongue" has been given to the first language learned and spoken by the child. When both parents are present in the home, it is usually the mother who is with the child most of the time and whose influence upon the child tends to be greater. It is the female who most often serves as the primary model for the child's attempts at imitation of language patterns. It is fortunate though, for the hearing-impaired child that fathers are now taking a more active role in their child's development. The acoustic characteristics of male voices are excellent for children with poor auditory reception. More of the auditory clues are available to the child when the father is the speaker rather than the mother. The acquisition of language by the child is essentially a learning process dependent upon feedback between parent and child — ideally both parents.

This process of language acquisition is three-dimensional. At first it is the child initiating "conversation" followed by the parent responding with tangible reinforcement. In his early days, for example, the infant cries. While it is difficult to always know what the baby's crying means, the adult quickly responds and usually can comfort the child with a dry diaper, a warm bottle or even just the comfort of cuddling. Importantly, this gets accompanied by "sweet talk:"

> What's the matter with Johnny?
> Oh, your diaper is wet!
> Here's the dry diaper.
> There we go!

Whenever the baby cries, the adult attempts to alleviate his discomfort. He coos and Mother comes and smiles and probably pats him. If the baby babbles, it is good for the parent to encourage him by joining in or imitating him in fun, so that in turn, the baby imitates the adult. In any event, he learns that vocalization pays off. His vocal efforts move people! Importantly, there is feeling in the adult's voice; there is warmth in the handling of him. The baby feels this warmth. The adult is telling him, "I LOVE YOU." It is so important that all early talk is positive in nature, that it not be, "Don't do that!" "No!" "I don't like that!" On the contrary, baby talk is "love talk." Love is the critical nature of the dialogue between parent and child. This interchange has a flavor all its own, and though the child doesn't understand all of the talk, he feels it and feels good about himself.

Implications

Regardless of the age of the child when the initiation of language learning is begun, the adult (perhaps the teacher) needs to make sure that:
1. vocalization or utterances pay off for the child;
2. the rudimentary semantic content of crying and cooing are recognized from the very beginning;
3. appropriate language is applied to all situations; and
4. the affective content of the adult's response is warm and positive — loaded, as it were, with messages that spell love in its intonation pattern.

The Home

The ideal place for all interaction is the child's own home. While in the home there are usually kitchens, family rooms, bedrooms, and bathrooms; there are no talking or listening rooms. Talking and listening (receptive and expressive language) are not confined to one area or to a special room. These processes are part of the setting, the home, where thoughts and ideas are converted to words and eventually shared with others.

The features of the home environment are readily perceived by the child through the senses. Too, these perceptual features have verbal labels associated with them which, in time, assist in the storage of the language (e.g., vocabulary) and the concepts. The concepts and vocabulary that develop from the child's perceptions are part of his actual experiences. Through multiple experiences with features in common, and with which similar language is mediated, a child's concepts develop. Through this process, language is absorbed. In this way, the child receives data from which to induce his linguistic rules. For example, "washing" (like previously mentioned labels) is a concept which has various linguistic forms:

> wash hands
> wash face, hair
> wash someone else's face, hands, etc.
> wash dishes, pots, pans, silver
> wash clothes
> wash the car
> wash the dog
> wash the windows
> wash the floors, etc.

The implements in the home are soap, sponge, washcloth, and mop. While the features in common are water, soap, and rubbing action, the most important feature in common is the word "wash." Furthermore, it has long ago been proven that any word (in this instance the word "wash") experienced in a wide variety of situations is more readily learned by the child than the same word experienced many times in only one situation.

Familiar, everyday situations are more conducive to language learning and concept development than any artificial and/or contrived ones in which emphasis is on vocabulary only. Basic perceptual and sensory experiences abound in any home. The home address and its decor, matter not at all. Well-furnished rooms filled with a variety of expensive, meaningless toys do not stimulate. The loving input by caring people in a very modest home is more important than stoic attention in a palace. It has been said:

> A house is made
> Of wood and stone,
> But a home is made
> Of love alone.

Home situations are the ideal learning places for the young child, and parents are the best teachers for a number of reasons. This is so for a variety of obvious reasons:

- Parents know their child better than anyone else. They become aware of his interests and capabilities early in his life.
- Parents or parent surrogates are available all day, everyday, year round. They can be there when the child's interest

level is high and when he is feeling happy. At these times, the child is apt to be cooperative and "ripe" for learning.
- Parents can be there when situations arise that are fun for learning.
- Parents can work with their child on a flexible schedule. They can achieve much when a child is in a receptive mood and wisely drop it when he is too fatigued to pursue it.
- Parents are available for constant repetition about things and happenings that are interesting and therefore important to the child.
- Parents have an edge in offering incentives and rewards. If the child is allowed to stay up a quarter of an hour or so later to "talk" with someone, this privilege will magically be mingled with the delights of talking.

Both the quality as well as the quantity of language input a child receives influences his speech. Children who are exposed to simple but stimulating experiences of day-to-day life achieve greater growth in language than those whose language input is parceled out in scheduled periods of the week with a limited amount of daily close personal contact.

Quality concerns factors such as appropriateness, need, as well as the affective aspect. Learning his "mother tongue" is an abstract and difficult task to be sure, but it is a deeply emotional experience for both members of the dyad, parent and child. This should, and does, increase the joy of sharing and learning.

For the child raised in an environment where the input is restricted, *the emotional content of the communication is of particular significance.* Nonverbal cues will be important ones in obtaining meaning. The real meaning of the messages may be conveyed not only by the words the parent utters, but by the silent language of her facial expressions and general behavior.

The child can quickly perceive without words how his mother feels about things and especially about HIM. Too often, he can interpret the dissatisfaction portrayed in his mother's or teacher's face as dissatisfaction with him. The hearing-impaired child is asked to observe minute movements of the lips and the slightest auditory signal to derive meaning. Yet, a facial expression is many times easier to interpret. He can read meaning into the parent/teacher's posture, the look in her eyes, and her body language much more easily than he can read her lip movements. The parent communicates her love and affection daily in many subtle ways. Hearing-impaired children experience adult affection and support just as their hearing peers do. They, too, enjoy hugs, pats, smiles, winks, and love touches. Hearing-impaired children probably need this positive nonverbal language even more than hearing children because they miss so much of the "love talk" which is auditory rather than visual.

The optimum condition for successful language learning is a continuous and affectionate relationship between parent and child manifested in frequent and appropriate communication. The reciprocity of the interaction is the essence of language learning. It is through interaction that the parent begins her language teaching. When she responds to his utterances, she is a language teacher. She teaches him the first step in expressive language viz. vocalizing pays off. Someone has read his thoughts. The listener has received his message. Conversation has begun!

Parents think so often that language means words. In the early stages, there are no real words and no real grammatical form to the child's language. It is basically pre-linguistic, or before true language has developed. The child's earliest language or communication consists of wiggles, squirms, eye gazes, pointing, hungry cries, painful cries, tired cries, whining, gurgling, and cooing. Although lacking true grammatical form, sounds exist, and they will increase in frequency as the months pass and will begin to take some shape. The point is that through all the sounds, motions, and gestures, THE CHILD IS TELLING HIS WORLD SOMETHING! He doesn't know yet that these sounds signal meaning to the people in his world. Parents learn to interpret these signals, to respond, and thus to assist the child in knowing he is, in fact, communicating.

In order for a child to have functional communication at any age or any stage of development, he must be able to communicate his intent. His intent can be a reaction to physiologic changes in his body. He feels discomfort from the feeling brought about by an empty tummy and he cries. It is through the consistent response and appropriate reaction to this cry by the parents that he begins to learn. He comes to realize his cries are functional and that they communicate specific messages.

Every communication exchange has content. The cry has content, i.e., discomfort. His mother communicates content when she goes to him thereby saying that she will make him feel better. The content of what the child needs to communicate to his parents is that his bodily needs must be satisfied. He needs to be fed, changed, rocked, held, entertained. The way he expresses that is through his cries — his hungry cry, his uncomfortable cry, his angry cry, his bored cry, and his whiney cry. He also communicates his needs through gurgles, coos, babbles and shrieks, waving his arms about, pulling on sleeves, and making faces. These are his first steps to communication. Through the parents' talking, laughter, singing and so forth, the linguistic foundation is being laid.

The adult talks about experiences appropriate to the interest level of the child, always keeping in mind that the young child is still very ego-centered. The adult talks about HERE AND NOW experiences. Since the child at this level is not yet understanding any specific words or sentences, it is imperative that the talk or reciprocal language spoken to him be tied to meaning. In other words, if his mother were changing the child's diaper, she WOULD NOT talk about the little blue bunny that the child left in the playpen in the next room. She WOULD talk about the dirty diaper, the clean diaper, the powder can she is holding in her hand, the child's toes as she shows them to him and so on. She WOULD talk about the food as she feeds him, the water as she bathes him, and the things outside as she takes him for a walk.

By the parent's appropriate and deliberate interaction with the child at varying times throughout the day, she is demonstrating to him that she values these exchanges with him. This happens all day long, not just one or two exchanges, not "lessons" in segmented times, but in natural interactions throughout every day. During these daily interactions, the parent is communicating her messages to her child through language, gestures, facial expressions, the manner in which she holds her child, and the sound of her voice. Since she is not struggling to master a new mode of communication, she can speak naturally, fluently, and spontaneously. These simple things that are often taken for granted are all crucial to the beginnings of communication. It is the total involvement of the child and definite interaction with his parents that furthers his development.

Summary

The goal for the hearing-impaired child is that he function in the real world as a contributing member of his community. This necessitates not only physical, emotional, and social growth, but cognitive and linguistic development as well. The foundation is laid in infancy in the child's own environment and his parents are his very first teachers. They perform the same role as parents the world over, whether the child hears or whether he does not. The steps for learning the "mother tongue" are the same whether it is Swahili or American vernacular. The hearing-impaired child, if given the opportunity, will proceed at his own unique rate in acquiring the linguistic tools necessary for functioning in our society as it is composed today. Reciprocity is the vehicle of learning which parents must master and it is through his total involvement with his environment — socially, emotionally, physically, cognitively, and linguistically — that the child acquires the concepts. The CHILD learns, not just his eyes, tongue or fingers! It is the CHILD to whom parents respond, care for, love, and watch grow into a communicating person.

Chapter 2

The Parents

Recently, education for parents of hearing preschoolers has received enthusiastic support across the country. There is a great deal of optimism about the potential of the parents' role, and numerous programs have been designed to teach and assist parents of normally hearing children. This enthusiasm is the outcome of extensive research in which the home environment was found to be central to the social, cognitive, and linguistic development of children. Researchers' findings have established the fact that the child's experiences in the first three years of life are critical.

When parents were involved in an intensive program with their children before they were enrolled in preschool, these children achieved greater and more enduring gains than children enrolled in child-focused group programs. Although parent programs shared the common goal of getting parents deeply involved with their own children, the variety of programs was considerable. While some focused more on the child than the parent, other groups emphasized the mother's unique role. Very few programs concentrated on the mother-child dyad but rather the focus was on either the parent or the child. Occasionally some projects included the entire family in the educational process. All of these programs were concerned with the non-handicapped child. All unanimously agreed that parents are their child's best teachers.

Educational agencies traditionally had not been enthusiastic about adding the emphasis on increasingly younger children until the research on parent education by Burton White of Brookline, Massachusetts, (White, et. al. 1973) was recognized. It was that research which was implemented by the State of Missouri's Board of Education. Four local school districts, two rural and two urban, initiated a three-year program for parents including home visits and group meetings (Winter, 1985). The findings of the Missouri project were indeed impressive. In all areas, especially in language, these non-handicapped children exceeded the growth of the control group to a statistically significant high level. In the process of the study, parents were assisted in becoming outstanding delivery agents for their hearing children.

Prior to the Missouri project, one of the most recognized evaluations of early education was that of Bronfenbrenner, (1974). He concluded that the strength of the parent-child approach was clearly impressive in terms of productiveness, performance and practicality. Bronfenbrenner generalized that the earlier intervention was begun, the more lasting were its effects. The more involved the parents were in the child's education, the greater and longer lasting were the child's gains. The interactions between the mother and child involved both cognitive and emotional components, which were reinforced by each other. Parent-infant programs that were begun before a child was three years old were far more effective than those begun later.

Historically, however, early intervention programs did not often emphasize the unique capabilities of families. Families were frequently treated as if they were a monolithic group with similar needs, values and abilities. They were considered to be homogeneous as to age, economic and social status, and family structure. The necessary one-to-one, family-to-teacher learning situation was avoided. Consequently, the staffs of these programs developed common models and goals for family involvement.

As a result of Bronfenbrenner's thorough study, he recommended that strong emphasis needed to be placed on the importance of the family and their interaction with their child in relation to a common task rather than the infant, the task, or both. For a program to be successful, Bronfenbrenner stated that it had to be seen as a *parent's* program for *parents* instead of a parent's program for children. This process was shown to be needed in order to enhance the parents' perceptions of themselves as educators of their own children and of their children as individuals capable of independent thought.

This psychologist warned that teachers, through their actions, often devalued the dyadic interaction by demonstrating concern over procedures or materials. When teachers stressed the activities or implied that the school could do a better job, parents abdicated their responsibilities.

Results were also negative when individualized instruction was sacrificed for group meetings and when parent education was secondary to preschool training for the child. Bronfenbrenner concluded that any force or circumstance that interfered with the formation, maintenance, status or continuing development of the parent-child system greatly jeopardized the child's development.

Parent Types

Unlike with children, when one can describe a "typical" two-year-old or an average eighteen-month-old, there are no tests, scales, or descriptions of a "typical" parent. Common sense tells one that, like children, parents are unique. Just as children differ as to age, social development, cognitive ability, and experience, parents differ also. They vary in age, socio-economic level, and cognitive ability. Parents have different cultural values, home environments, educational opportunities, and so forth.

Each family, each parent has a unique combination of strengths and coping skills. Some have more abilities than others. Some have innate talents while others require detailed education to develop adequate parenting skills. Some have definite ideas about childrearing which were passed on by their parents; whereas others are extremely unsure of themselves. There are books available with the child as the focus and suggested behaviors to make the child a "super child". Most of these books were written by pediatricians (Gesell, 1940; Spock, 1976; and Brazelton, 1987) which may explain the direction taken. Burton White (White et al., 1978), however, is one of the few who has written to help the parent become a "super parent".

White, too, was concerned with how a child became a "super child" and studied the child's early environment. He wanted to know what parents were like, how they raised their children, and what they did to develop children that were achievers. Early on, he found that it was not due to economic or social level, cultural or educational ability. *It was parenting ability.* Fortunately, he captured the pattern. From their observations, he and his colleagues at Harvard identified at least five distinct types of mothers (Pines, 1969).

The first type, the woman who usually produced an exceptional child became known as the "super mother." She educated the child constantly, but not in any formal or rigid manner. She taught casually as part of her daily routine and enjoyed and accepted her child at his level of development. She didn't try to teach her two-year-old to read, but she would show him how to drop wooden shapes in the correct holes in a drop box.

Part of this mother's success stemmed from the fact that she read, sang songs, and did a lot of talking to her child. She would look to see what had his attention and would say something like, "That's a big red truck. It's a moving truck. I guess new people are moving in there." She took an idea, elaborated on it and added bits of relevant information. These short but frequent episodes helped to increase the child's language and general fund of knowledge.

The second type of mother, the "almost mother," didn't reach the same high standards. Although she enjoyed and accepted her child, she often had trouble understanding or satisfying his needs, especially before he could talk. During the toddler stage, she missed many chances to teach. When her child observed the same truck, she might simply say, "See the truck." She seemed to lack the capacity for making spontaneous associations that heighten a child's interest.

The third type of mother, the "overwhelmed mother," was one who was beaten down by the difficult circumstances of her life. Her children spent a great deal of time in aimless, unmonitored behavior.

The fourth and fifth types were opposite in behaviors. The "smothering mother" pushed her child to achieve. As one researcher put it, "She was preparing him for Harvard at age two." She was so responsive to his every little need that he rarely had an opportunity to take the initiative or to express himself. This mother spent hour after hour drilling her child on how to perform and got some positive results for her efforts. Her child may have had high intellectual skills, but he was also whiney, clingy, and socially immature.

The "zookeeper mother," on the other hand, spent too little time with her child. She was too involved in her own life — clubs, organizations, hobbies, and classes — to find time to talk or play with her toddler. Her child was likely to be apathetic and spent much of his time alone, often in an immaculate crib in a nursery filled with the latest toys.

White and his colleagues (White et al., 1978) were quick to point out that many mothers do not fit neatly into any of these categories. Their project used these classifications only to help explain different maternal styles. However, the value of this study is that it does describe parental styles and is useful information for a program for parent education.

It was through White's influence that such a program was established in Missouri. The program, mentioned earlier, was entitled *New Parents as Teachers*, (Winter, 1988), and it used the "super mother" type as a model for parents of non-handicapped children from the last trimester of pregnancy to the child's third birthday. The value of educating parents to the role of "super mother" was proven. The NPAT project proved beyond a reasonable doubt that parent behavior can be shaped, and they can be successful as educators during their child's early learning years!

Fathers

Though mother plays a starring role in the drama of a child's development, his father, brothers and sisters, and grandparents have leading parts, too. Although some authors have addressed the issue, no definite pattern of the father role has yet emerged. Probably the most resourceful material is that of Klinman and Kohl, (1984) who gathered information on fathers across the country.

The empirical description of father's role is that they have fun, play games, and engage in physical activities with their child, whereas mothers are more verbal. One researcher attempted unsuccessfully to repeat the process White used with mothers, but the data were not definitive (Clarke-Stewart, 1973). She found that children were equally attached to both parents, but responded more to the play initiated by the father in structured situations. Fathers favored social and physical games but were not as verbal nor at the child's developmental level.

Schaefer, (1972), another researcher, believed that the father's importance is often ignored with less-than-happy results. He concluded that the healthy child needs both a mother and a father who are active and involved in his upbringing from the start.

A survey done by *Family Circle* (1988) showed that practices distinguishing parents of highly successful offspring from those of average children centered on the expenditure of parental time rather than money. It also found that respect for children's independence and individuality rather than force-fed lessons at an early age led to achievers. The authors concluded that fathers of superachievers played a more active role in their youngster's life than other fathers. Fathers tended to see their role as one of imparting facts and objective knowledge. Children seemed to flourish when fathers took part in the children's daily activities and this gave children the chance to learn from two role models. These authors, as did Schaefer, concluded that the ideal situation is one in which both parents promote ways to help a child know his world.

Idealistically, we can design roles for fathers as different from those of mothers, but pragmatically it is impractical. The incidence of one-parent households is high, and that parent is usually the mother. To be sure, a process as complicated, stressful, and rewarding as childrearing certainly would seem to go better when shared by two parents, but we have little or no hard evidence to support or refute this notion. It would follow that any and all parents involved need support and assistance.

The "Super Mother's" Role

In determining the role of the "super mother," White's investigators (White et al., 1978) looked into what experiences actually made up the small child's world. They considered how often his mother talked to him, what she taught him, what encouragement she gave him, what restrictions she conveyed. They looked at which member of the mother-child dyad initiated the activity and which member followed the interaction. They investigated the kind of toys which were available and how they were used. In short, the investigators wanted to find out what "super mothers" did differently to produce more highly competent children than did mothers of children who never seemed quite able to cope. The investigators also wanted to know when "super mothers" did what they did.

Interestingly enough, these researchers found no major difference between the management of children by the various types of mothers from birth to ten months, but from that point on, radical differences took place.

Surprisingly, the superior mothers didn't spend an unusual amount of time "interacting" with each child. They found that the mothers of eventually superior children did not give their child unlimited quantities of undivided attention nor did they do much deliberate teaching. Rather, they were superbly effective in three roles: Designer, Consultant, and Authority.

Designer

In the role as Designer, the superior mothers made the home safe for their children to play; provided a rich, but not necessarily expensive, variety of toys and household objects; and allowed the children to roam all over the living area.

The contrasting mothers, on the other hand, "protected" their children (and possessions) by ruling a large number of places out-of-bounds. They restricted the child's instinct to explore. Restrictions of playpens, gates, and high chairs over long periods of time stunted a child's curiosity severely and seemed to seriously impede intellectual development.

The superior mothers were not meticulous housekeepers. Freedom to explore did not, therefore, conflict with a spotless house. They were willing to tolerate the scattered pans, stacked cans, etc. Furthermore, the superior parents were always willing to stop and delay their household chores in order to respond to the child. In other words, superior mothers paid attention to the child's fingerpainting, not his dirty clothes.

Consultant

The mother's consultant role came into play when the wandering toddler ran into something particularly exciting, or an obstacle which he could not overcome. The superior mother then would pause immediately for the few minutes it took to assist. In that interval, she would:

- Talk to the child.
- Motivate the obvious curiosity.
- Provide the child with some related ideas which would start him thinking.
- Teach him the skill of using adults as resources.

One example, similar to those which all five types of mothers encountered in this study, readily comes to mind. In one of the author's programs, there was a table with a leg which was loose enough to fall off when a child touched it. When the inevitable happened, most of the children looked to their mothers for some explanation. The superior mothers were found to say:

> "What's wrong?
> Where does the leg go?
> Let's put the leg back on.
> Let's twist the leg.
> Here's the screw. Put it in.
> There's the hole for the screw.
> Turn the screw.
> Let's turn the leg."

Some mothers said: "Leave it alone!
                                Don't touch it!
                                Put it back!
                                It's broken!"

On the other hand,
some said: "Did you break it?"

Some even said: "You broke it!"

Others just ignored the incident and kept on talking to the instructor.

There are valuable times when the child confronts an interesting or difficult situation and turns to his mother for help. She should respond promptly. Importantly, these interchanges are focused on the child's interest of the moment rather than mother's interest or need. The initiative does not come from the mother, rather it comes *from the child*. The "super mother" simply encourages the child to master the tasks he gives himself. The talk, which might be considerable, is at the child's attending level. The talk will be about *his* interests at that time. Mother can then *match her language to his thoughts*.

Authority

Parents need to be an authority figure without being a disciplinarian. Children want to know their security boundaries. Obedience and firm control negate children's creativity. Part of being parents is understanding that children need to know how far they can go. The superior mother is not "namby pamby" but rather she "runs the show." Her child does not drift aimlessly because she sets realistic limits and is consistent in seeing that they are followed.

Consistency over time and in all settings is of great importance. For example, playing at the stove is off limits whether it is on or off. It remains off limits no matter where the stove is — at Grandmother's, Aunties', or even an appliance store. Superior parents would say, "The stove may be hot, don't touch it. No!" Some parents fearing tears may offer distractions instead. Some might overwhelm the child with a multitude of reasons. Some may pay no attention to the situation.

Parents need help with learning strategies for establishing confidence in the child that, "Mother knows best." The "super mother" model serves to help parents learn techniques which don't initially come easily.

The primary goal of a parent-oriented program should be to assist all parents to become "super parents". In being "super parents", they will provide the necessary experiences for the child's cognitive growth, see that he is motivated, and match language to his thoughts.

Parents' Role in Language Acquisition

Universally, parents need to understand communication and language. They need to know how language develops and their role in their child's language acquisition.

The infant's period of dependency is relatively brief, but the experiences within that period are of utmost importance. The emergence of language depends on the social stimulation during that interval. The power and potential of the parent-child interaction system has no parallel. Every child needs the warm, constant, and expanding reciprocal activity that is the basis of an affective and an effective system of interaction.

Language begins with the parent-child interaction at the earliest pre-language stage. His coos, smiles and babbles elicit useful feedback from the environment. That strong mother-infant matrix leads to eventual language competence.

There should be no doubt about the reciprocal effect between the parent and child. It is the belief of many researchers that the communication system can be understood only in the context of the parent-child dyad. This interaction becomes the foundation.

Not only is it important that parents talk to their children, but the manner and style in which they do so is of equal importance. Observations of effective mothers have provided information about "motherese" that needs to be incorporated into an understanding of language development.

Babies use facial expressions and body movements as well as vocalizations to communicate. If parents are expecting the first utterances to be words, they will tend to pay too little attention to the cooing, whining, smiling which are necessary precursers of real language.

Mothers need to use eye contact, along with other modes of communication, such as body posture and demonstrations, on which they build the foundation of the dialogue. The earliest communication system is primarily an affective one. The behaviors of parent and child are integrated through the expression, reception, and reaction to affective behaviors of each member of the adult-child duo. Although researchers are not certain about the child's affective messages, the behaviors of the parents undoubtedly signal the parents' interpretations. Some people feel that affect, that which arouses emotional response, is the organizing concept for parent-child interaction.

Parents talk more to young children than to their older siblings. They also use simpler syntax and a more concrete vocabulary of the here and now with these younger children. Most parents need help in talking, in knowing what to talk about, how to talk, and when to talk.

The speech of parents to toddlers is slower and has fewer disfluencies than when talking to the older siblings. They repeat their utterances frequently and single out phrases for emphasis. They use prosody to gain and maintain attention. It is a linguistically *responsive* environment rather than a linguistically stimulating one when parents are aiding in the earliest stages of language development.

The talking that parents do is at first "self talk." It is as if they were talking to themselves about what they are doing, i.e., "Mommy is tying baby's shoes." or "Mommy is sweeping the floor." or "I am washing your dirty face." Later, it becomes "parallel talk" when the actions of the child are labeled. "Baby is in the bathtub." "Oh, you want the rubber duck." Still later it becomes "modeling" of the concept the parent thinks the child has, i.e., "Johnny's balloon floated away."

Parents use talk to model, to bond, to entertain, but they also use speech for rewards. When the child achieves, they comment. When he puts the right lid on the proper size pot, the parents comment. The parents talk about the joint activity when they show him how to drop wooden shapes in the correct holes or clothespins in a bottle. In essence, parents talk often about the child's interests. He understands the meaning for the talk they use. His ideas get clothed in language all day long. It is not idle, meaningless talk.

Parent Intervention

Parent involvement is now seen as more than information giving. It should aim toward increasing the parents' understanding at many levels of learning. Just as children need experiences to learn, so do parents. They can gain from films, videotapes, pamphlets, books, and other parents, but most of all through experiences with their own child.

As a result of intervention, parents' personalities will not change, nor should they change. They must keep the integrity of their "selves." The desired changes would be changes in their procedures with their child. Probably, their behaviors as parents have their roots not only in their own knowledge but in their upbringing. These may need expanding or specific attention directed to them. Some parents have innate abilities, but others may require assistance to acquire adequate parenting skills. Wherever they are, parents need to know (only if in review) child growth, child curiosity, social development, and cognitive growth. Each child is different at any given time, and parents' reactions to that child may well differ from the reaction with other siblings.

Parents of Hearing-Impaired Children: Specific Factors

Parent involvement needs to be the same whether the child has normal hearing or has a communication problem. At the same time these latter parents are dealing with the infant's needs as a child, they are also coping with hearing impairment as a handicap. Few, if any, parents escape the questioning, "Why?" "Why me?" "Why my child?" It is the goal of this text to assist parents to move on to other questions, such as, "What do I do?" and "How do I do it?"

The interval of time between the asking of the "Why?" questions to the asking of "What to do?" and "How to do it?" can be shortened if strong positive guidance is offered the family and the mother in particular. The intervener can offer positive suggestions, firm directions, and effective models for tapping the child's abilities and for providing pertinent information to parents. The very moment the parent is ready for affirmative action, the process can begin. Formal language stimulation techniques, however, should not be recommended until parents are manifesting definite responsiveness to infant behavior and infant vocalization.

It must be remembered that the affective (emotional or response-evoking) condition between parents and their hearing-impaired children is often less than ideal. In a study at the Lexington School for the Deaf, Greenstein et al. (1976), stated emphatically:

Perhaps the most important finding of this investigation is the centrality of the affective aspects of the mother-infant interaction to language acquisition of the hearing-impaired child.

But they continued that:

> Specific aspects of the mother's language programming the child, however useful, pale in significance when compared to the importance of restituting the damage done to the mother-child bond. (Greenstein et al., 1976, p. 35)

Thus, teachers need to help parents learn to be the child's first language teacher. But as important as this is, it has low priority over establishing a warm, loving interaction. Of most importance is the bonding that parents must establish before great results can be accomplished. Greenstein et al. said:

> The main priority must be given to helping the mother adjust to her child's handicap and to facilitating the flow of communication between them.

They concluded by cautioning against putting too much stress on the child's achieving lest the mother might coerce the child and by so doing, impede the process. As a mother gains competence as a parent, she also gains confidence in herself as the primary agent of change for the child. The consequence of a positive parent-child relationship lasts beyond the duration of intervention and produces long-term results in the child's development.

There are inherent problems when the child is hearing impaired. He may miss signals from his parents and may emit signals to his parents which are misinterpreted. Parents may not secure the infant's attention and their efforts are then futile. The potential asynchronization may impede language development beyond the effects of the hearing loss alone. The important vocal reciprocity may get extinguished and this is difficult to reinstate. Not only has the habit been set, but the child may be toddling off to his own little private world. When a child's behavior is not easy to understand, parents may not develop attachment; and, therefore, they feel inadequate. This in itself minimizes the necessary reciprocal action and influences the warmth and affect of the process.

For most families, a hearing-impaired child creates stress, challenges, and demands to which each member must adapt. How families cope with this stress influences family functioning, satisfaction, feelings of efficiency, and the child's development. Yet, many families have great strength and excellent coping behavior. This is one of the many ways parents vary. Each individual must experience warm loving feelings. If parents cannot feel good about themselves using their own resources, they will need help.

The intensity of the feelings of disappointment because their child is not the idealized child they expected can mitigate against parents establishing a strong support system. However, some parents can cope especially well, as one young mother of a profoundly deaf boy was shown to do at a parents' group meeting.

In a discussion of goals for which she was quite ready, this mother said she felt like the Norman Rockwell magazine cover that shows Daddy at the hospital to see his new baby for the first time. He is loaded with football gear and is somewhat startled to see that Junior is a girl. Quite suddenly all of his dreams and thoughts of football are shattered. He now has to develop a whole new mental set. This mother said she had dreamed of her child being poised and strong, kind and gentle, quick to learn but not a smart aleck, courteous, thoughtful, generous and a good musician. After a thoughtful pause, another mother replied, "Why, not one of the those things, save musician, has a thing to do with being deaf." The young mother said, "Well, maybe he can use music for dancing, and I'll see that he learns how!" The goal for their child at which the above group arrived, was "a lovable child, a self-disciplined one, one who made friends, and one who was happy and well adjusted." A grandmother in the group concluded the discussion with: "Dream wisely and then as you express your love for your child in ways he can understand, you will find him seeing your vision and be just as eager as you to make it a reality."

Parents often mobilize themselves in the presence of professionals. If the staff sees the family infrequently, they may not recognize the problems parents are facing. This is also true if the program is child-centered rather than family-focused. It is not easy to provide individualized parent programs. The beneficial aspects of the 1988 Public Law 99-457 is that staffs are required to develop a *family* orientation because the law mandates that *the parent is the pupil.*

Even for the parental roles of bonding, interacting, and stimulating, parents will need to learn to compensate for the hearing problem of their child. Furthermore, the strategies of compensation must be individualized to the families' abilities. In addition, these strategies must be appropriate to the amount of hearing the child has, his age, his abilities, his overall development, and his interests.

Individualization to each family and their child is of the first order of importance. A teacher needs to be skilled in creating an atmosphere of ease, transforming apprehensiveness into creative energy, and helping the parent feel the need for interaction with her child. Since the parent may experience emotional problems because the diagnosis of deafness can throw the underlying personality structures into strong relief, the intervener must be sensitive to the psychological domain. It is also important that the professional persons be able to recognize the limits of their competency in meeting the parents' emotional needs. Sometimes family problems may be sufficiently intense to require referral to other resources in the community.

Having a handicapped child can magnify any personality pattern that already exists within the parent. Intervention is not an attempt to change the parents' whole personality organization. Rather, its goal is to change the parents' outlook while providing them with specific techniques which they can use to help their children.

In order to be sensitive to the feelings parents experience, it might be well to give some attention to the phases many parents experience as they recover from the shock of having been told that their idealized child is handicapped. Some parents have been anticipating such a diagnosis and may have a less traumatic reaction. Others may have been anticipating the diagnosis, but their structure breaks down, nevertheless. Other parents may have had no expectation of a problem and are truly shocked to hear their child is hearing impaired. *Again, we say each family is unique.* Many parents may experience each stage of grief briefly; others continue at one or the other phases. Not all parents move through the stages sequentially. *Again, we say each family is unique.*

Phases of Reaction to Diagnosis

Parents are individuals and do not move in a linear way nor at the same rate. Nevertheless, they do have one thing in common. They hurt and hurt badly. They have lost something. They are in mourning for the child who never was. The stages of grief each parent will face are real, but may vary from parent to parent in both intensity and sequence.

Believing your child is normal and observing him as an intact youngster, you experience shock when you later learn that he is hearing impaired and will need help. Fortunately, today doctors are diagnosing hearing impairment in children when they are very young. A few years ago, and tragically in some cases today, the medical personnel told parents not to worry. The child was "just slow to talk." It is an established fact that the earlier the diagnosis takes place, the better it is for the child in the long run. Furthermore, the trauma seems to be less for the parents if they learn about the handicap when the child is young. Whenever the diagnosis comes, there is, however, some element of shock. When the parents are experiencing their initial shock, they may retain little of the important crucial information given them. The implications are obvious. Not only must that information be repeated in the future, but all important points should be written down. Immediately following diagnosis is not the time to overwhelm parents with technical information. Instead there is need to focus on the "here and now." Such things as the mechanics of putting in ear molds and checking the battery of the hearing aid are, of course, basic. Emphasis needs to be placed on the lovability of the child to encourage bonding and interacting. It may be necessary for a time to de-emphasize the ears, and instead stress the role of the "super mother."

Parents may appear to be bitter, anxious or sad. Just listening to the parents with empathy may be the wisest thing to do. Guiding honestly at all times is essential.

At this stage opportunities for parents to talk to other parents might prove helpful. Parents of older deaf children provide an excellent resource. As one psychologist said, "Professionals are not the experts. Other parents are the experts and parents of older handicapped children are the oracles."

During the earlier stages following the initial diagnosis, parents tend to start shopping around for another diagnosis, another specialist. They even seem bewildered or confused about what they're hearing. An obvious problem for the parents arises when they meet conflicting reports. Consider the mental attitude of a family who is beginning to face the reality of the diagnosis and is thrust into all the conflicting philosophies of the profession. "Teach him the unisensory way." "No, lipreading is the route to go." "By all means use Total Communication." "Use American Sign Language." "Oh, no, use finger spelling." "Instead use Cued Speech!" No wonder parents feel confused and upset. An example of this confusion of parents is indicated by the following letter from M. J. Rhodes (1972):

When will it ever end? Why can't professionals understand that parents of deaf children cannot be constantly torn apart by a methods battle? Why must we and our deaf children be constantly in the middle of the "big experiment?"

Most parents are not linguists, nor do they want to be. Few understand what you are talking about when you say "sign in concepts." They only want to have their deaf child become as much a part of their world as possible with the least possible adjustment demanded on the part of other members of the family.

I have come to the conclusion that no one understands what it is like to be the parent of a deaf child except another parent of a deaf child. Professionals that I thought understood the confusing role of parents are apparently not really tuned in. I am tired of having these people blame parents for all of the ills in education and psychological adjustment of their deaf children. Many deaf adults find it difficult to understand hearing parents of deaf children because they have never walked in our shoes. Some take their frustration against their non-communicating parents out on the new generation of parents who are doing everything within their power to communicate with their deaf children.

I do not understand professionals and deaf adults who are so tuned out that they don't try to understand the needs of parents. My heart aches for mothers and fathers of deaf children who are being caught up in yet another methods battle. I could cry — and I do. (page 20)

When the situation becomes overwhelming, it is natural for parents to want to run away from it. Parents just want someone else to take over the task — a full-time school, a tutor or even the teacher. They have excuses: "I don't know how." "He doesn't pay attention to me." "He only responds to you." The message is clear that they want out. Parents can't be coerced into assuming this responsibility. They will eventually find out that the miracle they seek is the miracle of education and love.

The emphasis by the professionals can be on parenting with supplemental materials focusing on the strategies universally used by parents. Films, slides, and books help focus interest on how to be a "super mother." The intervener needs to de-emphasize the role of the mother of a *deaf* child. These parents need help in learning the charm and cunning characteristics of their *child*, who just happens to be deaf. Compassion is the key teaching strategy for the intervener. The cuteness, cuddliness, and the normalcy of the child should be stressed. Parents need to be guided to show *love* to their child.

By talking with the professionals and to other parents, confused, fearful parents become able to achieve realistic expectations. They then can give appropriate help to their child. With this acceptance, however, comes sorrow. Many parents report it as if "they had buried a friend." The weight is there, but the outlook is encouraging. This may not mean that they have overcome their own personality conflicts. They may still be sad and sometimes bitter. They will still question why it happened to them and indeed the intervener should help them get assistance from their doctor. They need the peace of mind of knowing the causes — heredity, rubella, uremic poisoning, etc. Parents at this stage, unlike at the earlier stages, will more easily understand and learn the techniques and rationale for auditory procedures and language teaching.

A great deal of positive reinforcement for the parents and lots of opportunities to demonstrate growth are now in order. In the parlance of an old World War II song, *Accentuate the Positive* is the approach that is most acceptable to the parents and most productive at this stage.

While the teacher is working toward creating the qualities of the "super mother," some parents tend to be "smothering mothers" when they reach this stage of acknowledgement of the handicap. It may be they want to make up for lost time, but in the process some are almost obsessively overprotective. These children are often denied the opportunity to think for themselves, to be independent. This parent behavior must be dealt with before the child can reach appropriate levels of maturity.

If the professionals are patient, wise, cooperative and capable, they will help the family through the periods of insecurity and fear. Eventually, the parents will be able to acknowledge the handicap of their child. They may never accept it, but they will acknowledge it. Once this occurs, parents can then "roll up their sleeves" and begin the process of becoming "super parents."

The Family

Often father and mother are not at the same stage of acceptance or experiencing the same feeling simultaneously, thus compounding the role of the intervener. Though challenging, it is important that the educator assess the various feelings and be sensitive to their presence in each parent.

The total family composition may be of such a nature as to alter entirely the paternal or maternal attitude toward any individual child. Sickness of the mother or in other family members, economic crisis, change of job or location, or changed marital relationships all have their effect. Children born at times of crisis within the family setting naturally put strain on the parents' attitude. If these strains are brought on because the child is handicapped, certainly parent-child relations can be affected.

In the family setting are also siblings and others who need consideration and inclusion in the total process. The handicapping condition is not an isolated occurrence but affects the entire family. Brothers and sisters must sacrifice some of the parents' time. Aunts and grandparents don't understand the problem. Even close friends need to comprehend the difficulty so that they can be supportive. Some parents may unknowingly deprive their family and social groups while they spend an inordinate amount of time with the handicapped child. This isolation of and by the parents is unhealthy not only for them, but for their child. The educator must strive to encourage total family participation. The appropriate balance between family and child needs is of great importance for the mental health and growth of all involved.

The number of children and the handicapped child's rank in the family also affect the parents' relation with the siblings and the special child. A handicapped child who is the oldest can receive more of the mother's time than one who is the youngest of a large family. It has been found that mothers of first-born hearing infants interact significantly more often with these infants than they do with the children who follow. Interaction is important for the child with communication problems wherever his rank of birth falls. Documentation of the early "enrichment" environment of first borns is particularly interesting in that the intellectual advantages of the first born and only children have been reported frequently. Wherever the handicapped child ranks in a family, the enriched environment of first-born children and only children needs to be replicated.

The lifestyles of parents at any given time can greatly affect their ability to deal with the demands of parenting a handicapped child, as well as their ability to accept intervention. Consideration must be given to the single parent still living at home trying to establish a mother-child relationship while she is still in the role of a child herself; to the single parent alone or living with a boyfriend and his children; to the single parent who is trying to build a future for herself and is going to school and must rely on day care; to the single father; to divorced couples with joint custody — each having the child for half of the week and both working. Though challenging for the intervener, these situations are reality, and many times these families are more in need of help in creating support systems for themselves and their child than the typical family constellation of the past.

For all these reasons and more, it is critical that each family be viewed as unique. Frightened and grieving parents should not be offered stereotyped solutions or be pressed for awesome decisions. At a time when they have not yet begun to come to terms with the diagnosis or to understand childrearing habits, parents should not be urged to choose a lifestyle for their child's total life span. Rather, they should be given support and help to know their child as an individual. Some parents begin sooner than others to accept the situation while mobilizing themselves to help the child.

This very uniqueness of families presents difficulties in a parent-child program. Some parents handle principles regarding their child's management quite well and make application easily. On the other hand, some parents seek and need specifics. They are the ones who want a "cookbook" telling step one, two, and three. For these parents, application and consistency is most difficult.

Some parents read and believe everything, simply because it is written. Others don't need to read at all to be good parents. Often parents find that great help comes from other families who have had similar experiences. For some, the generalization of the discussion to their own problems is only achieved by patient direction by the intervener.

Some parents tend to be selective listeners and some don't listen at all. It is not uncommon to hear a parent reply, after being told the same thing by the educator, preschool teacher, classroom teacher and principal:

No one told me that before.
I never heard that.
Why didn't someone tell me?
Oh, it's good to hear that at last.

That same parent very likely will ask the same questions for several years to come and will make similar replies for all those years. Aggressive attempts must be made to work on the basis of honest communication and to encourage questioning. By all means, however, educators need to respect the psychological defenses, including denial, which might be employed by parents.

Furthermore, many parents do not possess the information and understanding as to the importance of early stages of learning, nor the need for sensory stimulation. Frequently, parents lack knowledge of child development, are not informed about behavior management, do not understand the handicapping condition nor how to ameliorate the effects. Certainly, there are few who are aware of ways language is acquired and the parents' role in its acquisition. Contrary to the notion that parenting is instinctive, evidence is accumulating that it is, in fact, learned.

Because of these variables, each family group needs to be considered as an individual group for a large part of the intervention. Not only do parents have individual needs that must be recognized, but the identification of the handicap may occur at any time during a year. There can be no waiting until the child is six years or even six months. The parents need help IMMEDIATELY! The task of the educator is to enter into the parent-child transaction to modify the naturally-occurring dynamics and produce the necessary changes as soon as possible.

It is important that parents master the "parent-as-teacher" concept. They must at the same time become first-rate parents, not second-rate teachers. No, this is not contradictory. "Parents-as-teachers" means teaching as parents the world over teach. GOOD PARENTING IS GOOD TEACHING!

While the long-range goal of intervention should be for the child to reach the maximum level of which he is capable, the immediate aims must be for the parents to provide the stimulation necessary for that achievement. Just as a child is an individual who advances through stages of development at his own particular rate, so are parents individuals who are unique in their parenting behaviors, their abilities, their acceptance of their child, their priorities, and their attitudes. We do not want to change a child — only direct his development. Nor do we want to change parents — only shape their interaction with their child.

Parent involvement should help the parent be an on-going "designer" of the experiences, a "consultant" constantly, and an "authority" figure when needed. The various types of parents and the effect they have on their child's development were determined through studies of parents of normal hearing children. How much more critical is the role of the "super parent" in the life of a hearing-impaired child!

Summary

There are roles that parents must assume if they want their child to do reasonably well in our society. There are a few models which have been used successfully to raise parents to the role of "super parent." Each family, however, has a unique combination of strengths, vulnerabilities, and coping styles. Unlike assessing the child's needs, there are no tests to pinpoint the problem areas of parents.

The basic goals of parent education do not differ, however. Just as we want each child to achieve the most of which he is capable, we want parents to achieve their fullest potential. Just as teachers take children at their developmental stage and help them proceed forward, so must the intervener meet parents on their ground and help them advance. *Parents are the pupils when the child's language age is under three years.* The consultant must be the parents' teacher. Not until the child is speaking at the three-year linguistic level does the role change. Up to then, the intervener is a teacher educator. The parents are their students, as it were, "in training" to be their own child's teachers.

Interveners need to know the parents' innate abilities, the family's milieu and what strategies will be appropriate given their life style, availability and other factors that make up a "whole parent" and a "whole family." While there are no standardized tests to assess parents, let alone families, the teacher of the parents must set realistic goals for the parents just as a teacher of children does. That means they understand the pupil's ability and potentials and priorities. They then can set acceptable goals.

Parents of every deaf child can become "super parents". They need a sensitive, supporting intervener or teacher who guides them. Parent behaviors can change, parent behaviors can be taught and parent behaviors can be learned! In order to make it all happen, the educator's challenge is to be a "super teacher."

Chapter 3

The Child Has Much To Learn

The greatest learning task that the hearing-impaired child has is the acquisition of the language of his community. When he has language, nothing is impossible for him. A father of a young deaf man was interviewed upon his son's graduation. His son was one of only a handful of deaf medical students to have ever graduated in this country. This father said that he had wanted his son to develop oral language because he felt if his son could not talk, many doors would be closed to him. The authors of this text support this idea. The generalizations being shared in these chapters are based upon years of having seen deaf children who could speak and who could understand speech open many doors, from holding PhD's in biogenetics to becoming leaders in suburban communities.

There are certain fundamental principles critical to the child's acquisition of language behavior:
1. Early exposure to communication;
2. Hearing aid(s) as early as possible;
3. Appropriate and consistent amplification;
4. Parent interaction and ongoing meaningful experiences in which the speaker and the listener use the same code. (The language code is an auditory-vocal process in which the sender of the message speaks and the receiver of the message takes in the acoustic information.)

Whatever concepts a hearing child must form about sounds, words, and thought units, he makes at a very early age. Therefore, the process has to be an inductive one. Surely any other route would be impossible with an infant and toddler. Based on our current information, we are forced to reject any notion that language requires special processing of discrete elements.

It has been hypothesized that not only is language learning a tedious process, but it probably would not be learned at all if children had to learn it sound by sound and word by word. The critical processes are active listening and speaking in ongoing real-life situations. *There are no neat packages of techniques, devices, or objects. The process is simply that of daily experiencing to which the language forms are applied*; experiencing in which the child stores the concept with the language. The child perceives the content while the language form is superimposed simultaneously.

The authors believe that hearing-impaired children do not develop deviant language, but rather follow normal developmental stages. The rate of learning will differ depending upon how much use is made of the residual hearing, how much meaningful input is provided, and how the child's output is shaped. Although many people plan differently for children with hearing losses that are mild and moderate from those that are severe or profound, the authors do not. Obviously, the child with a mild hearing loss will progress faster than the profoundly deaf child. All other things being equal, all children progress along the same course.

Amplified hearing, while essential, is insufficient. When the acoustic input is not directed to the child nor related to his experience, he cannot discover the language structure. Children who have even mild hearing problems which go undetected until they are preschool age or older demonstrate grammatical confusion. Self-auditory feedback is insufficient to acquire language behavior. Children must hear speech related to them, to their own actions, and to their own interests. They need a model. Then, they need to be reinforced for their efforts at vocalizing.

While individuals differ in their degree of hearing, type of parents and kind of environment, there seem to be sequences of language acquisition that are characteristic of all children. However, the authors would like to emphasize that the hearing-impaired child does not necessarily reach the stages at the same age as a child with normal hearing. For the former, the stages may be later and each of the stages can be longer in duration. Nevertheless, it has been the authors' experience that the same language acquisition stages that apply to hearing children apply to deaf children as well.

We have assigned descriptive labels to the stages in the language development continuance:

1. Prelude to Language
2. Prelinguistic Language
3. Fundamentals of Language
4. Actual Language Begins
5. Language Becomes Sophisticated

1. Prelude to Language

Prelude to Language is to language behavior what a prelude is to a musical symphony. It introduces the audience to the theme. In this case it introduces the child to language development. The theme of language is communication, an exchange of ideas from the mind of the speaker to the mind of the listener.

During the Prelude Level, the parents prepare for the melody. They transmit the theme. The stage is set for the hearing-impaired child to receive suitable hearing aids and for an intervention program to begin. The theme of the adult's "talk" is interaction which is part of the bonding process. Through the natural, loving tones of the human voice, the parents respond to the child and meet his needs. The purpose of the "talk" is to relate to their child and set the stage for language interaction, not to teach words or phrases.

One would consider it ridiculous for the hearing infant, who is at this stage and is only four, five, or six months, to be expected to acquire lists of words and expressions. Instead, he would be surrounded with "LOVE TALK." He would learn to feel the security of the sound of his mother's voice.

The hearing-impaired child, however, may be at this beginning stage of language development but may have outgrown his six-month baby clothes. He may, in fact, be twelve, eighteen, or twenty- four months of age. He, nevertheless, has not outgrown his need for the very same kind of loving input from his caregivers. He, like the hearing child, needs the opportunity to learn the comfort of his mother's voice, have consistent amplification, and hear deliberate language input. He also needs to know *his* voice brings Mother on the run! Certainly, he may be hearing sounds with a hearing aid during these early months of listening and watching people talk. Like all children, he hears *sounds*, not words, phrases, nor sentences. Therefore, he should not yet be held accountable for any of these discrete language elements. He has much to learn about language and the act of communicating before he becomes aware of the language within the utterances.

Biologic sounds

During this initial phase of language development, the child's sounds are mainly reflexive or biologic in nature. The child has needs for food, comfort, and loving that must be met. Instinctively, he vocalizes as a reaction to physiologic changes in his body. He cries or makes rooting noises because he feels discomfort from hunger. He fusses because he experiences boredom from staying in one position too long. He makes a low cooing sound when he feels comfort after a bath and a bottle. He also whines to be changed and cries for attention. These sounds are important signals to his parents.

Differentiated cries

The hearing-impaired child must learn, as does the hearing child, that he can manipulate people through phonation. Only through immediate response and consistent meeting of his needs will he begin to understand that his sounds can communicate different things to his parents. His cries become functional, and they communicate specific needs. It is assumed, of course, that the hearing-impaired child wears his hearing aid(s) during his waking hours. As he hears himself vocalizing, he, too, can learn which sounds elicit what behavior. He can enjoy listening to himself and derive kinesthetic and auditory feedback as he makes the sounds, even the biologic ones. He receives an auditory imprint from his environment, and he is unknowingly storing it for his later vocal communication.

Absorption

During this beginning level, the child is listening, observing, and soaking up language like a little sponge. "Absorption" is a good term for this process because not only is he listening, but he is taking in this language experience. He is a very passive participant at this stage in the language learning process. He is like a passenger on a bicycle built for two, and the parent is doing all the pedaling!

Prelude to meaning

The child is still a long way from understanding the actual language or words being spoken. He may, nevertheless, be beginning to sense the meaning for some sounds and facial expressions, body movements and routines. The child seems to know that if his father is coming toward him with outstretched arms that he is going to be picked up. He may start to fuss when he sees his mother putting on her coat because he may remember the last time when she left without him.

As he absorbs the talking of the adults around him and to him, he may begin to sense the meaning in their intonation. The quality of their voices may take on significance: Their voices might be soft and pleasant, or loud and harsh. They can be laughing, coughing, or singing. Each of these voices may sound different to him. He may note that each is used in different situations. He may notice that certain intonations or voice patterns accompany different body positions, different facial expressions, each having different meanings.

A difficult stage for parents

The early period of exposure to speech is likely to generate tension in the family. Some parents have expressed the feeling that they receive no positive reinforcement from their child for all their efforts. They may respond to all his needs, talk to him as much as possible, and the child still may not pay much attention to them. Other parents have a difficult time with this level because they, by nature, may be quiet, non-talkative people. For whatever the reasons, the *Prelude to Language* period is recognized as a difficult stage, but a very important one. A normally hearing child has eight to ten months or several thousand hours of exposure to language before he begins to demonstrate the understanding of the words which are said to him. The hearing-impaired child can have no less time to go through the similar period of language exposure.

Thus, the *Prelude to Language* stage seems to be one of continual input about the child's immediate environment. That input needs to be high in varied phonologic features such as intonation. Furthermore, that intonation needs to have positive affect as in "love talk." Parents and teachers are communicating that the world is a fine place to be: even better because they love him.

It may appear at this stage as if the child is not learning, if one's concept is academic learning. The fact is, this is the most critical phase of all language learning. While it is the prelude of what is to come, it is also the strong foundation on which the skyscraper of language is to be built.

First of all, the child learns that he has a voice, and he can use it. He learns that by using it he can control people. He learns he can be tuned in to his parents much as the pilot of a plane is tuned into the radio tower. He can get the message from the tower through his *amplified* hearing and through his vision. Finally, he learns what communication is all about. He learns that the first role of language is its function, and those functions are love and security. Parents do all of the work, but the child does all of the learning.

It is not *how much* parents work or talk with their child, rather it is *what* is said, *how* it is said, and *when*. Through the *what, how,* and *when* of his parents' talking, the child has begun to learn many basic language skills.

Objectives

All teachers should provide behavioral objectives for every family because the intervention must be planned and systematic. However, with the introduction of legislation that causes teachers in intervention programs to be accountable for the services they are providing, objectives are mandatory. Therefore, some objectives are suggested throughout this text. Since the teaching is individualized, the appropriate objectives for each child, the time envelope for mastery, and the criteria for achievement are left up to the teacher. The objectives which the intervener might project for the child at this stage could include:

- Child will vocalize.
- Child will turn when the parent comes in the room.
- Child will watch what the parent is doing.
- Child will smile at parent.
- Child will watch parent's face.
- Child will interact with parent.
- Child will make frequent eye contact.
- Child's vocalizations will increase in frequency.
- Child's vocalizations will become differentiated when wet, tired, in pain, when happy, etc.
- Child will attend to parent's talking.

2. Language at the Prelinguistic Level

The Prelinguistic Level is just that. It is how the child communicates prior to the emergence of linguistic forms.

Awareness

The Prelinguistic stage seems to be characterized by the child becoming aware of speech. For the parents, this stage is more rewarding and reassuring because of the feedback the child gives them. The child appears to pay attention. His eyes begin to seek the speaker's mouth and he appears to watch the people in his environment talk to him. Some parents report a feeling of "thereness" when the child begins to show that level of awareness when something is being said to him.

Purposeful vocalizations

The reflexive nature of the child's vocalizations at the previous level is now replaced with what seems like more purposeful utterances. These vocalizations may include vowel-like sounds such as "oo," "ah," "uh," and some of these sounds will be paired with an initial back consonant like "g" or "k." These are not words, but the child may "coo" and "goo" to a friendly, familiar face. If that person responds consistently, the child's expression of humor and enjoyment begins as laughter and chuckling. The period of babbling or "chatter" has definite patterns of intonation. There are pauses and starts that may resemble the rhythmic use of sentences by adults. He utters patterns of sound and uses them in ways in which people can reinforce him by making the sounds function for him. As the child progresses, his consonant-vowel syllables ("guh" or "duh") will increase in frequency, and they also may begin to be in the form of repetitive babble ("guh-guh-guh-guh-guh"). The child may point to an object or person he wants with grasping gestures while vocalizing, "uh-uh-uh." This is definite communication! He is "saying," in no uncertain terms, that he wants something or someone! This communication could cease unless responded to by the adult.

Early meanings

There is evidence that the child at this stage has begun to

understand the meaning of spoken language. The child may stop or pause in his activity and give a knowing glance toward his mother when she says, "No!" He may respond appropriately to some routine phrases. For example, if his mother says, "Let's go bye-bye," the child might start to wave. If Grandpa says, "Grandpa's boy is so-o-o-o-o big!" the child may stretch his arms up over his head to show his "bigness." Or if his father says, "Give Daddy a hug," the child may throw his arms around his father's neck. He appears in tune with his environment and the people around him.

The child has become responsive to facial expressions, gestures, and some situational clues. He may seem to respond to *what* is said, but it really is a response to *how* it is said. His reaction may be happiness, interest, or fright. It all depends on the intonation the adult uses, the facial expression she has, and the child's familiarity with the situation.

The "what" of the language input the adult provides is about the things the child sees, tastes, smells, hears, and does. The adult points and describes:

> "There's the puppy."
> "Look at the kitty."
> "Let's get the milk."
> "Here is your cereal."

The objects are very much here and now. They are all within the child's perceptual range, and significantly, they are his possessions or have to do with him. The "how" of the adult's input is animated vocal expression. The "why" of the child communicating is to get a desired adult response. He can move people!

Skills

At the Prelude to Language level, the child was compared to a passenger on a bicycle built for two, and the parent was doing all the pedaling. At this Prelinguistic level, the child is still a passenger, but is beginning to give reinforcement to his parent. He, too, is starting to pedal!

As the parent and child "pedal" down the road to language development, the stage is being set for full language competence. While these skills are prelinguistic in nature, they nevertheless are critical to the give-and-take of the communication exchange. The critical feature of getting and maintaining appropriate eye contact is being established. Understanding meaningful intonation patterns is a precursor to effective communication.

These and other "extra" features of language are being stressed in the first three levels of language development. These aspects of language develop naturally as the child grows and experiences language. They are very difficult to "teach" a child later. The importance of allowing skills to develop in the proper, natural sequence cannot be overemphasized.

Objectives

Some possible objectives for the child at this level are:
- Child will make frequent eye contact.
- Child's vocalizations will include changes in loudness and pitch (cooing).
- Child will play reciprocal games with mother using eye contact.
- Child will vocalize consonant-vowel combinations.
- Child will babble repeated syllables.
- Child will demonstrate comprehension of "no" by responding appropriately.
- Child will demonstrate comprehension of a few routine phrases without accompanying gestures ("Give Mommy a kiss." "It's time to go night-night." "Wave bye-bye.") by responding appropriately.
- Child will vocalize and gesture to indicate wants and needs.
- Child will watch the speaker spontaneously.

3. Fundamentals of Language

The fundamental aspect of language that develops at this stage is comprehension and meaning. Meaning provides the undergirding upon which future structures are built. Through much repetition, the child develops an understanding of the sounds having primary stress patterns. These are usually the names of familiar people, objects, and actions. By now, hearing aid(s) are being worn all day providing the child with auditory and/or multisensory experiences.

Beginning skills

At this level, the child is becoming more aware of his world. If the child has been wearing his hearing aid(s), he may start to echo some exclamatory expressions. If his mother drops a sandwich and says "Uh-oh!" the child may imitate, "Uh-oh." When his father is reading a book to the child, and says, "The doggie says, 'Bow-wow,' " the child might imitate, "Wow-wow!" This imitation is rewarding for both the child and the parents because it is fun and the parent-child dyad (duo) is engaging in a verbal exchange. The emphasis, however, must continue to be placed on developing the child's *understanding* of the language rather than his imitation abilities. If the child does not have the basis of meaning, he may start imitating things in a parrot-like fashion.

The imitation skill parents helped develop earlier now begins to be used independently. While the child is responding, he may be observed mouthing the words and mimicking the speaker. For example, his lips may come together accompanied by the wave of his hand as his response to "bye-bye." In reply to questions such as "Do you want a cookie?" he may move his lips in the "oo-ee" position.

Comprehension

During this stage the child may identify part of what is being said but may not comprehend all of it. He may still need help from situational clues. He may pick up the shoe when his mother tells him, "We will put on your shoes and socks." He may get his coat when his mother shows him that they are going outside.

In his understanding of language, the hearing-impaired child has progressed from the perception that someone is communicating with him to understanding simple directions, "Show me your eyes." "Give the ball to Mommy." "Blow your nose." His simple responses show the beginning of comprehension of speech. He has learned to get ideas from the situation. This skill is essential to language comprehension and must be encouraged.

By now the hearing-impaired child should be responding to his own name and the names of the people and the pets in his immediate environment. He may even recognize and attempt to use the names of his favorite objects. However, he understands far more than he says. Comprehension will always exceed expression.

Spoken language efforts

Even though he may attempt some words, the child continues to babble and chatter. Some people call this jargon. It is more elaborate than earlier babble with a wider range of sounds and intonation patterns. The child may use it when interacting and when alone.

Some parents observe jargon in role-playing. For example, the child may be pretending to be Daddy and "scold a doll" for getting all muddy. In this situation, there may be a long string of babbled sounds with meaningful, "scolding" intonation that makes it sound like a normal conversation.

Other hearing-impaired children's parents report that they hear their child babbling when he awakens in the morning. It is as if he were practicing the vocalizations he has acquired and the intonation patterns he has heard. The quality of the hearing-impaired child's spoken language efforts is directly related to his use of amplification and the parents' skills in using normally intoned speech and presenting intonation patterns in playful exchange.

First labels

The child communicates his wants and needs by vocalizing or babbling as well as pointing. If he wants a cookie, he may point to the cupboard and say, "muhmuhmuhmuhmuh" or "dadadadada." If parents consistently respond to this attempt to communicate by giving the cookie and modeling the language for what he is trying to say, the child's first true words will eventually appear.

More often than not, a sound or syllable the child says just happens to sound like the label for the object he wants. The child may say "Dah" as his father walks in the door. His mother responds with great excitement and says, "Daddy! You said, Daddy." That little syllable "Dah" has been interpreted as the word "Daddy." The positive reinforcement the child received will encourage him to try it again. Very soon, this syllable becomes *his* word for "Daddy." He might say "baw" for "ball," "poo" for "spoon," and "wah" for "water." As his parents imitate and begin to shape the sounds, the child's attempts at words will gradually become closer to the correct form.

First labels are unique for each child. They are difficult for teachers to predict; thus making it impossible to "teach" a set of labels meaningful to every child. The family and his environment influence the choice. One of the author's oldest children spoke the word "dog" as her first word. There was a beloved dog in the household, and a great deal of discussion was centered about and around the dog, i.e., about feeding the dog, not dumping the dog's food or water, petting the dog gently, not pulling the dog's tail, letting the dog outside. It is easy to see why the word "dog" held the interest of this child and became her first word.

Objectives

- Child's vocalizations (babbling, jargon) will increase even when playing alone.
- Child will demonstrate understanding of the meaning of familiar, simple expressions, i.e., "Come here." "Get your coat." "Show me your eyes." "It's time to go bye-bye."
- Child will observe turn-taking in imitation activity.
- Child will echo sounds and expressions such as, "Uh-oh," "bow-wow," "bye-bye" with appropriate intonation.
- Child will demonstrate understanding of the meaning of many common things and people in his daily life.
- Child will respond to his name when called.
- Child will communicate his wants and needs by pointing accompanied by vocalizing or babbling.
- Child will use jargon — a string of babble that is sentence-like in form with meaningful intonation.
- Child will observe his turn to talk and vocalize when Mother pauses in her talking.
- Child will start to identify people and some of his possessions.

4. Actual Language Begins

Like all children, the hearing-impaired child proceeds from the thought (whole) to words (parts). All of the language preparation up to now has dealt with the *function* of language. *The child's first step in speech production is not learning phonemes and words. Rather, he learns to communicate in order to control people in his environment. He learns the function of communication before he learns the language itself.* He acquires language as a means of getting attention and regulating activity.

The beginnings of spoken language are gradual. Even though vocabulary often gets primary attention, the labeling process has been developing throughout the previous stages. "Teaching" words does not insure the meanings needed in spoken communication!

One linguist (Crystal, 1986) addressed the rate at which hearing children speak new words:

On the average, the children understood fifty words before

they were able to produce ten (words), and they did not arrive at a corresponding number in their speech until five months later. (p. 67)

Earlier, another linguist (Bullowa, 1964) examined the interval of time required for a hearing child to learn a common word such as "shoe." That particular word, used naturally with a toddler, required eighteen months from the initial use as in, "Let's put on your shoe," to the spontaneous use of the word by the child. It must be noted that never did the mother in this study use the word without the object being associated with it. Obviously, there was much repetition of that word. Furthermore, it was considered to be "learned" only when the child used the word when the object was not present, i.e., he would ask for his shoe when he couldn't find it.

At all times the child experienced the word in the richness of its linguistic environment. The word "shoe" can have many modifiers, i.e., Mother's shoe, white shoes, tennis shoes. It can be used with a number of active words, i.e., put on, take off, clean, tie, polish. The perceptual characteristics and the linguistic function of the word as a noun must be acquired simultaneously.

The same theory needs to be applied to all labels, whether they are nouns, adjectives or verbs. It is not the single word that is to be stressed, but the comprehension of the concept in all of its dimensions.

Single words

The first spoken words of children are basically what are called "dada words." They have loose referents and may even appear to have babble-like qualities with no referent at all. Instead of "dada words," deaf children tend to use those with lip movement of the "bababa" variety because these can be seen. Parents must be cautioned, however, not to read too much meaning into the interpretation of these utterances. They may merely be imitations.

While hearing children do, deaf children do not move quickly into the second type of word which linguists call "label" words. Hearing children easily use the label word, but it takes more time for the hearing-impaired child to do so. Nevertheless, his comprehension continues to grow and precedes his expressive language.

Even though the acquisition of new words continues to be rather slow, the hearing-impaired child does begin to express his ideas in single words. Often one word can represent a whole concept or sentence. For example, if the hearing-impaired child comes to an adult and says, "Ball," he could be indicating any of the following:

> Where is my ball?
>
> Give me the ball.
>
> Roll the ball.
>
> Throw the ball.
>
> Jenny took my ball.
>
> Let's play ball.

Because the child is in the environment where the meaning is clear and because his parent has been tuned-in to him, she can rephrase his single word "ball" into proper sentence structure and respond accordingly. Since he is capable at this stage of imitating two- to three-word phrases, this parent of the hearing-impaired child can ask for this type of imitation in order for him to "process" sentence structure.

The hearing-impaired child tends to use mostly nouns spontaneously. These are concrete items from his daily environment, i.e., foods, toys, vehicles, and of course family names and pets.

He also begins to use a few adverbs spontaneously, i.e., "there," "all gone," and "no." He uses "down" when he knocks his blocks over or falls. He uses "up" when climbing steps, but does not necessarily extend the meaning to pulling up a shade or putting a toy on a high shelf. Some routine phrases may occur such as "ee-a-oo" for "Peek-a-boo" and "atteecake" for "Patty Cake," but usually it is the activities of the "here and now" which are verbalized. They may spontaneously use expressions to manage their situations: "Get up." "Open the door." "I want a turn." "Go home!"

Chained single words

The hearing-impaired child, like the hearing child, likes to add length to his sentences. After considerable imitation of two and three word phrases, he begins to use them spontaneously. He uses a word, pauses, and then another word to create a novel utterance, i.e., "ilk...(pause)...ooie," meaning he would like to have milk and cookies. "Bye-bye...(pause)...car," means "Let's go bye-bye in the car." He may say, "Tie...(pause)...shoe," meaning "Tie my shoe."

Function words

While the *learning* of important structure words takes place at the next level, the *practice* begins at this stage. The child comprehends the meaning and should imitate the parent's expansion of his telegraphed utterance. Now, parents can respond to "milk" with the liquid, but soon after, the response can change to "more milk," and then to "I want more milk," and finally "Please pour some milk." The appropriate emphasis for the child is the content or the actions to be achieved by the phrase. Responses to questions about milk should proceed from "No" to "I *don't* want *any* milk." In this way, functors occur in their natural position, not as objects for drill. Here, as at all levels of language, it is *meaning* that is stressed.

As the child learns that language works for him, he begins to generalize. He will find that he can get the milk passed, can get his coat zipped, can have more candy, can go outside if he uses phrases. *Language functions for him.*

Objectives

- Child will learn that he can manipulate people with language.
- Child will learn that he can obtain objects by vocalizing.
- Child will learn that verbalization pays off.
- Child will learn to imitate parent, thereby shaping his utterances.
- Child will begin to understand words in context.
- Child will identify several items from the same category.
- Child will search for several items from the same category when they are not present.
- Child will play "Where is the — — ?" game.
- Child will use content words as single "sentences."
- Child will use words in his jargon.
- Child can identify words without situational clues.
- Child will comprehend ideas with situational clues.
- Child responds to the labels for foods at breakfast, lunch, snack time, dinner.
- Child will call siblings to dinner.
- Child will call pets to their dinner.
- Child will use question intonation and label when hunting for his toys.
- Child will imitate two and three word phrases.

- Child will identify sentences about his experience through audition only.
- Child will use expressions to manage his situations.

5. Language Becomes Sophisticated

As the child enters and progresses through this stage, it is impractical to describe all that the "typical" hearing-impaired child may say or understand. The range of language abilities becomes more pronounced as well as the rate at which the child progresses. If given the opportunity and assistance, the child at this level is able not only to comprehend, but to acquire a great deal of new vocabulary, when presented in the context of phrases and/or sentences. Unlike at a younger language age, the child now uses function words in his language after only a few presentations. It was at this stage that a preschool hearing-impaired child was heard to respond to "What is the matter?" with "(I) ange wid Dadee."

The child can tell what he has seen, what he found, what he did, and what he has. He can, if given opportunities, *think with language*. He can tell how he thinks a story will end. He can figure out situational clues from pictures and relate a story. He can answer *why* questions, i.e., "Why do you want more blocks?" "Why do you want blue socks?" "Why do you want a nickel?" He can respond to other questions such as How—? When—? Where—? etc. He can *ask* the questions when *he* is seeking information. He can also develop strategies for seeking information when he doesn't understand someone. Instead of over-using "What?" or "Huh?," the child should know when to say: "I didn't understand you." "I don't know what — — means." "I didn't hear you."

At the Sophisticated Language level, approximately 60 percent of the child's utterances are in the form of statements, 28 percent in the form of questions, 7 percent requests, 4 percent in greetings, and 1 percent in calls. He has control over the prosody of speech both to convey meaning and to indicate syntax. His grammar advances from simple sentences of subject-verb or subject-verb-object to more complex structure.

The child at this level should begin using synonyms for many of the words he knows and be using a variety of ways of expressing an idea. Instead of always using simple language as in, "John went to his closet. He got his coat. He went outside," he should be encouraged to use other ways of expressing the same thought:

> John got ready and went outside.
> After John got his coat, he went outside.
> John got his coat to go outside.
> John got his coat from the closet before he went outside.

During this stage, a child will develop all the grammar he needs for the rest of his life. The task from this point on is no different from that of hearing children, that is, extending his concepts, enriching his vocabulary, and refining his sentence structure. By the five-year-old linguistic level, the child is a skillful speaker. His use of syntax or sentences is complete. His vocabulary exceeds two thousand words. His phonologic skill of intonation, phrasing, and stress should be established. He moves into the abstract. He knows time, both past and future. He can talk about ideas. No longer is he bound to the here and now.

Through modeling and imitation of the model, the hearing-impaired child learns syntax. He, like the hearing child, searches the language behavior of others and the models given him until he locates the rule or rules that hold the key of language structure.

The child can give evidence of knowing the rules of grammar by responding with the correct morphemes. Many children can demonstrate this with "nonsense" sentences which measure their knowledge of morphemes.

> If this is a wug. Here are two — . (wugs)
> A man is baying. Yesterday he — . (bayed)

It is not, however, the mastery of the rules themselves that hold the key to the development of new structures. It is, instead, the connecting of these rules with real-life situations that gives the child control and mastery over language. Language teaching, if based upon the *functions* for speaking, can enable the hearing-impaired child to achieve a complete language repertoire and reach the *linguistic* age of five years in the same way as the hearing child.

This stage is one of developing and solidifying the basics. There will always be more to learn. There are new *concepts* to explore. There are different ways of saying things that need to be incorporated into spontaneous language. There are ways of combining words that have to be experienced and tried. There are new and exciting ways the child can learn to express himself as he moves along the language development continuum toward sophisticated language.

Chapter 4

The Parent
Has Much To Learn

As has been discussed earlier, the parents are the most effective educational delivery system in the life of their child. Yet most parents have so very much to learn about parent skills and behavior. As Burton White has often said, "Parents get more information with their new automobile than they do with their baby." Superimpose upon this lack of knowledge the finding that the child has a hearing loss and, therefore, needs special attention. *Parents need help!* It is an established fact that the *earlier* this help is given, the more lasting are its effects. The more *involved* the parents are in their child's learning, the greater and longer lasting are the child's gains.

The notion that parents are important has always been true; however, the urgency of the parenting role has been evolving during the last three decades. The program of intervention being described in this text began in the fifties, 1958 to be exact. It was found that social, emotional, cognitive, and linguistic development hinges upon the child's interaction with his environment. Parents are the process by which that interaction takes place.

The long-range goal of a parent program is for the child to reach his maximum level of competence, but the immediate aims of the program are for the parents to provide the necessary stimulation for that achievement. Language competence is then the goal for each child, but the dominant aim is for the parents to achieve reciprocity with their child. The strength of interaction depends upon the parents understanding their child and his problems, along with sensitivity to his needs. Parents world-wide help their infants learn to listen, to communicate, and to learn. Parents of children with a communication handicap are no different.

The understanding of that task must be built upon a solid foundation of knowledge and appreciation of their critical role in their child's development.

Simply programming parents to provide specific listening experiences, learning tasks, and communication exercises is insufficient and frequently premature. The teaching of strategies which elicit language should not be encouraged until parents have demonstrated harmonious interaction with their child and definite responsivity to him and his behavior. In all probability, time will have to be allowed for adjusting to the hearing loss itself.

Our advice to teachers is to listen to the parents. This listening enables one to learn the stage of emotional acceptance at which the parents are operating. Depending upon that stage, one can proceed along the continuum as described or, if deemed necessary, remain at a level until the parent has had adequate support and information from the teacher. In our age of instant cooking, instant recording of news, and instant travel, educating an oral hearing-impaired child is a slow process.

Knowing the parent will enable the teacher to provide the information she wishes to impart. That includes the background the parent has and her experience with children. The teacher should not assume, however, that because the parent nods and seems to agree, that he or she understands. Frequent discussion of the same topics in a variety of ways is often necessary for a parent to understand. Then, too, during the early periods the material needs to be in written form as much as possible. The emotional stage of a parent can interfere with only one presentation. They need repetition.

Although interactions between parent and child are considered to be the antecedents of social, cognitive, and linguistic development, there is no set pattern to the process. Unfortunately, the parents must become involved in a *process* rather than a *curriculum*. The latter would be easier if it only worked.

Process acquisition is much more difficult for parents to learn and teachers to teach than stereotyped lessons. It is not something achieved through set toys, games, or certain experiences. Rather, the natural environment and the activity of the home are the necessary "teaching media." The home is rich in the necessary tools of language learning and cognitive experiences.

Unlike the programs of old, the authors do not believe that words and strings of words make up the whole act of communication. Rather, there is much involved in the act that is learned by a hearing child at the non-verbal level from his interaction with his mother. This act requires listening when someone talks, attending to the speaker's feelings, focusing on the topic, and responding to someone else. These are all part of the patterns established during the first level of language-skill learning. These are important skills definitely taught by parents and more easily learned by the hearing-impaired child at the earliest level. In the authors' experience, *patterns* of communication are presented as parental love and attention before any consideration is given to actual language or thought.

A problem exists when attempting to describe the sequences necessary for the flow of interactive behavior — the *process. Where* priority should be assigned and *which* particular patterns are beneficial are still somewhat empirical. However, we have learned from the plethora of studies of "motherese" more about the parents' role with hearing children (Simmons-Martin, 1983). There is a continuum of interaction found to exist with parent-child dyads (twosomes) when the child was deaf (Anderson, 1979). The items that are in the repertoire of successful parents tend to fall into five discrete categories, each with sub-units of desirable parent behavior.

The five levels of behavior are:
1. Nurture the child
2. Tune in to the child
3. Talk *to* the child
4. Talk *for* the child
5. Talk *with* the child

1. Nurture the Child

Fundamental to successful development of children is a parent knowledgeable about growth and development. Knowing the stage at which their child is performing enables parents to select and provide appropriate stimuli at the proper time. For example, melba toast to the small infant is as inappropriate as is eating with a spoon before he has eye-hand coordination or the ability to grasp the spoon. Therefore, the parents need a thorough briefing on the abilities and needs of a six-month old, a two-year old, or a three-year old. Obviously, the parents' greatest concern is their own child's growth and developmental abilities and the needs of children that same age.

The complex role of nurturing parents is not instantly learned. This is true particularly when the child does not respond to verbalization or meet the parent's overall expectations. The important and necessary bonding between the child and his parents is disrupted and may even become non-existent.

Intervention must seek to prevent or repair the break in reciprocal action. It is hoped that the intervention begins before the negative habits become established. Focus, then, is set upon parents learning their role as parents, and only when that is acquired can they learn the special skills necessary for parenting a hearing-handicapped child.

The areas of particular concern include:

> Bonding
> Responsivity
> Watchfulness
> Affection
> Authority

Bonding

Children need first and foremost warm, constant, and expanding responsive behavior from and interaction with their parents. It requires diligent, consistent, and concentrated emphasis. Bonding comes about at first through parents simply being available. Such things as prompt response to his cries, his distress calls, his whining, and his cooing tells the child the parent is present and available. When his "calls" are recognized, he needs to get the physical security of the parents, usually the mother's presence, and her reinforcement of handling him, patting him, picking him up, or merely giving him his fallen rattle. The security serves to intensify the essential bonding. Needless to say, the parent uses her voice to reinforce as well. In fact, the parent must learn to talk to her child with the same purpose as does the parent of a hearing child. She will reassure the child with, "Mommy's coming. She will be right there!" just as a "super mother" does. She will, however, of necessity go to the child in the next room, in his crib, or wherever he might be.

Physical contact is a powerful bonding device. Patting, rocking, singing, carrying, and even massaging add to the feelings of closeness. The first step in communication learning is the parent and child engaged in mutual enjoyment and accompanying talk.

Responsivity

There is no general agreement about which are the most

desirable bonding traits, but the mother's responsivity seems to be related to the child's overall competence. The hearing-impaired child is less able to elicit reciprocal responsive behavior. While the parents' natural interactions with the child will grow out of the bonding process, the hearing-impaired child may not respond in a visible manner thereby possibly thwarting the parents' overtures.

To assist parents in receiving this much needed response from the child, the educator can have specific objectives for the child, i.e., "He will turn when mother comes into the room." "He will smile when mother leans over his crib," etc. As the parent becomes more and more aware of the responses wanted from the child, she will develop her own devices for obtaining them, i.e., making frequent eye contact, smiling at her child, or returning his smile. *This initial mutual responsiveness between parent and child is so basic it can easily be overlooked.*

Watchfulness

The parent can monitor the child's activities by sound and sight. By monitoring she is able to synchronize her interaction initiatives with his actions. While she is aware of what her child might be doing in the other room, her child does not know this. Therefore, this parent-child behavior should be made *obvious* to the youngster.

Mother really should make a point of bringing the child to the room where she is working. The bonding intensifies as the mother watches the child. By watching him, she becomes more and more familiar with his actions. She learns what triggers them and what actions certain stimuli produce. Watching, therefore, continues whether Mother is otherwise engaged or whether she is involved in intense conversations. The baby knows he is being watched and grows more secure and the bonding intensifies.

Knowing what the child is doing, why he is doing it, and what will be his thoughts on the action is of top priority in the task of teaching the "mother tongue." Mother needs to watch sufficiently so that she can imagine what it is that *the baby is thinking*. That is the material that needs language. It is the *child's thought* that has *meaning* for him. Parents, by watching, can learn those thoughts. It is so important that they do this in the early stages when the child's thoughts are transparent. By succeeding at this time, the ability to know what a child is thinking increases and at a later developmental stage, Mother can give language to his more abstract thoughts. It is very true that, "mothers should read their children like books."

Parents must become very familiar with their child's feelings, moods, and thoughts. These are the bases of his eventual language expression. It is these to which the parent will give linguistic form as the child develops. As the parent watches, she can identify actions and feelings and appropriately respond, "Do you want Mommy to get your teddy bear?" "Oh, did you pinch your finger?" These verbalizations plus handing him the object or giving a hug for the hurt can begin to teach the child that he is understood.

What security a child must feel when the parent responds to his feelings by tender contact for a hurt, a calm countenance for anger, a happy facial expression for joy. The deliberate attention given to his needs and his thoughts is a critical step to language development. As the parent watches, she will become more and more in tune with her child and will understand him.

Affection

Though tactile communication — a hug, a pat, a squeeze — is strongly advocated to display affection, tonal devices must be used as well. While sound, as *we* know it, is denied the hearing-impaired child, he can derive value from voice quality and intonation. These are available to him even before he has amplification. This is especially true in the early period when the child is physically close to his parent.

One of the early tasks for parents to become aware of is the realization that the child can learn the value of praise. The message of, "That's a job well done," provides a strong basis for developing a positive self-concept. Showing pleasure is another important task for parents to experience. All dyadic interaction between the two should not be just pleasurable but *obviously pleasurable*. It is futile to pretend and use a plastic smile. Children very soon differentiate sincerity from insincerity.

A mother sometimes needs lots of help to display love for her handicapped baby possibly because of her own unmet needs for responses from him. Furthermore, until the parent learns the appropriate response to match the child's behavior, the child may cry all the louder and completely thwart her affectionate response.

Teachers need to realize parents need the same kind of help as the youngster. Knowing the parent's stage of acceptance is crucial in helping her. A teacher must remember that an angry parent, a depressed parent, or a hungry parent will have difficulty seeing what is occurring in the demonstration of love to her offspring. He may not seem cute and cuddly or smart to her at that time. Needless to say, the *teacher* observes the same caution given parents. The concern and affection they show for the parent as well as the child *must be sincere.*

There is a familiar song that has a powerful message — "I can't live without love." The child or his parents cannot live without it either. Basic to bonding is a mutual expression of LOVE.

Authority

As discussed in Chapter 2, authority is an important role for parents to learn. They need to assume the role as an authority figure as early as possible. This provides the child with a secure framework within which to develop. Even though parents are encouraged and assisted in demonstrating affection, they must learn early that they "run the show." The child needs this security. Regardless of how permissive the parent might feel inclined to be, this is not the child with whom he can be indecisive. The hearing-impaired child needs a parent who gives him a secure framework in which to operate.

This does not mean, however, that the parent is a disciplinarian. In fact, if the child's behavior is such that he needs repeated discipline, parents have already abdicated their parental role. They have not communicated their LOVE. Their smiles, their hugs should have reinforced the good behavior. Deprivation of those positive forms of support should be more than enough discipline for most children. Parents can set limits through affectionate displays of acceptance and rigid faces for rejection of misbehavior.

Critical to the role of authority is consistency. *Consistent over time*: What is wrong today because Mother has a headache, must still be wrong tomorrow even though her tolerance level is up. *Consistent across members of the family*: Even though Dad is home less time than Mother, his limits are just the same as her limits. *Consistent across places*: What works at home must also work at the store and Grandma's house as well, even though on-lookers may seem to disagree.

Be loving but firm is the motto. If Mother maintains her watchful eye, the child will not be able to drift aimlessly, explore carelessly, or behave indifferently. He will know he is under the loving care of his parent because the parent both shows it and says it.

The principle tasks of the parent at this level are to become knowledgable about child growth and development; bond to the child in a secure relationship; be responsive and watchful; show and feel affection, yet maintain authority; and above all else, be sure to *talk* when near the child.

Objectives

The academic climate is such today that all teachers need to prepare behavioral objectives. Therefore, these are some suggestions for this level. Since the teaching is individualized, the appropriate objectives for each parent-child dyad (duo), the time envelope, and the criteria for mastery are left up to the intervener/teacher.

- Parent will be aware of growth and development of children the same age as her child.
- Parent will provide appropriate playthings for the child's age.
- Parent will see that child is wearing his hearing aid(s) during all waking hours.
- Parent will respond promptly to child's distress calls.
- Parent will interact with the child.
- Parent will bring child to the room or place where she is working.
- Parent will watch child even when otherwise engaged.
- Parent will anticipate child's interest.
- Parent's talk will match child's thoughts.
- Parent will respond to child's gazes, smiles, sounds, and gestures.
- Parent will make frequent eye contact with the child.
- Parent will smile frequently at the child.
- Parent will return the child's smile.
- Parent will frequently demonstrate affection.
- Parent will use "love talk."
- Parent will display pleasure in interaction activities.
- Parent will set limits.
- Parent will demonstrate consistent authority over time.
- Parent will respond in a positive way to the child's positive behavior.
- Parent will handle the child with confidence.

2. Tune in to the Child

"Tuning in" is a term borrowed from telecommunications. Just as we want sharp reception from the television, so, too, we want sharp reception of the spoken word by the child. We want to know what he is thinking because it is those thoughts that need language labels. By understanding the child's moods, his interests, and his incentive for action, parents can "tune in" to what *he* needs to say. *This crucial task of tuning in to the child is the basis of the theory of language development in this text.* This is the way a child learns language. He has the meaning, and the adults supply the language. *The child learns language from meaning. At this stage, language does not give him the meaning, experiences do.*

Rather than viewing the parent's role as doing things to and for the child, it should be seen as a process of reciprocal interaction. Initially, our concern is with good parent behaviors. As we move along the continuum to our goal — the child's maximal achievement of his innate abilities — we become more concerned with communication. The first order of importance rests with the *ACT of communicating.*

The actual act of communicating requires certain types of behavior. It is a two-way maneuver. It can be prompted by an outside event, or it can be a response to a spontaneous thought. Verbal response to an action, to a person, or to speech is a basic language skill.

Review, if you will, the act. Think of social conversations you have had recently. Something happens and conversation ensues, i.e., the meal elicits conversation, someone moves, stands, or does something and talk follows. Even silence from a companion can initiate conversation, i.e., "A penny for your thoughts."

Conversation requires two-way behavior. Responses are a language skill. Responding is learned behavior, and it is learned at the pre-linguistic level. Parents need to learn how to foster these behaviors in their hearing-impaired child.

The levels of behavior falling in this category are more interrelated than at the previous stage. These levels dealing with "tuning in" to the child, which is the essence of communication, are:

> Face-to-Face Contact
> Eye-to-Eye Contact
> Turn-Taking
> Matching Language to the Child's Thought
> Responding to Vocalizations
> Reinforcement

Face-to-face contact

Face-to-face communication requires the parent to position herself and the child so as to enable the infant to see the mother's total face. Not only does he perceive the mother's looks of pleasure, but he can also observe her lip movements as she speaks endearing terms or meaningful phrases.

Learning how effective this physical position could be led one of the authors to develop a program for parents over thirty years ago. The author had an opportunity to meet a twenty-month-old, profoundly deaf child and his mother. The author was asked by the toddler's mother if she could show parents how to stage situations for acceptable lipreading experiences. (This was before hearing aids for infants were available and before audiologists thought anything could be done for the "under-five-year-olds.")

Coincidentally, it was at a time television was also in its infancy, and the manufacturers were advertising "No Stoop, No Squat, and No Squint." This advertising slogan seemed to be appropriate for parents of the young potential lipreader, and the author tried to demonstrate it. This child could understand whatever was said to him as long as he could watch the speaker's face. He could not understand, however, if the speaker covered her mouth. The author was a stranger to the child having met him just prior to the "demonstration." Nevertheless, this child responded appropriately when the author directed him to do such things as manipulate toy people and furniture: "Put the red chair in the living room." "Put the dishes on the kitchen table." "Daddy is in the garage." This author was amazed at the lipreading comprehension of this child.

Promptly, the author looked into the background of the child to see why he performed as well or better than most hearing children his age. Yes, he was profoundly deaf. Yes, he was born deaf. But he was the third child in the family, and the two older siblings were deaf. Hence, the parents suspected that he might also be deaf. Before the mother and child left the hospital, she had him in a face-to-face position every time she held him, which was often. This mother's practice was to talk normally, always demonstrating her affection for him. The author reasoned that it was because of this behavior that his receptive language had kept pace with normal developmental patterns. It was this experience that led this author to dedicate herself to the proposition that *the parent is indeed the child's first teacher*.

Parents need to become skilled in positioning their child for the best face-to-face contact and listening conditions. For example, if the child is an infant, the parent needs to hold him so he is facing *her*, not the world. When she needs to be free to cook, wash, or clean, she can put him in an infant seat. As the child grows older, he might be put in a moveable highchair or booster seat. If he becomes a typical two-year-old and runs about the house, the mother will need to devise ways to get to his level. Her knees must work well. Some of the reinforcement talked about earlier might also have to be given for the child's attending behavior.

The important message is that the parent must face the child for the act of communicating. Communicating takes place throughout the day. When dressing, feeding, bathing, and cleaning, the "super mother" will face her child when communicating with him. This emphasis on face-to-face contact *does not* negate listening, which must be stressed, but points out that we *communicate* face-to-face most frequently.

Eye-to-eye contact

Eye-to-eye interaction is less overt than face-to-face contact, but equally powerful in developing communication. It is the forerunner not of what is said, but of the act of reciprocity: I talk and you react. Conversation is reciprocal. I look at you, and you return my look — a similar reciprocal act and an early step leading to conversation. Even averting my gaze has significance. These are essential skills for language. This fundamental act is rarely included in curricula, but is critical to the social aspect of communication.

Unlike the hearing child who gets clues auditorily and turns and looks to his mother, the majority of hearing-impaired children need to learn to observe faces as well as listen. Parents need to understand that eye contact is a precursor to auditory attention. They need help in learning how to respond to his looking and subsequent gaze aversion.

Parents also need to learn that they can make frequent eye contacts while "on the run." When doing this, they need to reward the infant for looking — a smile, a look of pleasure, even a wink will suffice. Eventually, parents will learn to respond to the child's gaze with words, but first they need to realize how important the eye-to-eye interaction is. The child needs to know his mother cares about him before he finds out that she has a message for him as well.

Teachers must make sure that the mother stops her conversation about hearing aids, batteries, books, or whatever, the moment the child looks at her. Mother needs to respond to the child's gaze *immediately* — nothing is more important. She may only smile, but it would be even better if she said something to him and demonstrated that she was responsive to him. At another time, the child may do something and then look at the parent. That look must be rewarded! While the parent is smiling, she may say, "You pushed the truck." In time he will respond, provided that he is given the pause and then the words to do so. Hopefully, Mother should now know, from watching her child, what he wants to say. She has now "tuned in" to her youngster, and the communication is in process.

Turn-taking

Turn-taking develops naturally from the eye-to-eye contact. It is the reciprocal interaction which can be observed in any dyadic situation with two people — "You talk, I talk, you respond, and I talk more." Turn-taking in eye-to-eye contact, babbling, and play are important forerunners of verbal communication. Children need to acquire the knack of playing the conversation game. It has a ping-pong like pattern which each member of the dyad (dialogue) displays. Mothers need to know why they should alternate appropriately with their child in eye gazing now and in verbal activities such as "Peek-a-Boo" later.

At this stage if the child is babbling, adults should babble back. In this way, the parent is demonstrating imitation. The child is part of a turn-taking experience, and he is being exposed to prosodic features of language which are essential for speech intelligibility.

Matching language to the child's thoughts

Because parents, through watchfulness, will know what to say when the child is playing, eating, dressing, and so forth, he will acquire meaning for language. The content of the parents' communication will be about his objects, his actions, his possessions. To those thoughts, parents will give the language structure. The child has the meaning already in his mind, and it is to that meaning to which the parents match language. It is the match of his ideas to the parents' words that is the key to content learning.

Children are communicating thoughts, ideas, and feelings many times throughout the day. The challenge is to recognize these thoughts, ideas, and feelings and model appropriate language for them. It is important to remember that the language must match the child's thought. For example, a child has been hurt from a fall on the playground, and he comes to the adult in tears. Many adults would say, "Oh, you'll be all right. Don't cry." It is doubtful that the child is thinking *that!* In order to match the adult language with the child's thoughts and feelings, the adult would need to model something like, "Oh, you fell down. Let me see. *Ouch! That hurts!* Do you want me to kiss it? Let's get a band-aid for your knee." The more often the adult is able to communicate with the child by reading his thought or figuring out what he is trying to say and then matching those thoughts with an appropriate language model, the faster he will progress in language development. This cannot be confined to a couple of isolated incidents during the day, but it should be on-going, all day long, in a variety of situations and locations.

This approach to learning language is in stark contrast to drilling on words or labels someone has ordained as a child's first words. Parents must avoid "working" on names of objects or actions that are not present and not within the child's current thoughts! This *is* the time, however, for *one particular word to take on great importance, and that is the child's own name.* Every time the child looks at the mother, she should respond in some way such as, "Hi, Tom, how are you?" She should preface many of the activities with, "Tom, let's go night-night." When she looks at him, she uses his name. When she wants him to look at her, she calls his name. When she wants to play with him, she uses his name. In short, the child's own name is the most important word he will acquire. Knowing his name is basic to his self-identity.

Responding to vocalization

If we were asked to give a priority rank to all the areas thus far discussed, response to vocalization would probably head the list. While tuning in to the child's thought gives him the content of verbalizations, and turn-taking shows him the pattern of communication, responding to his vocalizations gives a child the *why* of speaking. Through the response to his oral efforts, he learns the function of communicating.

Developmental linguists believe that the child's "mewings" are his first steps to spoken language. They are critical to effective oral communication. "Mewings" are the baby's way of phonating his feelings, his needs, his pain. He cries when he is hungry. He has another cry when he needs a fresh diaper. He coos to be played with. He whines when he wants to be picked up. These cries, whines, and coos are the child's communication. He must learn that communication can function for him. He must see that his communication moves people; his efforts produce results.

Parents must recognize the vocal efforts and respond to them promptly and appropriately. The *promptness* is crucial. Ten minutes later, a child won't know that his whimper brought Mother running. Ten minutes is an eternity to a small child.

By three months of age, the baby with normal hearing has his parents jumping in response to his demands as if they were puppets and he, the puppeteer, controlling the strings. When that hearing child wants to be fed, carried, played with, or made comfortable, he says, in effect, to the parent, "Jump," and she, in turn, responds, "How high?" So, too, must the hearing-impaired child learn the value of vocalization. The *meaning* of his vocalizations precedes formal speech production by many months and sometimes years.

Too often, adults get busy and tune out the noises a child is making. No discussion with the teacher or news sharing with neighbors is worth reducing the motivation of a child to vocalize. The parent must "tune in" to her child regardless of what she may be doing. The young child has no waiting power. He needs instant gratification.

Up to now, screams and shrieks have not been mentioned. Too often, we as teachers see children whose only means of getting a response has been obnoxious vocalizations. It is not difficult to realize how that came about. Although the child in a parent program may be older than three months chronologically, he is still at an infant language level if he hasn't learned the power of acceptable vocalization. Part of the teacher's work is to help the parents know what the child's utterances mean and recognize them correctly. They, then, need to know to respond promptly and allow their deaf child the thrill of being a puppeteer and "moving his puppet." In this way vocalizations have positive results, and inappropriate, obnoxious vocalizations will not develop nor will they need to be extinguished.

Reinforcement

Another aspect of the teacher role is to alert parents to the role of reinforcement and its value in the emotional and educational growth of the child. For some children just getting the parent's prompt and undivided attention is sufficient. For others it may take additional positive reinforcement such as patting, love talk, smiles, and obvious pleasure on the part of adults. It is just like the advertisements for a financial advisor, E. F. Hutton: "When E. F. Hutton speaks, we listen!" So, it needs to be with a hearing-impaired child. When he vocalizes, we listen!

Not only are appropriate reinforcers necessary, but consistency is in order. If a behavior gets a response and is rewardable one day, it must not be ignored the next. In time, the intensity of the reinforcement diminishes, but behaviors get positive attention until they are firmly established. Eventually, reinforcement will be used for specific language learning, but at the outset, it is for more global (general) behavior.

On the subject of reinforcement, there are two areas that should be considered. First of all, it needs to be stressed that reinforcement is not a task only for parents, but for all members of the family. Everyone needs to know why and how the child's vocalizations must be reinforced and eventually shaped. Not only is this reinforcing to the child, but is rewarding to all family members who share in the young child's life.

The second area is the parent reinforcement. Since they receive little, if any, response from their hearing-impaired child, parents need to be encouraged. Just as the child needs to know his vocalizations pay off, so must the parents, through support and encouragement, know they are doing the right thing. Who reinforces whom in the parent-infant dyad, duo, is a question of considerable magnitude. Is it the child reinforcing the parent or the parent encouraging the child? With a hearing-impaired child, it is less likely to be the child, so mother's reinforcement may have to come from the teacher. The instructor must find ways to help mother get the child to look, to smile and to vocalize. These tasks are easier for the parent when she feels she is understood and appreciated in her efforts. Reinforcement from the teacher and the child make the mother's task easier and more rewarding.

Objectives

It is helpful for some parents to have specific objectives. The following might give them direction in knowing how to help their child:

- Parent will see that child is wearing his hearing aid(s).
- Parent will face the child frequently.

- Parent will hold the child in front of her when she talks to him.
- Parent will make eye contact with the child.
- Parent will follow the child's eye gaze.
- Parent will smile, wink, or give a look of pleasure when she gets the child's eye gaze.
- Parent will talk and use the child's name when she gets his eye gaze.
- Parent will play reciprocal eye-contact games with the child.
- Parent will play reciprocal, imitative games with the child's vocalizations.
- Parent will match language to the child's feelings and moods.
- Parent will match language to the child's ideas and interests.
- Parent will use the child's name whenever talking to him.
- Parent will use the child's name to get his attention.
- Parent will stop activity to respond to the child.
- Parent will respond promptly to the child's crying, cooing, or babbling.
- Parent will use reinforcement effectively.

3. Talk *to* the Child

The concept that a child develops language from birth is a relatively recent consideration. Most psychologists and teachers long assumed that language began after the child said his first word. It is that assumption that possibly led parents to be unduly concerned about the "first word," "what words," and "how many words" the child knew. The reality is that parents have many skills to teach their child long before the first words appear. This over-concern with words can be compared to starting to build a skyscraper from the penthouse down. A firm foundation must be laid in language, just as in the skyscraper, so it, too, will be a lasting structure.

Attention to a child's utterances facilitates his linguistic progress. Shaping those utterances into linguistic form lays the foundation of a fully-developed language system. "Super mothers" usually respond to and *shape* their child's utterances without being aware of the important job they are doing. For other parents, the strategies may have to be learned.

The input to their child is part of the process which

investigators are calling "motherese." What mother does and says and how she says it have proven to be critical factors in language development.

The tremendous complexity of language is overpowering, however, the model set by the "super mother" gives an orderly procedure leading to its development. After having set the stage for communication skills and the art of interacting, she proceeds to incorporate the following components:

> Intonation,
> Prosodic patterns,
> Imitation,
> Immersion of the child in spoken language,
> Repetitions.

Intonation

The most salient feature in the language addressed to children is intonation. Intonation patterns are used to carry syntactic, pragmatic, and semantic meaning.

The syntax of spoken statements is indicated by a rising intonation contour, a falling intonation contour, or an explosive tone. Is it a question (a rising contour), a statement (falling contour), or a command (flat contour)? Each pattern will elicit a different response from the listener. Though this appears to be a sophisticated language skill, interestingly it is heard in the babble of five-month-old hearing children. If the language addressed to hearing-impaired children observes the syntactic principles natural to our language, these children, too, can be found to use syntactic contours in their babble. The urgency is that they have amplification and that parents utilize every opportunity for natural *sentence* input — not single words, not "pigeon" English, but appropriate, linguistically correct sentences which possess meaning for the child in age-appropriate content.

From the data being gathered on language input to a baby, it is evident that parents use shorter sentences with a child under two years than they do with toddlers and preschoolers. There is a high percent of simple statements, with questions next, and only a very small percent of commands. From hearing these voice contours, babies produce syntactic intonation of statements and questions long before their first word. The hearing-impaired child must have the same opportunity to hear intonation spoken to him as often as does the normally hearing infant!

Intonation serves in a social exchange. Its function signals when it is the listener's turn to speak or respond. The drop in the speaker's voice indicates that it is the listener's turn. This is the linguistic skill that is being built when engaged in the ping-pong type of play. The important turn-taking that was identified at an earlier stage was the beginning of this pragmatic aspect. Learning this social linguistic device begins with verbal play between parent and infant.

When a listener responds to a speaker, he needs to have abstracted the speaker's feelings about his topic. The speaker may even be using a foreign language, the words of which are not understood. Nevertheless, knowing the syntactic principles which are universal, the listener would know the speaker has paused in his discussion to allow him to respond. He would also know how the speaker felt about the topic under discussion. Did he like it or hate it? Is he excited or calm? The speaker's feelings are perfectly clear from the universal intonation patterns used.

Intonation can change the meaning of the same words used differently within a given language pattern. Suppose a speaker used the four words: "He is a good man." He could indicate much about that man. He might be saintly, but on the other hand, he might be a crook. It might be a truthful sentence, or it might be sarcastic and cynical, or it might even be a question. The interpretation is not within the knowledge of knowing the meaning of "He" or "is" or "a" or "good" or "man," but rather the knowledge of the suprasegmental — the intonation. Suprasegmental means that the sound covers all the segments of the sentence. No, language is not taught by teaching words! How would a child ever learn the suprasegmental tools if language were discrete segments having static meaning? It cannot be done!

Suppose one takes a phrase such as "Oh, my!" and sees how many meanings can be derived from it by changing the intonation pattern. Differing intonation patterns could convey surprise, disappointment, happiness, sadness, concern, anxiety, and love. Yet, the words remained constant. Intonation contours carried the meaning.

Love is the first and fundamental meaning that should be conveyed to a beginning-language child whatever his age. Does a person ever cuddle a baby and shout imperatives to him? Of course not! No one demands, "Look at me." "Say it again." Instead, one would hear, "Aw, you are so sweet." "Aren't you a cute baby?" "Look at you!" "You are a sweet boy." A child learns the contours and semantic content through the earliest bonding, clothed in language.

In the delightful movie *Three Men and a Baby* (1987), there are many good lines relative to child rearing, but one in particular is worthy of noting here. Actor Tom Selleck is holding the baby and reading aloud from a sports magazine when his friend yells to him, "The baby doesn't understand that." Selleck's response was simply, "It doesn't matter what I read. It's the tone I use that counts" and the camera closed in on a very happy baby.

Not only do parents need to have love in their intonation, but they need to show it as well. Their facial expression must be appropriate for the meaning being transmitted. The hearing-impaired child needs to have the tones clarified by his parent's speech. Just as it is not appropriate to talk in a monotone, neither should speech come from a stoic, expressionless face.

In order to check on the very early age at which children learn the power of intonation, one could experiment with an infant at play. If vocal tones indicating negative feelings are used, the effect on the child is obvious. The child will become restless and possibly cry. If, however, warm and loving vocal tones are used, they will bring smiles and cooing.

There is appreciable evidence that children under six months of age respond to the intonation of syntactic signals, particularly imperative forms. At the same time, they react differently to vocal tones which indicate feelings. Responding to a rich intonation input, babies produce intonation contours in their babble long before their first word — intonation contours establish the basis for sentences used at a much later stage.

Prosodic patterns

There are other devices such as pitch, time, intensity, rhythm, and accent to clarify the spoken messages. These devices, including the global or suprasegmental intonation, make up the prosodic or melodic aspects of speech. Meaning is conveyed more by HOW something is said than WHAT is said. Take, for example, the word "Daddy." The intonation will vary when: (1) He is outside, and he is called in for dinner ("Daaaadeeee!"); (2) He has been denied permission to buy a new bicycle and disappointment is apparent ("Daaady"); and (3) He has come home unexpectedly and there is excitement ("Daddy!"). The difference is embedded in duration, stress, and pitch, not in the word itself.

A speaker may also employ pitch and stress to communicate

an infinite number of meanings. Suppose he says, "Where are you going tomorrow?" The responses will vary according to his pitch and/or stress. If his voice rises and falls on the word, "where," he is primarily seeking destination. If, on the other hand, he stresses "tomorrow," he wants to know the plans for that future time, not today. If the stress in on "going," he may be giving a message not to stay.

The prosodic patterns transmit meaning in very poorly articulated speech, whereas precisely spoken speech without rhythm and with exaggerated time is not as intelligible. Deaf children denied auditory opportunities lack prosodic features which clarify meaning. Silverman (1982) translated the following:

As we all know, hearing exerts a very significant influence on speech which is most evident in a person who has been deaf since early childhood. His or her speech appears for the most part harsh, without any modulation... and not always easy to understand. (p. 73)

This was a statement made by Victor Urbantschitsch in 1895. Unfortunately, close to a century later, similar statements could be made about many deaf speakers. Studies continue to cite poor breath control, restrictive voice pitch, longer duration of phonation, and inappropriate overall speech rhythm as some of the significant factors affecting the intelligibility of deaf speech (Ling, 1978).

It is known that deaf children who have only sensitivity to sound at 500 Hz can perceive the melody of speech. It has been demonstrated also that these children can perceive pitch, stress, and duration. Not only do the prosodic nuances enable speech expression to be clear, they also aid in the comprehension of speech of others through lipreading.

Emotional states can also be received through amplification. Therefore, the role of the parent is to provide the auditory stimulus but not necessarily ask for its recognition. Parents can do this by honestly conveying their feelings. For example, if the child pinches the new baby, the parent should not say, "Be nice," in soothing, soft tones, but rather she should show her true feelings. "Don't hurt the baby! That makes me angry!"

How long the hearing-impaired individual needs to "hear" the suprasegmentals before he understands is unknown, but we do know that hearing children can discriminate between intonation contours of speech while still in the crib. Attempting to instruct a hearing-impaired child to impose these features on his already developed speech patterns is inadequate, at best. Experiences with vocal pitch, intensity, and duration need to be prominently included in the language the parent associates with a child's daily routines from infancy onward.

Parents also need to engage in interactive play with games such as Peek-a-Boo and Patty-Cake providing many prosodic features. These games that they play with linguistically young children are ideal for developing intonation, stress and rhythm. Furthermore, they are one-to-one, parent-to-child, and are usually face-to-face. They can be repeated very often and continue to secure bonding.

With amplification, the hearing-impaired child can hear the intonation and nuances in the adults' voices. It is important not to use exaggerated speech; not to talk in single words. Beginning-language children need exposure to the full spectrum of "meaning delivering" tools. These tools need to be practiced frequently in the beginning through imitation and later in spontaneous speech.

The authors recall a four-year-old who was sent to residential school because there was no facility within miles of his home. Because his siblings always attended camp, Mark's parents referred to the school as "camp." Mark was not making much progress until one morning his frustrations with school surfaced and with perfect intonation, he exclaimed, "Damn Camp!" His teacher showed extreme pleasure at his expression of feelings with proper intonation. Today, Mark is a high-powered trouble shooter for the Federal Reserve Banks traveling across the country to check on failing institutions facing much bigger frustrations today than "camp" was to him twenty-two years ago. His parents had taught him that language was to convey feelings — *his feelings* — not just to label or describe non-personal things as is too often the case.

Imitation

Imitation, unlike intonation and prosody, is a non-meaning-bearing device. The only meaning to be derived is "I have someone's attention." "She loves me." Appropriate here is the old saying, "Imitation is the highest form of compliment." If we imitate the infant, we are paying him a compliment. His efforts are worth our attention.

Imitation does more than that, however. It initiates the child into an important speech strategy. No better device has been developed to help a child, any child, acquire the phonemes of language. Teachers use imitation throughout the child's school life to perfect the articulation of speech sounds.

Previously, interaction and ping-pong play were discussed. The idea was to have fun and learn one-to-one techniques. If these features are being observed, the emphasis can begin to shift to the imitation act never forgetting the intent of communication mentioned earlier.

Parents can seize the child's vocal efforts and imitate them. Beautiful reciprocity! Child vocalizes and parent vocalizes back using the child's utterances. Of course, this could be called "shaping" the utterance, but there is more concern at first with the child learning the strategy of imitation. With hearing children as early as five-months old, the babble reflects the language spoken in his home. Parents — Chinese, French, Russian — did not consciously shape the sound of their babies' voices, playful imitation initiated the process.

Immersion of the child in spoken language

The hearing-impaired child needs to "hear" talk for many of his waking moments. That talk is connected language which puts words in their syntactical order. This is the way a child learns which words follow others in order to convey meaning. We know statements such as, "The green grass sleeps silently," are not meaningful but are grammatically sound, whereas "The sleeps grass silently green," are not. Sentence diagrams or analysis aren't necessary. The ear just allows the listener to accept one and reject the other. That is possible because the listener has stored syntactically correct sentences and has not been exposed to the incorrect ones. The hearing-impaired child must have the same opportunity if he is to develop a sense of the syntactic order of language.

The involvement between the parent and child should be TALK. This is not meaningless chatter, nor is it baby talk. Neither is it adult conversation. The savvy parent uses SELF-TALK instead. It is as if she is talking to herself while tuning into what is interesting to her child but not expecting him always to understand. "Here's the teddy bear. Cute teddy bear. The teddy bear is so soft. Aw, the teddy bear is on the floor."

One parent involved her six-month-old, hearing-impaired child in the activity of grocery shopping. She pushed him in the supermarket cart, and as she went along, she talked about what she was buying, weighing, counting, and stacking in the cart. At the time, shoppers did give her strange looks, but when this child spoke in full but short sentences at age two, the looks became those of admiration.

The hearing-impaired child has a continual need for talk. Talk should be blended into nurturing times as when he is being fed, held, rocked, carried, bathed, cuddled. Parents can talk on any subject: "Feel the soft teddy bear;" "Do you want a cookie? Mmmm. It is good!"; "Now let's wash your hands . . . now your foot." Then, of course, there is lots of love talk, "Hi there, Tim. You are a big boy. Mommy loves you!"

The parent should say something whenever the child's eyes are on her. If nothing else, she could talk about what the child is observing:

"Johnny is sitting in his high chair."
"Johnny broke the cracker."
"Johnny is drinking his milk."

If the child's attention goes to persons or pets in the environment, something should be said about what they are doing:

"Grandma is fixing some toast."
"Mary is playing with her doll."
"Mommy is drinking coffee."
"Spot is barking."

The same activities occur and reoccur in a household, and these give numerous opportunities for valuable *repetition.*

Parents will need support and assistance to overcome the self-consciousness they feel when talking and getting little reciprocal response. It is not an easy task to keep up an ongoing conversation with one's self. Nevertheless, this directed talk stores the information upon which the child will draw for the rest of his life. He will develop a feel for which words follow which, for how language is organized, for how he is to express himself in language.

Mother uses relatively short sentences that focus more on the idea than on the object. She tells about what will happen. She talks about things past. "Daddy will take you to Grandmother's this weekend." "We had fun at the park yesterday, didn't we?"

In all of this input, the child is receiving information about the notion of time and how we express it. He is learning how Mother feels about things from the intonation in her voice. He is being exposed to pronouns with their abstractness. He is getting vocabulary, not just label words — park, daddy, and Grandmother — but also structure words — will, take, this, at. He is seeing how these thought-connectors are used and that they have meaning only in structure. *Therefore, it is important that complete phrases and sentences are used at all times and that the meaning grows out of shared experience.*

Repetitions

Parent repetition can sustain interest, present information in small doses and facilitate language learning. Repetition is bound to occur if parents talk about ongoing activities.

No parent can deny the great value of spaced repetitions. Piano playing, dancing, and baseball all need practice to perfect those physical skills. Linguistic skills need practice too. Think of the grocery cart scenario. How many times did that mother talk during that and similar activities — probably several times a week. These linguistic development skills are not something to do occasionally. Neither are they something done at a set time as a "lesson." On the contrary, they must be interwoven into the fiber of the dyad's (twosome's) day. True, the life of a mother of a linguistically young child can be monotonous, but such is the challenge of "super mothers." Repetition at this stage focuses upon reciprocity, intonation patterns and imitation. Later, the repetition will be for attention — "Where's the ball? The ball. Where's the ball?" Or it may be repetition of similar language structure for several experiences, i.e., "Wash the dishes." "Wash the doll." "Wash your hands." or "Wash the dog." Each of us heard these multiple repetitions in order to learn our language. So must the hearing-impaired child! With daily routines, these repetitions occur naturally.

While the hearing-impaired child may not be using "full sentences" at the *chronological* age of three years, with help he can be talking at the *linguistic* age of two years! While linguistically he may be two, he can be five or more years old chronologically. Linguistic age means the level at which *he functions in language*. Some people go so far as to say the child is at zero linguistic age until he gets the hearing aid(s), however old he might be.

The principle task for the parent at this level is that she surrounds the child with spoken language and uses animation and appropriate intonation to convey her meaning. Following her daily routine, the language input is repeated throughout the day and day after day. The exposure the child receives to lexical and structural vocabulary ordinarily comes in the form of simplified, repetitive, and idealized dialect. It is always and forever in sentence style. Further, not only is the language said frequently, but usually it is also very much about the hearing-impaired child himself.

Objectives

The behavioral objectives in a systems approach might be similar to the following:

- Parent will see that child is wearing his hearing aid(s).
- Parent will use appropriate intonation prominently in her talk.
- Parent will utilize statements, questions, and exclamations in her self-talk.
- Parent will read child's signals regarding turn-passing.
- Parent will wait after vocalizing, using stress and intonation to signal to the child that it's his turn to talk or vocalize.
- Parent will express feelings of love, surprise, sadness, joy, with appropriate tone etc.
- Parent will play games such as Patty-Cake and Peek-a-Boo providing intonation and prosodic features.
- Parent will use a <u>variety</u> of the prosodic features in length, pitch, and loudness in her talking.
- Parent will imitate the child's intonation in her vocalizations.
- Parent will imitate child's utterances.
- Parent will use relatively short sentences.
- Parent will speak more slowly than she does with an adult.
- Parent will say something when the child's eyes are on her face.
- Parent will repeat the self-talk frequently.
- Parent will repeat activities and language about the activities often.
- Parent will apply similar language to a variety of situations.

4. Talk *for* the Child

As stated earlier in this chapter, there is a continuum of interactions which lead to language development. All children move through sequences which are absolutes, but proceed at their own rate. It is not a hit or miss situation, but rather a smooth transition from stage to stage. No more than we expect a child to ride a bicycle before he can walk, can we expect a child to communicate before he learns the basic devices. He must learn the important skills of vocalization, turn-taking, emphasis through intonation, and meaning as the basis of communication.

Teachers and parents often want to start immediately on countable things such as vocabulary. This can be done with a parrot, but *not* with a child. It is extremely counter-productive. Communication precedes language just as in math, addition precedes calculus. *Long before the child learns words or even simple sentences, he must learn the FUNCTION of language, the purpose of communication, if you will.*

As a review of the previous sections will reveal, the first three stages focus on the *why* of communicating. This may take weeks or months depending on the parents' strategies, as well as the child's abilities, and the critical use of amplification. Most of the early categories are auditory, but *available* even to the profoundly deaf child if he has proper hearing aid(s). It also must be remembered that it takes at least ten waking hours a day of listening for a normally hearing child to say his first word by approximately twelve months of age. Twelve months or three hundred and sixty-five days of ten hours a day means something close to four thousand hours of listening prior to the emergence of a word. It is another four thousand hours before word-like sounds begin to appear, and it is equally long before language strings are used. Realistically, it takes eight thousand hours of good listening before the hearing child is communicating!

Teachers and some parents must learn a hard lesson. They cannot go against nature and condense those eight thousand hours of listening and interacting, as we described in the three earlier categories, into a lesson presented a few times a week. Parents must build the firm foundation day in and day out or rather, hour in and hour out. Our empirical data indicate the sad negative results when language is taught as discrete elements of sounds, words, or even sentences. We do not want the deaf children of the future talking like those who had the atomistic, separate and fragmented, unnatural approach to language.

When language is perceived as a subject rather than a highly abstract interrelated process, the deaf child will show poor communication ability. When a teacher perceives the *child* rather than the *parents* as her pupil during the early stages of language development, the deaf child will be deprived in his overall development. It is he who will suffer because of the lack of bonding, eye-to-eye contact, reinforcement, intonation patterns, responsivity, affection, and interpretration of *his* meaning.

The skills of communication were begun at the nurturing stage. Now the parent is approaching the specific teaching tasks of:

Labeling
Parallel talking
Modeling for the child
Expressing the same ideas in many different ways
Asking and answering questions

Labeling

During the early stages, the child has been learning *why* we communicate, and parents have been developing the strategies to ensure that message. We want to tell the child in effect, "Come on into our culture; the water is fine." The pre-linguistic stage tells the child we love him, he has security, and it is fun. He uses the vocalizations, intonation, and babble to get adults "to jump" to his command. Parents have to make a special effort so that he knows they are responding to his orders! It seems logical, then, that we call these stages *function* levels. To be sure, we will continue this phase as the child's language usage grows. Nevertheless, we recognize the importance of the early stages as the foundation.

Once the child sees that he can manipulate his environment through vocalizing, progress is underway. He should learn that he can obtain food, drink, comfort, and most importantly attention from vocal "symbols." Thus he gains his first control over his environment.

He is now ready to move ahead. The child is not learning merely to speak or to understand words or to build up a stock of words. He is learning a whole mode of behavior, the *linguistic* mode, which is prior to any particular symbolic acts in which he may engage. The acquisition of these symbols is a tremendous intellectual endeavor. The principle achievement in learning the symbols is that the child learns how to represent the external world through those symbols established by simple generalization. No small task!

The symbols come from his whole world — his social, emotional, and physical world. They relate to the things he is doing, seeing, tasting, feeling, smelling, hearing, wanting, needing, liking, finding, and on and on. Understanding of the *meaning* of the symbols precedes understanding of the words themselves.

In order to process the information and generalize to symbols, children need a broad base of concrete experiences from which they can derive reliable concepts about their environment. However, a single experience, no matter how successful, is not enough to build valid concepts. A child must make many approaches from many angles over a period of time before a concept has some measure of stability.

Consider the concepts to be acquired with the symbol *WATER*. You can:

drink it	go boating in it
bathe in it	fill an aquarium
cook it	sprinkle the lawn
pour it	wash hair with it
boil it	wash windows with it
clean the car with it	wash the baby in it
wash the car with it	wash the clothes in it
water plants with it	freeze it
wash pets in it	splash in it
wash dishes in it	make ripples in it
swim in it	float in it

Other concepts connected with water are:

It is colorless.
It looks blue when there is a lot of it.
It takes the shape of what it is in.
It seems to magnify things.
It is tasteless.
Little drops go together to make big ones.

These are all concepts that the parents can ensure occur in their home. The rich, diversified, concrete manipulation can be part of the parent-child interactive activity, and parents can see that through his sensory perception their child learns.

The generalizations at first are easiest, *water, ball, shoe,* but increase in difficulty as the child's cognitive ability increases. He will need to learn categorization, i.e., "dogs," "cats," "cows" are *animals.* Later, "dogs," "cats," "gerbils" are *pets.* Still later, "cows," "horses," "pigs" are *farm animals.* Then there are concepts related to words such as soft and hard, big and little, sweet and sour, thin and fat, small and tiny. Language topics are not just nouns, but include all content words as well. Adjectives, adverbs, and verbs, like nouns, are topics also.

Parents must provide the experiences. These are simple, everyday activities, but involvement in those experiences aids the child through his perceptual process to acquire the language symbols if presented to him at the right time.

The sensory mechanisms respond to such characteristics as size, shape, weight, color, texture, temperature, odor, loudness, pitch, distance, movement, spatial and temporal relationship, and body position. Sensory input, however, is only one part of the perceptual process. The labels must be stored with other stimuli, matched with previous experience, and put into meaning.

The perceptual level of input follows the sensory-motor level in which children handle the concrete materials and learn the labeling of objects and actions. At the perceptual level, children make discriminations at a gradually increased level of difficulty and sophistication. As a result of his perceptual processes, the child discovers meaning, and it is that *meaning* which has the language symbol.

The features of a home environment are highly perceptual, and those perceptual features have verbal labels associated with them. The verbal labels, in turn, assist in the storage of both concept and language. If the parent provides the information at the appropriate moment, the child will receive the data by which he can induce the language rules. For example, *pulling* is a concept which has linguistic form:

> Pull the toy.
> Pull the shade down.
> Pull the chair.
> Pull your socks up.
> Pull your sweater down.
> Pull the drawer out.
> Pull the string.
> Pull up the doll's socks.
> Don't pull Mommy's hair.

The action is a tugging motion which all of the above expressions have in common. The hypothesis is that the word "pull" experienced in a variety of situations can be more readily learned by the child than the word experienced many times in only one situation. We recently observed an adult who was giving the command, "Pull" to a child about three times a minute. The intended response was for the child to separate pop-it beads. When asked, "What is the purpose of the activity?" the teacher's reply was, "To teach 'pull.' " One action using one concept does not ensure linguistic nor conceptual stability. What could be of interest in such an activity with a young child? Wouldn't he have been more interested in pulling the wagon, pulling his sweater off, etc?

With very young children, formal teaching situations are less effective; the natural approach is appropriate at this age. All parents have many opportunities in their homes, moment-by-moment, for shaping language behavior. There is dressing, washing, feeding, playing, cooking, dusting, etc., etc. Children move from gross perception of objects and their functions to salient features of the objects. The more a child comes to see the characteristics of an object, the stronger imprint the word makes.

There is a classic study in which the investigators wanted to know how vocabulary was acquired. To two groups of Russian hearing four-year-olds, the English word *doll* was given fifteen hundred times. To one group the word was used in four sentences, none of which marked any salient features: "Show me the doll." "Get the doll." "Where is the doll?" "Point to the doll." To the other group, all of the perceptual characteristics were pointed out: "The doll's hair is long." "Where is the doll's thumb?" "The doll has blue eyes." "The doll has two feet." Both groups knew the word *doll* at the end of the study. (Koltosova, 1962)

When tested again at the end of six months, however, they still knew the word. However, when told that, "That is not a doll," the first group became confused and quickly extinguished the word. Not so for the second group. No matter what was said to them, they "stuck by their guns." Nothing could shake their confidence. They became angry with the experimenter but never doubted that the object was a *doll*. Learning the word by having the salient features pointed out established the word very confidently in their cognitive mechanism.

The fact that objects have different names also facilitates their being perceived as separate objects. A washer and a dryer, although both white enamel, are given different names, and this causes them to be discriminated as different objects. However, if the child has not been around either object nor seen it in relation to other stimuli, "washer" and "dryer" would have no meaning. It acquires meaning when he sees dirty clothes, water, and soap going into one; and clean, wet clothes going into the other. These are perceptions that neither pictures not toy objects provide. Yet, these clear, non-ambiguous perceptions are important for learning.

For a child to differentiate "cookie" from "ball" or "milk" is equivalent to adults learning about mitochondrial biogenesis and that mitochondria is present in every eucaryotic cell. (Which one of the author's former hearing-impaired students wrote recently in his Doctor of Philosophy studies.)

For the child to incorporate "cookie" into his language behavior, he needs to have concepts similar to his listener. He needs to know cookie can be something that he wants or of which he wants more. It can be baked, iced, eaten, broken, crumbled, stacked, counted, saved, shared, passed, stored. It can be bought at a bakery shop or received from Grandma or a neighbor. It can be in a box of the same kind or a bag of different kinds. It can be round, square, oblong, or shaped like an animal. It might be chocolate or chocolate chip, chewy or crisp. While usually it is "mmm good," sometimes it might not be so. Such are the perceptual features which expedite the learning of a concept as simple as *"cookie."*

The object should be very much "here and now." The cookie is within the child's perceptual range. He can hold it, smell it, and, importantly, eat it. So the features should be addressed. No, not at the same time, but each time he wants a cookie, the parent phrases her question differently:

> Do you want a cookie?
> What kind of cookie do you want?
> Where are the cookies?
> Would you like a chocolate cookie?

Even though the parent may pull the word out of context to identify the object more clearly, she should put it back into its sentence form, i.e., "Do you want a cookie? A cookie? Yes, a cookie. Do you want a cookie?"

Parents should learn to say something about things that will be repeated often:

> Eat your cereal.
> Let's make your bed.
> Let's wash your hands.
> Get your white shoes.
> Put your toys away.

The most mundane things are repeated with a great deal of frequency. Similar language repeated often accompanying the experiences teaches concepts in a spontaneous natural manner.

The authors toyed with calling this chapter, "The Elephant in the Living Room" for obvious reasons. The new, the strange must be *present* for the child to learn the meaning. Probably there is little need for "elephant" in the vocabulary of the linguistically young child. However, there is also little need for "fish," yet in many programs one can still see "ball," "fish," and "shoe" being given the child from pictures or toys. Note, the authors didn't say "taught." Artificial objects do not help teach anything at this stage. Children must move from the *concrete to representational* in steps. Meaning precedes naming. Perceptual characteristics assist in acquiring the meaning. Yes, if "elephant" is critical language, can we borrow the pachyderm from the zoo? *Language in its earliest form must be reality-based.*

Parallel talk

The labeling now is unlike "self-talk" which was for the child to absorb. The child took in the total language picture and stored it. The mother talked almost as if she were talking to herself. With parallel talk, she is talking to make her child aware of language. This includes the language, the situation, the intonation, and other linguistic features.

The talking is neither formal nor rigid and it grows out of the daily routine. "Super mother," however, makes an effort to see that she has the child's attention, she enjoys the talking, and accepts her child at his level of development. Actually, the reason the child becomes alert is because his parents learned to "tune in" to their child and his needs.

Parallel talk takes many forms. The savvy mother may sing songs, show the child how to do things such as fit wooden shapes in a form board and even "read" to him. Reading, in this sense, is telling short sentences about the pictures. The parents will be surprised when they encourage the child to select the story he wants "read." He develops preference early, just as do hearing children.

Another important type of behavior, from the standpoint of future success, is the mother's engaging the young child in mental activities. Her ability to talk to her child in ways that help him define and master tasks influences his cognitive growth. Contrast the mother, who, when playing with her child simply says: "Put it there," with another parent playing the same game who says:

The red circle goes in this hole. See, it's round also.
No, the blue squares have four sides. They go in this
place. It has four sides, too.

The latter mother gives information as well as a model. She not only gives the child specific information, but by telling him she provides immediate feedback on how well he has done.

Actually, parents have several roles to learn, but those of MEDIATOR, MODELER, AND REINFORCER are probably the most important at this stage. The parent MEDIATES the environment through the strategies of vocalizing, labeling objects and activities, playing games, and, in general, talking most of the time. She MODELS by coordinating the experiences the child is having with language. When sorting the laundry, for example, she can utilize categories as well as identify the items, e.g.:

Daddy's shirt is blue.
Your shirt is blue, too.
Here is a blue towel.
Where are your blue socks?
This is a blue washcloth.

Finding a caterpillar in the yard, the parent might model:

Look, Billy, here's a caterpillar.
Feel how soft the caterpillar is.
Look at the caterpillar crawl.

The parent should REINFORCE continually, using a positive feedback system most often, e.g., praise and encouragement rather than a nod or an "okay." She can also reinforce by helping the child accomplish his desires because he vocalized or imitated.

Parallel talk describes everything the child does, but frequently, it is modeling. The parent gives the language for the concept she observes the child developing. She might model for him while on a walk:

Look, there's a dog.
That's a big police dog.
I think the dog will protect the house.

The parent takes an idea, elaborates upon it and adds a bit of relevant information. These short but frequent episodes help to increase both the child's language and his general fund of knowledge.

Modeling for the child

Modeling expressions they want the child to use is familiar to all parents from their own experience. It can run the range of, "Tell Mrs. Jones you had a good time," to saying, "Thank you," "Excuse me," and, if old enough, "Please, may I be excused?" More than likely, that was modeling that the grandparents used with the parents. Now, they must do the same for their children.

We want parents to be reality-oriented at this time, however, and model language that is *needed* by the child. He needs language to obtain things, to express his feelings, and control his environment. Therefore, parents need to program for the child those expressions he needs: "Oh, you want some ice cream. Say, 'I want some ice cream.' " Because he may imitate only time and/or intonation, the child may need many models for a while. However, parents must reward the child's first attempts by giving him the ice cream. In time, they can ask for a closer approximation, but they should never discourage the child's efforts!

Similarly, the child needs models for his feelings, his likes and dislikes, and his reactions. He needs the tools to tell when he's afraid, when he is happy, why he is unhappy, and where it hurts. No one can teach these "feelings" words of: to want, to need, to wish, to like, and to hope better than the parent who is with her child and knows him well. Often, she provides at the proper moment such models as:

> I don't like that.
> My finger hurts.
> Johnny hurt me.
> Stop that!
> Let's go home.

Expressing the same ideas in many different ways

While care must be taken to use sentence structure, parents and teachers need to express the same idea in as many different ways as possible, taking care that the experience is appropriate and of interest to the child. It is far better to prevent the habit of "rubber stamping" language patterns (Simmons-Martin 1971) than to extinguish the habit after it is formed. "Rubber stamping" means that the same code is used time after time. Children who only use simple sentences, few if any adjectives, and only prepositions of place, may not have been given the opportunity to experience other, more descriptive language. Children need to be exposed to:

> I see an apple. It is red.

There comes a time, however, when they need to hear and experience:

> I found a red apple.
> Here is a big, red apple.
> I see both red and yellow apples.
> After we buy some apples, we will bake a pie.
> In a few minutes, we will bake an apple pie.
> There is only one red apple, but there are several yellow ones.

Specific, colorful, and interesting language only develops if the child is exposed to such language while he is experiencing the concept and at the appropriate time, using the language himself.

Questions asked and answered

The deaf child needs many opportunities to answer routine questions such as:
> What's that?
> Where is Daddy?
> Where is your nose, eyes, mouth, etc.?
> What does the doggie say?
> Where is the ball?

In asking the child the questions, the adult is developing the prosody for questions and doing it in a playful manner. By the next level, the adult should be asking questions for answers of location and purpose. At this level, she may ask "Where?" but may have to model the answer herself.

The main tasks at this level are to provide experiences through which the hearing-impaired child can gain a wealth of perceptions about the topics he is acquiring and to supply the missing language for his ideas. His hearing is utilized more and more for acquiring new information, and therefore, parents must provide the necessary auditory input.

Objectives

The objectives for this stage are obvious, but we will list a few to indicate the level of achievement the parent will have accomplished:

- Parent will see that the child is wearing his hearing aid(s).
- Parent will label in complete sentences the child's food, clothing, playthings, body, actions, feelings, perceptions (smells, tastes, sounds, etc.).
- Parent will point out perceptual characteristics of object.
- Parent will provide activities at the child's interest level.
- Parent will provide linguistic models for the child through parallel talk.
- Parent will make a special effort to include structure words in her language models.
- Parent's utterances will deal with the child's interest in the here and now.
- Parent will participate in verbal activity with the child such as reading, singing songs, or playing games.
- Parent will give the child the linguistic form for what she believes to express his thought and wait for him to imitate it.

- Parent will use prosodic features prominently to help the child imitate.
- Parent will reinforce the child's efforts in a positive manner.
- Parent will express the same idea in many different ways.
- Parent will see that experiences are repeated.
- Parent will ask questions.

5. Talk *With* the Child

Up to now, the child has learned how his parents feel about things from their intonation. He has had the model for expressing how he feels about things. He is receiving the language of his environment and has been exposed to some of the most abstract aspects of language. He has learned the words for objects, actions, properties of those objects and actions and their relation, and phrase structure. Putting the words into phrases to describe meaning requires the use of structure.

There is a large segment of language that only gives structural meaning. Over 30 percent of our language has no meaning out of context. Its sole purpose is to carry the meaning in structure. The function words, as they are called, are words like "a," "the," "will," "can," "to," etc. None of these words can be held up and labeled. This is the important reason why parents must talk in simple but *complete* sentences. The meaning of the total sentence grows out of experiencing the vocabulary modified by the structure words. Note the great difference in meanings in:

Take the medicine IN AN HOUR.
Take the medicine ON THE HOUR.
We will be there FOR A FEW MINUTES.
We will be there IN A FEW MINUTES.

The exposure the child received to the global language came in the form of simplified, repetitive, and idealized dialect always in sentences. He has been given the opportunity that all children need, and that is to INDUCE[1] the language principles which he should begin doing by this phase.

During this advanced stage of language comprehension, parents need to give the child opportunities to learn the meaning created by words which defy definition, i.e., "if," "because," "may," "of," etc. These are few in number, less than two hundred, but frequent in use. They are words in linguistic categories sometimes called

[1] Inferring a general principle from specific instances.

connectors, intensifiers, determiners, auxiliaries, and prepositions, which give the meaning to symbolic utterances.

A parent can note that when a child distinguishes *a* from *the* in "Get *a* ball," and "Get *the* ball," he should be given opportunities to use others such as in:

Can you get *another* cookie?
You *may* get *some* cookies.
You *may* have *some more* milk.
You *may* play *with the* ball.
If you get *the* ball, you *may* have *this* cookie.

While parents often prepare lists of these structure words or Functors, it doesn't really help. The children do not seem to induce the principles from non-functional language. Nevertheless, if parents use natural, non-stilted, language in its global application, the structure words fit into place easily.

Meanings of the structure words, such as prepositions, need to be extended beyond the one-to-one correspondence level of object to words. Parents should find lots of opportunities to use such expressions as:

We will go *in* just a minute.
Mommy's *in* a hurry.
Don't walk *in* the rain.

Of course, the usual positional use will surface constantly, and the parent should wait for the child to follow through:

Put the dolly *in* the crib.
Look *in* the box; your airplane is there.

Furthermore, prepositions other than *in*, *on*, and *under* occur often and must be used, i.e., above, for, by, over, to, etc.

Similarly, attention can be directed to auxiliaries in order for the child to develop a sense of time — past and future. By now, parents may be using little drawings or stick figures to illustrate experiences outside of the child's immediate environment. These can be shown to the child to illustrate meaning:

We will go to the store.
...............candy shop.
...............toy store.

Later with the same drawing, the parent may recall, "Mommy and Jim *went* to the store." This drawing can accompany other experiences in his environment. Sentences like, "We will bake a cake," becomes "We baked a cake." in later conversations.

Questions can follow activities, and parents can wait for answers and model the correct form. After the store, she can ask: "Did you buy apples?" or "What did you buy?" After the cake: "Did you eat some cake?" "What did you do?" "Did you lick the spoon?" Questions where the questioner does not "know" the answer should be asked frequently, e.g. "Where did you put your doll?" Those requiring choices, e.g., "Which do you want, an apple or a pear?" and demanding a description of a procedure, "How did you make the cake?" help the child establish cognitive organization.

While putting the topics into sentence structure or *global* form, parents must be cautioned to express things in as many different ways as possible. "Rubber stamping" was mentioned earlier and refers to a circular procedure. The child knows the expressions and even uses some of them, yet the adult continues to model the same expressions over and over. Parents need to be helped to move up the ladder of accomplishment. When the child knows one level at the usage stage, input should be at the next level for comprehension. The child must have opportunities to store the language of comparisons, causality, inference, generalizations:

> The red ball is bigger than Daddy's golf ball.
> The water leaked because there is a hole in the bag.
> The strawberries were in the freezer.
> We bought fruit — apples, oranges, and bananas.

While parents are describing the topics, the child can *induce* its many properties, i.e., a ball can be thrown, caught, rolled but NOT worn, and only eaten if it is a "meatball." A ball can be round, but so can a cookie, but a ball isn't flat, whereas a cookie is. A cookie can be broken, baked, frosted, crumbled, etc., which a "ball" cannot. Never, never would we gain mastery over language if we had to have language taught atomistically (in separate, isolated components).

Reality-based language

This stage of talking with the child is excellent for providing input at the conversational level. In order to detect underlying patterns or rules, hearing-impaired children need frequent exposure to reality-based language models so that the meaning is clear. The daily life of a parent-child dyad (twosome) abounds with opportunities for conversation. During these important exchanges the adult needs to introduce the child to sophisticated language features.

These natural communicative interactions provide opportunities not only for communicating experiences and ideas, gaining information and manipulating the environment, but for stimulating the child's more sophisticated language learning process. It is frequently in his home environment that the child acquires:

- Time relationships: Grandmother is coming tomorrow.
  Tell Aunt Susie what we did yesterday.
  After dinner we will watch television.

- Locations: The big ball is on the middle shelf.
  Please put the pan on top of the stove.

- Causality: The egg broke because it rolled off the table.
  You need your cap because it is cold outside.

- Contingency: We can eat when Daddy gets home.
  If you pick up your toys you can go outside.

- Categorization: Let's put the white things in the washer.
  Stack the cups on the counter.
  Put the spoons in the silverware drawer.

- Classification: Get your jacket from the coat closet.
  I have something good to drink.

These are just a few of the examples within the home to help the child lay the groundwork for more advanced language features. Children need to have speakers who know and use the rules of language. These adult models provide the input for the learner to induce the rules.

Language enrichment

The first four stages should not be short circuited to move into this phase. It is the equivalent of giving the child Shakespeare rather than nursery rhymes at age three years. But at this stage of talking *with* the child, parents should be telling nursery rhymes, traditional stories, and stories from the books they get at the library. Parents may need some assistance in telling these to hearing-impaired children, but by now, it should be mostly help in positioning the book and using the pictures. An experience of this type needs to be done often.

Nursery rhymes can be used for listening. They have nice

rhythm and prosody and are wonderful times to share. In fact, many parents routinely do bedtime stories with the favorites repeated often. Each repetition maintains the same idea, but with the language slightly changed.

Refining and expanding the child's language

The parent continues to talk, but it is more than just talking. While language-training up to this point has been reciprocal and playful, parents are now responsive to the *child's idea* and develop it. When the child says "puppy big" the adult engages in a conversation about the puppy. "Where are his eyes, his nose, his tail?" "What does he like to eat?" "What is the puppy's name?" "Where does he sleep?"

Talking with the child may be facilitated with a scrapbook story of his experience. Time and again, the mother and child can review the things they did together. Other scrapbooks may deal with categories, their family, their friends, foods they like, clothing they wear, and animals they have seen. All of these can be items for conversation, the sophisticated ping-pong game. Similarly, trips to the zoo, fire station, ride on a bus, picnic, etc., can be shared with the other parent and others who were not along. Language for telling is important conversational material. By this time, parents should be including causal relations, contingencies, time, and other ideas with linguistic signals in their conversations. They must remember that: *Language comprehension precedes language expression by at least one level.*

Probably at this point, the child is to be enrolled in a preschool with the parent in a supportive role while the classroom teacher directs the language activities. A shift has been made from one that was *parent-centered* to one that is now *child-centered*.

It is up to the parents, however, to provide input as to the child's communication needs outside of the classroom. They need to be aware of such issues as: How does he communicate with his friends? Is he able to make himself understood? Does he understand his friends? Does he interact with friends and playmates appropriately? Does he talk with other adults, in addition to immediate family members? Does he greet people appropriately and respond to their "social" questions? Does he understand and use the slang and common expressions used by his hearing peers? Many of these issues never come up in a classroom situation, but they are real needs if the hearing-impaired child is to develop communicative competence.

In concluding this chapter, it might be helpful to review a longitudinal sequence from our files. Debbie was a severe to profoundly deaf infant of ten months when we met her. Her parents were people with average intelligence and modest means. While their hearing son gave them some insight into parenting, they were hesitant to do anything for Debbie. They did not know *what* to do. After a few months, we observed lots of self-talk from Debbie's mother:

> Here's your cereal.
> I'll cut your egg.
> Eat your bacon.
> Here is your toast.
> I'll butter it.

For a few weeks Debbie looked blankly, smiled sweetly, or fussed furiously. The educator kept reassuring Mrs. J. that Debbie was absorbing the language so necessary to that developmental level. In a matter of months, however, Debbie watched the speaker's mouth. Her mother reported that Debbie attended for about four words. The family then shifted to asking *if* she wanted cereal, *if* she wanted toast, bacon, jelly, etc. The objects were there, of course. Debbie still watched.

Several weeks later, she began imitating the key word ("ba," "toa") which had strong intonation. Very shortly thereafter, she was nodding to "Do you want some bacon?" but shook her head "no" to "Do you want toast?" She had really meant "No," because when served the toast, she threw it. When on a grocery trip later the next week, her mother told Debbie she needed eggs whereupon Debbie darted off to the dairy department to return with a carton of extra large ones.

By her third birthday, Debbie not only attempted the words: "eggs", "toast", "bacon", "juice", and "milk", but also put them in context, "No oo, mih ee." translated into "No juice, but milk please." Her mother modeled immediately: "I do not want any juice, but may I have some milk, please?" Debbie was in preschool six months after her third birthday, and her parents supported the teachers beautifully. By the time Debbie was nine years old, she was using language equivalent to her normal hearing peers.

This example is one of hundreds which support the fact that *the hearing-impaired child follows the same universal developmental steps to linguistic competence as do hearing children*. This may occur at a later chronological age, but sophisticated language levels can be reached. The hearing-impaired child can achieve communicative competence if teachers understand language development and guide parents accordingly. If parents are helped, they *can* be "Super

Parents." They *should* be their child's first teacher. Experience of the authors supports the fact that skilled, involved parents *do* "create" listening, talking deaf children!

Objectives

The objectives for the fifth level, "Talk With the Child," seem too obvious to list, but just as a guide, they should include:

- Parent will take child's utterances and expand them into complete and/or correct language.
- Parent will expand child's sentence to include appropriate structure words.
- Parent will model new ideas related to the child's utterances.
- Parent will keep a scrapbook.
- Parent will use drawings to serve as a reference.
- Parent will point out perceptual characteristics (e.g. smell, touch, taste, sight and sound) while talking about items.
- Parent will expand the child's experiences by trips into the community.
- Parent will provide experiences that naturally promote active learning and talk about the concept of *classification*.
- Parent will provide experiences that naturally promote active learning and talk about the concept of *causality*.
- Parent will provide experiences that naturally promote active learning and talk about the concept of *contingencies*.
- Parent will provide experiences that naturally promote active learning and talk about the concept of *spatial relations*.
- Parent will provide experiences that naturally promote active learning and talk about the concept of *time*.
- Parent will ask questions (information-seeking, open-ended, and choice questions, etc.)
- Parent will provide experiences to further the child's social development.

Chapter 5

Hear Ye! Hear Ye! More To Do!

The philosophical orientation in this text is that the hearing-impaired child is first and foremost a CHILD. Therefore, as a child, he follows normal developmental stages and has needs similar to all children. In addition, he has a great need for auditory stimulation so that his auditory modality can develop, and speech can be acquired in its sequential steps.

From observation of deaf children and adults who have developed excellent spoken language, it was apparent that they had these factors in common. These were early detection of their hearing loss and amplification during the critical early years. These children were surrounded by auditory stimulation *in the form of speech* not only early, but almost continually. Finally, they had accepting parents with strong parenting skills who learned that training their child to listen was part of every parent's role. Such are the supports which we desire for all hearing-impaired children.

Early Detection

Fortunately, pediatricians, otologists, and audiologists today are referring parents to early intervention programs. This is unlike former times when enrolling the child for habilitation was delayed until he was about three years of age. Some medical personnel continue to dismiss parent concern about speech delay with the classic statement: "The child is young. He will outgrow it."

With early detection comes responsibility. The teacher, therapist, educator, or consultant must be concerned with audiometric procedures and be able to interpret findings to the parents whether the determinations were made on Evoked Response Audiometry or with Play Audiometry. The results of the testing must be related to the type of amplification selected. Furthermore, the instructor, whatever he or she is called, must take on the responsibility for conferencing with the audiologist at frequent intervals and assist in decisions concerning amount and kind of amplification for each child.

Usually, the initial selection of appropriate hearing aid(s) for a very young child is primarily through inference from the audiologic data. Thresholds of speech detection, pure tone, and/or noise band measures tend to be the data for that early testing, not necessarily the child's overt response to listening. The first hearing aid needs to be monitored to see that it is functioning appropriately, and that the amplification is providing neither excessive nor insufficient power. Parents need guidance in observing this phase as well as reporting the information to the audiologist at subsequent and regular testing periods.

Hearing

For far too long, the prevalent idea in education of the deaf child was that the residual hearing of children born deaf was of little value in enabling them to talk. This idea led to the almost total disregard of the possibilities of using their remnant of hearing. It is known today that there are extremely few, if any, children who have no hearing at all. Even those children with minimal amounts of hearing can still receive important information about the spoken message.

Deaf children who have sensitivity to sound only at 500 Hz can perceive the melody of speech. They can learn to recognize pitch, stress, pauses, and duration. They can differentiate strong patterns from weak ones, short sounds from long ones, and loud sounds from soft ones. All of these components occur in intonation, prosody, and even with the vowel sounds of speech.

These speech components are the variations which indicate meaning to the child. Saying, "*Oh* boy" with stress on the first word differs from the meaning conveyed by "Oh *boy*" with stress on the second word. Vary the accent or stress within the question: "Why did you come today?" Immediately, the response differs:

Why did you come today?   *Because* there is a conference.
Why did *you* come today?   *I* was invited.
Why did you come *today*?   This is the day _____ is held.

Why *did* you *come* today?   I wanted to be *here*.

A large quantity of *meaning* is conveyed in the sounds of speech. It has been our finding that all hearing-impaired children have significant amounts of residual sensory capacity to learn the clues for meaning, if it is trained. Gross time and intensity patterns represent meaning, and children develop meaning prior to perception; namely, they understand what is being said before they identify the specific language.

As a child experiences the meaning of situations, the wise parent interacts with language that is appropriate. By being exposed to the language as in "parallel talk" and later in "one-to-one" talk, the deaf child becomes more easily attuned to spoken language through amplification.

Hearing Speech

The use of residual hearing is far more complex than just placing the hearing aid(s) on the child. Unlike practitioners of old, today's educators do not use drums, whistles, bells, cymbals, or any other noise-making objects to develop real listening. Instead, they recognize that the important medium for learning to hear is *spoken* language. In order to learn to listen, children do not need noisemakers, but rather a listening experience provided by a loving parent who makes time to play with and enjoy her child. This loving relation is the strongest incentive for a baby's learning. The deaf child who is spoken to often becomes attuned to sound and language much earlier than the child whose mother is silent or talks infrequently. A parent may be inarticulate or unaware of the need to provide stimulation or unable and/or unwilling to do so. But with supportive, definite guidance from professionals, the parent *can* learn to talk to her child!

There is evidence that *when acoustic input is relatively random in relation to events of importance to the child, as is the case when it consists almost entirely of radio or TV, the child is unable to discover the structure of language.* These inanimate objects have been proven ineffective with normal-hearing children when there was little or no spoken input by significant persons. These children were shown to need human interaction. Unfortunately, some did not receive this oral input to any substantial degree until they entered school, where they needed language training. Their progress was very circumscribed. *It is necessary for language development that a child hear speech as a part of interpersonal interaction.* Those children who had language delays did not have this experience.

Infants reared in institutions, staffed by few and inconsistent caregivers, demonstrated severe language defects. The tremendous lag in language as well as overall development was attributed to the lack of dyadic[2] interaction. The staff had neither time nor possibly the disposition to establish bonding nor were such things as turn-taking accompanied by conversation present. The one-to-one input so critical for language development was absent.

Critical Period of Learning

While there are steps of language behavior, the important early language learning begins with the love talk of adults. Language learning does not begin when the child says his first word, rather it starts months and months prior to that. Frequently, people assume because the infant makes no overt response that he is not absorbing. There is evidence that the child hears in utero, but it is the teaching that parents and loved ones do that enables him to learn language. This begins in the very first few hours of life. There is a critical period for acquisition of language behavior.

Audiologists have noted this critical age phenomena. They have reported children who, at an early age, had losses of only 15 dB experienced through serious otitis media, failed to develop normal language skills. This lack later resulted in poor school achievement. Others have reported that a mild hearing loss in infancy can cause poor speech and pitch discrimination when no auditory training is provided.

We know that hearing-impaired children with less severe hearing losses who were deprived of amplification until they were school age, later demonstrated responses similar to children with a profound loss. Getting children to accomplish various auditory tasks is much more difficult after several years without good auditory development than when listening was started within the first two years of their lives.

Scientists have presented considerable evidence that a failure of normal development of the central nervous system can occur with sensory deprivation. Several experimental studies of animals support the concept that sensory deprivation early in life causes impairment in the organism's later functioning which may be

2/ **Dyadic in the sense of personal, one-to-one.**

permanent. There appears to be truth in the hypothesis that nerves do atrophy with disuse.

Infant children as young as eight-months-old make discriminations and exhibit preferences for intonation, rhythm, loudness, and familiarity. They prefer the voice of their mother to that of a stranger. They like speech directed to them rather than speech used from one adult to another. The findings regarding "motherese" correlate with the listening preferences in the language learning infant. Even when infants' speech discrimination was tested, it followed a developmental progression that interrelated listening with experience.

While we do not want to be tyrannized by the threat of "use it or lose it," we, nevertheless, must look at the learning that takes place during the first twelve months of life. Since children learn their language from speech around them, deaf children should be stimulated in a manner similar to that of normally hearing children who are at the same *linguistic* age. Note, we did not say chronological age! We believe that sound can be made available to the deafest of children; that speech does not develop in a vacuum; that the child must have speech experiences in the natural home environment. Spoken language supported by amplification is essential if the child is to develop the listening and language to which we are dedicated.

Acoustic Facts

Relevant to the use a child makes of his residual hearing is how available speech is to him. It is a significant acoustical fact that the sound level of ordinary conversations at a distance of one meter from the speaker averages only 70 dB. This speech level can become 90 dB with a shout or raised voice. It can become 120 dB to 130 dB with hearing aids that have a high gain capacity. While that amount of amplification is rarely used, it indicates the possibility that amplified conversational level speech can be available to the very profoundly deaf child.

Our data, albeit empirical, has been accumulated over a long period of time with profoundly deaf children wearing hearing aids. Currently, data is being collected on children with cochlear implants. This, in effect, performs the same function as a hearing aid by bypassing the middle ear and delivering the message directly to the end organ or auditory nerve. While these findings are encouraging, young children should first be exposed to consistent, quality auditory input prior to decisions on a surgical approach.

Vibro-tactile aids are another means of providing the spoken message to the profoundly deaf child. Again, these aids should not be used until an accurate evaluation of hearing is made and after learning to listen is a "fait accompli." Whether feeling the message through taction can deliver information meant for the ear is still in the experimental stage.

Acoustic phonetics add to our growing understanding of speech perception. The presence of important speech information in low frequencies is valuable for auditory development and for speech production. Presence or absence of sounds such as voice in consonants, stress of syllables, and other prosodic features can be signaled by time and intensity available in those low frequencies. These are attainable even by a child with a very profound loss.

Hearing Is Learned Behavior

Repeated experiences are learned in time. Behavior that is reinforced tends to be repeated. Behavior that is instrumental in bringing about favorable or rewarding changes is inclined to be repeated. Experiences of hearing language at times of significance to the child such as feeding, being changed, being held, being stimulated through any sense modality will be the early basis for learning to hear.

Input to children is repetitive. Phrases are repeated to a very high degree. Repeated behavior is learned. It is through this procedure that the process of learning to hear becomes established. Learning to hear consists of learning to recognize sound and interpret it. Spoken language must be heard over and over before it takes on meaning.

The hearing-impaired child is free to employ any acoustic cues he likes provided they do the job of differentiating sounds. Learning to recognize speech is a matter of organizing the information that reaches the brain. While the amount of information conveyed to the brain from the hearing-impaired ear may be less than normal, it is what the brain *does* with this information that is important in learning to recognize spoken sounds.

The profoundly deaf child may never receive the same particular acoustic pattern a hearing child does. Nevertheless, he can substitute the cues he *does* receive and accept them as meaningful if they accompany meaningful experiences. There is some interesting research relative to the cues a deaf child uses. For example, a name like "Marianne" was heard by deaf subjects as one very long syllable rather than the correct three syllables. However, one very long syllable, in time, became a very important signal to Marianne when her name was called. His own name is probably the first learned response a hearing-impaired child makes. For this, of course, he must be reinforced or rewarded.

Listening is not intuitive, but rather something that a child learns just as he learns to perceive in the other sense modalities. His experience of reality will at first be global and undifferentiated. Because his perceptions are to the total message, training in listening should be to whole patterns of speech. Discrimination drills on sounds and words should not be used until years later. While a child will alert to a single sound and have fun playing with bells and drums, these toys do not contain the nuances of speech. Speech, therefore, must be the nucleus of auditory training.

Children as early as three months, if provided good auditory stimulation, utilize the prosodic features of sentence types in their babble. Declarative statements, questions, and imperative sentence patterns can be identified in their jargon. This is long before the child will recognize differences between noisemakers or between words, e.g., "boy," "toy." Intonation introduced to him as "love talk" shows up in his spontaneous utterances later.

The ideal time for learning to listen is the time that all sensory learning is developing. From the total experience of perceiving through the senses of vision, taste, touch, and smell, a child will learn perceptual characteristics. As his parents point out the salient features of an experience, a child acquires concepts and stores them in his memory. Forms such as bitter, sweet, warm, cold, rough, smooth, big, little, can be learned as the experiences arise. In time, these same concepts can be attached to other items having the same characteristic. At another time, he will experience the same item having different characteristics:

The ball may be *big*

and *round*

and *red*

and *smooth.*

BIG	ROUND
The chair may be *big*.	An orange may be *round*.
A hat may be *big*.	A balloon may be *round*.
A balloon may be *big*.	A pancake may be *round*.
A boy may be *big*.	A cap may be *round*.

The language input must be the natural language of the child's environment, sometimes colloquial, sometimes ungrammatical, but always the complete *idea*. The input should always observe the integrity of the meaning to be conveyed. However, parents use reiteration and segmentation in their interactions in a fascinating way. For example, if the parent wishes to direct the child or have him give her the red truck, she may say, "Give me the red truck . . . the red truck . . . red truck. Give me the red truck." Such segmenting of a fairly complex sentence is appropriate, but note that the "super mother" always puts it back into "global," complete form: "Give me the red truck."

Contrary to most general practice, it is the authors' philosophy that the natural setting of the home, while informal, is superior to structured type programs. In the home, listening becomes an integral part of all activities. The content can be infinite, but it is usually redundant. It centers on the here and now, the child's things, what he is doing, wants, or needs. The form is usually short sentences or phrases but may be meaningful single words. It is this input that must be processed through the auditory mechanism. A child must learn to hear the simple language that gets repeated day to day in the average home and which is tangibly associated with meaning.

Prior to delineating the parental tasks of helping the child listen, it might be well to review the ear and its functions.

The Ear

As part of the child's initial audiological examination, the audiologist usually explains the mechanism of the ear to the parents. By understanding the ear's function, parents can have a better grasp of how it can malfunction. For a thorough description of the ear's mechanism, one may read *Hearing and Deafness* (Davis and Silverman, 1970). In the event that parents did not receive that information, it will be reviewed here.

The ear is divided into three parts: the outer ear, middle ear, and inner ear. The outer ear is important since this is the area into which the ear mold of the hearing aid is fitted. The outer ear consists of the pinna and the ear canal, and as such are part of the child's anatomy. Just as all of the rest of his body grows, so does the outer ear. Periodically, the child will outgrow his ear mold; the aperture will become too big. It is important that there be a tight seal between the mold and the auditory canal; otherwise a squeal or whistle, called feedback, will occur. It is *not* appropriate to simply turn the aid down until the squealing stops:

new ear mold(s) will need to be obtained so the child can wear his aid(s) at the volume setting prescribed by the audiologist.

From the pinna, the sound enters the ear canal, which serves two basic purposes. One, to screen elements from the eardrum and the other to increase the loudness of sound. The canal is a resonating chamber because of its shape and thus conducts the sound to the eardrum. If the canal is filled with wax, sound cannot be delivered as it should. Occasionally, natural wax will build up and serve as a deterrent to sound traveling easily through to the eardrum. Parents should not try to remove the wax if it does occur, but rather have their doctor remove it.

The middle ear is made up of the eardrum, ossicles, and the eustachian tube. The eardrum is a delicate membrane stretched tightly over the end of the auditory canal. The eardrum is highly sensitive to vibration, and sound is vibrating air. After the eardrum picks up this vibration, it passes it along to the ossicles. The vibration activates these three small bones called the hammer (malleus), anvil (incus), and stirrup (stapes). The ossicles transmit the vibrations to the inner ear by way of the footplate on the stapes.

Air is furnished by the eustachian tube to the air-filled environment of the middle ear. The eustachian tube opens on one end in the middle ear and on the other end in the back of the throat. Usually, the tube drains off fluids that accumulate inside; however, when the fluids become thick, they can cause the ossicles not to vibrate. The mucous-like fluids can be caused by allergies (frequently milk in young children), colds, and any respiratory illness. If the ossicles do not function, sound cannot be delivered to the inner ear. At those periods when the child's ear is "stopped up," parents must make special effort to see that the child *sees* them. He may not be able to hear them at that time.

Evidence has mounted to indicate that normally hearing children, who had multiple middle ear infections during the critical years, did not acquire the amount of language of children who had no infections. Unfortunately, infections in the middle ear can go unnoticed in a young child for a long time, so it is important to have routine medical examinations. Antibiotics can help clear up the infection and restore middle ear functioning. Otitis media can not only block sound transmission, but can also become very painful. This is most difficult for a child who cannot verbalize the situation. Furthermore, it can be frustrating to him because he can get little help from his hearing aid. Parents need to learn the signals of middle ear build-up and supplement the audition with vision.

Middle ear blockage can cause what is called *conductive hearing loss*, meaning that the outer or middle ear does not conduct sound as well as it should. Some people have had successful surgery to loosen the ossicles so they again vibrate. These are usually adults who began to have ossification of the malleus, incus, and stapes in their early adult lives.

The inner ear consists of the cochlea (Latin for snail), the semicircular canals, and the endings of the auditory nerve. The base of the cochlea and the footplate of the stirrup meet at the oval window, a tissue-covered opening that separates the middle and inner ear and transmits vibrations. The semicircular canals do not affect hearing, but they do help an individual to maintain balance. They sense the position of the fluid and give the body a method for telling if the fluid is level.

This is the same fluid that is in the cochlea. The intense vibrations of the footplate set up a wave in that fluid. This wave sets in motion tiny hairlike projections inside the cochlea, which are in contact with the nerve endings. These nerve endings, or hair cells, translate the motion into nerve impulses, which are carried through the acoustic nerve. This nerve delivers the signals to the brain for processing. When the nerves do not function correctly in transmitting sound, it is called a *sensorineural loss* or sometimes "nerve deafness." This type of hearing problem can cause decreased capacity in sensitivity and discrimination.

Sensitivity is measured in decibels. In order to have an idea for the levels of loudness described by decibels, the measurements of some common sounds are:

0-10 decibels (dB): The softest sound a typical ear can hear.

10-15 decibels (dB): A faint whisper.

35-45 decibels (dB): Soft conversational speech.

45-55 decibels (dB): A quiet automobile.

55-65 decibels (dB): Ordinary conversation at about three feet.

65-75 decibels (dB): City traffic.

100 decibels (dB):   A loud factory.

140 decibels (dB):   A jet engine at takeoff.

Discrimination has to do with frequency of the sound. It measures how well an individual understands speech. If he were an adult, words and sentences would be used to measure how well or poorly the person understands. However, with children, measurements will be made of the frequencies, i.e., how many decibels of power are needed for the child to hear the high pitched and low pitched sounds. The loudness level where the child demonstrates that he just barely heard a sound at each single frequency across the range of frequencies indicates his threshold. His threshold is pictured on an audiogram.

An audiogram is a graph of an individual's hearing. It displays how loud sounds must be at each frequency or pitch level for the individual to hear them. It also shows which sounds a child hears best and how loud they had to be for him to hear. It is the audiogram that directs the audiologist's selection of hearing aids.

A hearing aid helps make sound louder and brings it directly to the individual's ear. Some audiologists will talk about the child's audiogram and also his aided audiogram. While they may differ, the hearing remains constant. The hearing aid cannot change the child's hearing. It can make sounds louder, but it cannot make them more clear. As he learns to listen, the child will learn the spoken signal he receives as the code of English, and it will become his code.

A hearing aid cannot enable the child to hear extremely soft sounds nor will the child be able to hear well when there is a great deal of background noise. A hearing aid does not amplify just speech; it amplifies everything. To sum up, hearing aids cannot restore normal hearing. They can, however, help the child make the most of whatever residual hearing he has, enabling him to function in a fairly normal way even though he doesn't hear normally. The child with a minimum of residual hearing can, with amplification and training, learn to use that hearing, however little it is.

The basic assumption of successful auditory training is that the human mind has a great capacity for organizing information. While it can do nothing if the end organ supplies no information about sounds, auditory training can assist the hearing-impaired child if he is exposed to sounds that are amplified and occur often enough. Language which is recognized indicates an auditory pattern is stored in the child's memory. The auditory memory assists in code learning or language use.

Hearing Aids

Much parent counseling regarding parents' important role in auditory management, should center around hearing aid usage. Obviously, parents need to understand the value of the hearing aid. An important role is to see that amplified speech is provided at all times; therefore, the child must wear his hearing aid(s) *regularly*. Parents need to check the aid(s) daily, using their own ear. Furthermore, they must maintain the aid(s), cleaning and inspecting the ear molds for fit and cleanliness. This is to ensure that the child hears the same acoustic signals over time. Since he is developing his own cues, the cues must be consistent from day to day.

A difficult concept that parents must master is the inverse-ratio principle. Increasing the distance from the microphone causes the volume to be diminished by the square of the power of the instrument. Parents need to know about distance from the microphone and realize that they must go to the child, not talk from another room. They need to know about masking noises, about signal-to-noise ratio, and about recruitment and attenuation. Above all, they must learn:

- What hearing aids *can* do, and also what they *cannot* do.
- About batteries and their monitoring.
- About ear molds and how to keep them clean.
- About the frequency with which new molds must be made.
- Hearing aids must be turned on to function; in the "off" position, they do not amplify.
- Hearing aids need batteries that have enough voltage.
- Dead or weak batteries do not amplify.
- Hearing aids must be worn by the child. Aids in purses or in dresser drawers do not help the child.
- Ear molds clogged with wax do not transmit sound.

Parent Objectives for Auditory Training

Parents must assume the crucial role of training their child to listen. Listening skills are prerequisite to the development of language. Auditory perception develops from an awareness of sound and progresses through alerting, discrimination, recognition, and eventually comprehension of sound. Hearing-impaired children need to be guided through these steps, while stressing that listening needs to be meshed with his developing language. Parents must keep in mind that whatever signals the child receives consistently can take on the same meaning for him as the auditory spectrum does for the hearing child. For example, if the sound for "ball" for the deaf child is "aw," with repetition "aw" can be spectrally complete for *him*. Thereafter, whenever he hears "o u aw" it has meaning, just as "Throw the ball." has meaning to a child who hears.

Hearing aid use

The manner in which the child uses his hearing aid(s) has a direct effect on the benefit derived from amplification. Unless the hearing aid(s) is worn by the child all of the time, he will not be able to build up his listening repertoire of sounds, intonation, stress, and prosody. The parent must monitor the hearing aid(s) conscientiously: otherwise the efforts to capture, train, and utilize the child's hearing will be futile. Therefore, training about the hearing aid(s) must be an integral part of parent education.

The child should be wearing his aid when the parent and child meet the teacher. The hearing aid(s) should be working. The parent should be able to talk intelligently about the life of the batteries and describe the problems if the hearing aid is not functioning. The behavioral objectives for parents might be:

- Parent will understand the importance of wearing hearing aid(s).
- Parent will establish consistent hearing aid(s) use during all waking hours.
- Parent will maintain hearing aid in good working order.
- Parent will respond promptly to questions about hearing aid function.
- Parent will respond appropriately to questions about the workings of the aid(s).
- Parent will describe the problem when the hearing aid(s) is malfunctioning.

Structuring the environment

The parent must set the stage and create optimal conditions for auditory interaction by utilizing environmental factors effectively. When the child's auditory perceptual system is so seriously impaired that speech can be analyzed only as gross patterns, he must not be limited in the *quality* nor the *quantity* of his daily auditory experiences. A noisy home can make it very difficult to learn any language through audition; hence it becomes the parent's role to structure the home situation in order to provide the most ideal setting possible. This task includes checking the home for "quietness," keeping unnecessary noises to the minimum, judging proximity necessary for listening. They, like all parents, should engage in humming, singing, and otherwise playing with sound in the quiet rooms of the house. Also, the parents must work to slowly increase the distance from the sound of their voices to the microphone of the child's hearing aid(s).

In order to foster the child's auditory sensitivity:

- Parents will provide the child with the best listening environment.
- Parents will close the doors, turn off the TV or radio, shut off mixer, etc., to cut down on ambient noise.
- Parents will be close to the child when talking to him.
- Parents will get the child's attention before speaking.
- Parents will speak at the child's ear level.
- Parents will call the child by name and wait for him to look.
- Parents will continually increase the distance from child when calling him by name.
- Parents will provide verbal auditory input with affectionate intonation.
- Parents will hum, sing, play games with sounds with the child.

Awareness of sound

Attending to sound is an early stage of auditory development. The signals can be either non-linguistic or linguistic. The auditory non-linguistic signals should be identified and talked about when the child is interested or alerts to the sound. As environmental sounds often effect what is said, i.e., "I think the lightning hit the tree," the parent should tell the child the cause of the comment, i.e., the crashing noise. To the degree that sounds from the environment stimulate subsequent conversation, children should be alerted to them.

Certainly, the informal training provided by the parent in the home is insufficient to train the child's hearing to the maximum, but it is in keeping with our global approach to development. The parent should not have to provide "listening activities" that require full-time involvement. That can become part of his skill learning later.

In order to maintain the child's interest and motivation, we suggest that the listening experiences be embedded in ongoing daily schedules. These include associating all sounds with their source, reinforcing the child's responses to sound, repeating sounds that please the child, and playing with noisemaking toys. The value of pots and pans as a source of sound and fun should not be overlooked.

Some possible objectives are:

- Parent will recognize need for child to have pleasurable experiences with sound.
- Parent will notice what sound the child is seeking and show him. She will label the sound, i.e., "The dog is barking."
- Parents will associate meaning with the noise. "The telephone is ringing. I'll answer it."
- Parents will call attention to noise such as popping of popcorn in popper.
- Parents will start and stop mixer, blender, vacuum, etc., to get child's attention; not as a learning situation.

Awareness of speech

The auditory signal of greatest importance is the *human voice.* Therefore, the primary job of the parent of the hearing-impaired child is to assist him in attending and responding to speech. Parents communicate with children in a manner which reflects their belief that the child is capable of reciprocal communication. This attitude is the basis of the turn-taking model. From this model, the foundation for reciprocity is created, and the context for learning is provided. Anderson (1979) discusses in depth the need for turn-taking experiences with the deaf child. The implication of this for a child's listening is obvious.

Intonation patterns play a basic role in language development, and are available even to profoundly deaf children. Intonation is the most salient feature in language behavior addressed to the child. It may also indicate the semantic aspect since the emotional content of communication is so marked. The syntactic signals are also thus identified by rise or fall of the speaker's voice. In fact, it has been said that intonation is the vehicle a child rides to syntax. Most importantly, intonation serves as a social function. One must pay attention in a conversation in order to know when it is one's turn to speak, and the turn termination is indicated by the drop in voice.

The tone of the parents' voices should be rich in rising and falling contours appropriate to the message as well as tones that are of a positive affective nature. Vocal play can be connected with just talking, with babbling, with imitation, or with spontaneously articulated structure with terms such as, "What a good boy!" "I like that!"

The objectives for intonation might be:

- Parent will use voice rather than non-voice auditory or sensory stimuli.
- Parent will rely on voice as attention getter.
- Parent will use child's name in positive vocal tones.
- Parent will call attention to the speaker.
- Parent will engage in vocal play with the child.
- Parent will *consistently* use the child's name as a means of getting attention.
- Parent will *expect* the child to respond to his name.

Auditory recognition

Auditory recognition, though not involving comprehension, is a preliminary step in developing audition. It proceeds from the general to the specific, as does all learning in small children, and may be very gross for some profoundly deaf children. Ideally, auditory recognition can be viewed as a unisensory event, but in reality it may be through looking as well as listening, that a child recognizes the parents' verbal stimuli.

Some children can recognize only a small amount of information through audition alone. They, therefore, should not be forced to listen without looking. Many profoundly deaf children would be at a tremendous loss if only one sensory channel, e.g., audition, were available. On the other hand, other profoundly deaf children can make surprisingly good use of an aural approach.

The role of the parent is to provide auditory stimulus, but not insist upon its recognition through hearing alone. She may playfully give the child vocal play with intonation, babble with him, and present prolonged vowels for enjoyment.

The parent may have a set of nursery rhyme cards with pictures which the child recognizes from the parents' auditory input when the cards picturing the rhyme are in front of him. When the parent places the cards in front of him she gives him many opportunities to see (lipread) and hear the rhyme. After much practice over time he may be asked to identify what the parent is saying.

Objects may be asked for in a closed-set situation, e.g., when getting dressed to go out, Mother may say, "Get your coat." turning her face away at the last word. Other closed set opportunities might be: "Let's wash your foot." "Now the other foot." "I have the milk. You get a glass."

Scrapbooks of meaningful experiences can provide other "closed sets" for auditory recognition. Sometimes parents may ask the child in natural situations for a toy, a utensil, or an action, e.g., "Throw a kiss." "Wave bye-bye." or "It's time to go to bed." These listening games can be done with the parent covering her mouth, or, if necessary, with a combination of listening and looking.

The behaviors teachers might expect are:

- Parent will give child intonation patterns.
- Parent will wait for some response such as cooing or a smile.
- Parent will ask child for one or two items child has among his playthings, clothing, food, etc.
- Parent will use certain phrases such as "Turn the light on/off," "Get your coat," and expect the child to recognize them.
- Parent will *expect* the child to respond to words, phrases, or sentences within a restricted set.
- Parent will expect child to comprehend freely from unlimited numbers of rhymes, objects, and sentences about experiences.

Speech Perception Through Lipreading

Although the emphasis has been on auditory information available to hearing-impaired children, attention must not be reduced to lipreading as only a supplementary avenue for language input. If only one sensory channel, e.g., audition, were available for learning spoken communication, many profoundly deaf children would be at a tremendous disadvantage.

For example, lipreading gives children place-of-articulation speech information. By watching the movement of the lips, tongue, and jaw, they can attain valuable information. If at the same time, they are receiving complementary voicing, manner-of-articulation, and vowels through their residual hearing, these children can achieve high levels of communication. By obtaining through one sensory system that which is not available through another, children with severe hearing losses usually comprehend quite well. Most children with profound losses need to receive considerable lipreading information in order to comprehend speech. This does not say that profoundly deaf children do not benefit from auditory perception, but rather they understand spoken language better when they look as well as listen. The pattern of intonation which is auditory, supplemented with place-of-articulation information, aids language acquisition.

The task, then, is to ensure the use of residual hearing and allow the child to "eye" the speaker. This way he perceives both acoustic and visual information. Perception is not innate any more than language is. The child must learn to perceive visually just as he must learn to listen.

Structuring the visual environment

Development of lipreading ability requires knowledge of environmental factors which can enhance or detract from the development of the skill. Specifically, the skill requires active attention to the speaker's face, to the lips and mouth particularly. It requires that the speaker's face is visible. If the speaker is between the hearing-impaired child and the light, either the window or artificial light, the speaker is just a shadow. Adequacy of light is another important matter. Children cannot be expected to lipread in darkened areas.

The eye-level of the child needs to be fairly close to the speaker's mouth. If both speaker and listener are standing and one is a young child, the distance can be over five feet. Three feet is recommended as the desirable distance from the microphone. This can still apply in lipreading. It would entail the "six footer" squatting or kneeling or raising the child to get that close to the lipreader's eyes.

The other "commandment" is that speakers do not give optical competition to the mouth movements. Therefore, they should refrain from engaging in distracting gestures and movements when speaking. Furthermore, a speaker should not compete with any other movement, e.g., television on behind her. This also includes elimination of distractions such as dangling jewelry.

Some of the objectives at this stage could be:

- Parent will see that she always faces the light — with the light at the child's back.
- Parent will see that there is sufficient illumination for lipreading.
- Parent will get to the child's eye level or bring him to hers.
- Parent will present to the child the full view of her face in order for him to perceive the place-of-articulation.

- Parent will minimize distractions.
- Parent will turn off the television when she is talking with the child.

Parents' speech patterns

As has been pointed out, the profoundly deaf child can get categories of place and manner-of-articulation information from the lips. This is a critical point because the data raise questions about the amount of content that is available in the optical realm. It is not known how and what children really lipread, but it is known that visual recognition of consonants is possible through lipreading. This recognition is closely related to general lipreading ability (Heider & Heider, 1940).

The contribution of the visual form to speech development must not be overlooked. Therefore, parents must present the best speech patterns possible to their deaf child to assist him in his eventual speech production. This includes speaking clearly without exaggerating. It means speaking more slowly than to older children or adults. "motherese" studies show that the speech of mothers of hearing children is slower for the young child. Parents need to stress the content words just as parents of young hearing children do. This appears to be a natural device used to develop lexical and referential information which, after all, is one of the tasks of communication.

The emotional and attitudinal features of speech should be marked by appropriate acoustic tools of pitch, stress, duration, and intensity cues so that the child can perceive the phrase structure unit of speech or the "gestalt", if you will. Lipreading is part of listening. They function together, not separately!

Therefore, the objectives in this section might be:

- Parent will speak clearly.
- Parent will not exaggerate nor slur her speech.
- Parent's overall rate of speaking to the child will be slower than with an older child or adult.
- Parent will make longer pauses between meaningful units of speech.
- Parent will stress the content words.
- Parent will use prosodic features prominently.
- Parent will mark emotional and attitudinal aspects of her utterance by stress, intensity, and other intonational devices.
- Parent will use proper intonational terminal to mark questions, statements, and commands.

Summary

The whole process of learning to communicate is not a passive stage of growth, but rather an immensely dynamic and energetic enterprise that calls upon the highest capabilities a hearing-impaired child can mobilize.

Research in infant perception has confirmed the hypothesis that auditory and visual functions, like other sense perceptions, are learned. Furthermore, they are normally learned in infancy and relate to listening experiences. The necessary stimuli are the parents' voices and faces, and the critical reinforcement is the affection that they extend. These facts remain the same for hearing-impaired children. They may not distinguish spectral features of speech, but they can differentiate gross variations in the acoustic pattern. The material must have meaning and be of importance to the child. Also, his attention should be rewarded promptly. This is the formula for programming the mind of the hearing-impaired child to comprehend and use speech.

There are no stages or set procedures for parents to teach their child how to receive speech. Rather, parents must be alert to the auditory task, provide appropriate listening environment and give their child language to which he can listen. They must integrate speech sounds with meaningful language. Receptive language, which precedes expressive language at every level, is achieved by a strong linguistic interaction between parent and child.

Chapter 6

The Teacher

While this text is primarily directed to parents, some attention must be given the teacher. Parents, in addition to being their child's first teacher, must also be their child's strongest advocate throughout his educational career. Possibly a parent's most critical task is that of selecting the agency, center, clinic or school which will assist them with their child's education. In order to do this, they must learn to be selective shoppers, not only for their child's program but for their own program.

Excellence in teaching in the home must be tied to excellence in the professional setting in order for the deaf child to reach his ultimate level of achievement. That program which will accomplish this excellence must have strong professionals who have appropriate orientations to their task and, above all, proper training for this involvement.

Throughout this text, this person who is to guide the family in the habilitation of their hearing-impaired child has been referred to as a teacher, instructor, intervener, counselor, or a combination of these as teacher-counselor. This very critical professional person may be all of these and more.

Task of the Professional

As Simmons-Martin (1975, 1976) has written on a number of occasions, this person's "job description" may require her to be:

A Teacher. She sets educational goals for the child and teaches parents to achieve them with their own child.

An Instructor. She talks with the family about a particular topic that is relevant. For example, the focus of the period of instruction might be on the value of residual hearing, it might be

117

specific suggestions on relevant play experience, or it might be on language growth.

An Intervener. She intervenes in the life of the family and helps them become knowledgeable, goal-oriented parents. It is she who knows effective results can be guaranteed through parent intervention. She will not only get the parents involved, but will educate them so they are their child's first teacher.

A Counselor. She guides parents from the periods when they question, "Why?" "Why me?" "Why my child?" to the level when they ask, "What do I do?" and "How do I do it?" It is she who must recognize the moment that parents are ready for positive action and lead them through the learning process.

This multi-skilled professional may be any one or all of these persons at a given time. More likely, she is a combination of several of these *most* times. Nevertheless, she must be prepared to fill each pair of shoes. It goes without saying that she is at all times a professional. Most of these professionals should have had training or experience in early childhood education or a related field, but all should have at least a bachelor's degree in deaf education. This must be the firm knowledge base that administrators seek first. Furthermore, ongoing inservice training and supervision should be available.

The feminine pronouns are used when referring to this person because of the closeness of mother and child to this person. This in no way implies a conviction that only women are qualified to offer guidance on child-rearing issues, but simply it has been found that mothers are often more comfortable with other women during this emotionally charged period.

If possible, programs should avoid "experts" or "theoreticians." Parents resent "authorities" who are armed with knowledge but no experience. It is certainly true that the difficulties of listening to a baby cry are different for someone who has been up with him all night than for someone who understands only that young babies frequently suffer from colic. It seems important that the teacher is able to identify with problems and concerns *as a parent*, as well as on a professional level. Therefore, it is recommended that all of the teachers serving families during the early months are also parents of young children. There is an old saying that certainly applies here:

> Before I was married, I had six theories about bringing
> up children, now I have six children and no theories.

Role of the Professional

There are certain characteristics that a competent parent educator needs (Simmons-Martin, 1978). Namely, she should be:

A Listener. She tunes into parents as they talk out their uncertainties. Parents often need to discuss their concerns about the way their child is developing, about their own sense of adequacy as a parent, about a feeling of isolation from the rest of the world, and any of a myriad of other issues.

A Responsive Person. She deals not only with the child, but the parent-child dyad. The one-to-one duo cannot be separated out from the rest of the child-rearing system, and, therefore, the most immediate needs of the parent must be addressed. Since the parent is the real deliverer of services to the child, the professional must often be able to adjust the planned lesson and acknowledge and respond to the pressing concerns of the parent.

A Modeler. She demonstrates through her interactions and activities with the child the role or roles she hopes the parents will emulate. This is *not* the time for "Do as I say, not as I do." Rather, it is "Show and Tell" of a sort.

A Reinforcer. She supports everything positive that the parent does. She remembers that the hearing-impaired child is often not as reinforcing as his hearing siblings. Therefore, as reinforcer, she supplements this lack.

An Activity Director. She gives ideas and support to the parents as they progress along the continuum from trauma to acceptance. Knowing *what* and *when* to recommend is a skill critical for the professional. One of the authors recalls observing a teacher giving the rationale for an excellent activity complete with details of executing it. She suggested that "Pat" needed to learn to make choices. Therefore, on a shopping expedition, Mother should let him choose whether he wanted bananas or apples. If he chose apples, he could pick red or yellow ones. He could further choose a paper or plastic bag. He also needed a concept of weight, so he could hold the bag as he put one and then another apple in the bag. Suggestions made were that he could carry them or push them *in* the cart, and the checker would *weigh* them. He would see money being exchanged, and when home he could help peel and core the apples and help cook them into applesauce. After getting the activity so well described, the mother responded, "Do I have to? We don't like applesauce!" The poor teacher didn't get the message and proceeded to go through a similar activity suggesting that they go to the store to buy beans. The mother this time simply stated, "But I use frozen foods." That mother was emotionally still at the stage of, "Why me?" "Why my child?" and was *not* ready for "What do I do?" and "How do I do it?" Maybe just *fun* in the bathtub, which was a regular need, might have been a wiser activity at that point.

A Reality Tester. She helps parents test out the reality of a situation as it concerns themselves or their child. They need support getting their feet on the ground, and to face facts as they really are. The dream of a parent for a child who could be a concert pianist may have to be tempered to the reality of a child who can learn to enjoy watching, feeling the rhythm of music, or moving in time to it.

A Resource Person. She keeps abreast of the latest information on child development, hearing, amplification, medical advances, community resources, and assistive agencies. She will need to address parents', grandparents', or neighbors' concerns the minute a "cure" or a device is reported in the media. Of course, the parent will need to understand the various systems of communication used throughout the country. A resource person needs to give accurate, up-to-date scientific and educational information in terms parents can understand.

Thus the role of that professional, by whatever title she is addressed, is multifaceted. It is true that the term, "Working With Parents" has a very appealing sound, but making adjustments in order to adapt a program to the individual family's needs as well as the child's is not simple. Family service programs mean a flow of ideas, energy, creativity, and leadership in an interactive way. Effective relations demand a free and easy give-and-take between the family and the intervention personnel. It is not a one-way authoritative role.

The success of the Early Intervention Program is to a very large degree dependent upon the one member of the staff who has the critical role of teaching, counseling, intervening, listening, and reinforcing.

Personal Qualities of Interveners

It has never been definitely determined what personal qualities are critical for the professional in an intervention program, but the following are necessary and important:

A Basic Liking for People. Parents, as well as children, are not all sweetness and pleasure. There are those who prize their children and want the best for them. There are those who never make appointments and seem not to care. There are the usual extroverts and introverts, the whirlwinds and the indifferent ones. It is important that the professional be tolerant and not impose her values on these families. She must like each and every one and identify the strengths of each parent that needs nurturing.

An Understanding of Family Life. The teachers selected for parent-infant programs should be parents of young children themselves. First-hand knowledge of the day-to-day reality of raising children is vitally important.

Empathy for Parents of Handicapped Children. While the professional does not require a psychology background, she does need to understand that parents may react in different ways to having a hearing-impaired child. It is important that the intervener assess these feelings and be sensitive to their presence.

Ability to Accept Parents at Whatever Level They Happen to Be. The intervener must be sensitive to what is said by parents and what is left unsaid. Some parents may want help and advice; others want ready answers and recipes for success. Some want services as much and as often as possible; others want to be left alone until they request help. The intervener must be aware of these levels and work toward bringing parents' expectations into alignment with the program and her own ability to meet them.

Understanding of One's Own Abilities. The intervener must understand her own boundaries and be able to make them clear to the families. Assuming more expertise than she has, or more responsibility than she is trained to provide can be both misleading and dangerous. The professional must remember that she is not a medical person, nor a psychiatrist, nor a social worker, nor a family counselor. She is a professional educator in its broadest sense.

Teacher Preparation

Throughout the text, we have stressed the need for personnel preparation to address family intervention rather than child-centered education. Obviously, the teachers need preparation for the language training they will give families. Of course, they need great competence in auditory training and hearing aid usage, but most of all, they need to understand the role of audition in language development. They must be experts in blending auditory input and spoken language into meaningful experiences at the child's cognitive level. Furthermore, they need skill in developing this ability in parents. These interveners must, therefore, be teachers of the deaf first and always.

One outstanding directive of the report to the President and Congress by the Federal Commission on Education of the Deaf (1988) reflects the above orientation. That directive emphatically stated that: "Individuals working with young deaf children and their families should be professionally trained in the area of deafness and early intervention." (p. 99) Federal mandates for Individualized Family Service Plans in early intervention raise significant issues which must be addressed by the program serving young hearing-impaired children.

Administrators would be wise to ascertain that the person who is to do the intervener's tasks is competent in the areas of deafness and early intervention. The Council on Education of the Deaf (CED) has established widely accepted standards developed by professionals within the field. (CED, 1975) Any teacher assigned the responsibility of the early education of young hearing-impaired children should be certified in Parent, Infant, and Early Education by that certifying body.

The person who is to guide the family needs substantial preparation to assume that important role. Unlike child-centered programs, teachers must now work with adults. While they could say a great many things with confidence about children such as, "Twos are into everything." "Fours find it hard to wait." "Sixes need a lot of activity." "Elevens think the sun rises and sets on their friends," such information is not available about parents. Therefore, teachers will need to learn what parents are like, why they are anxious and worried, what they tend to reject, what they know about listening and hearing, what information they have about language, how clear they are on speech development, what they and their child can do, and when they can do it.

Today teachers, educators, interveners can no longer enjoy a simplistic linear approach to language and cognition. They must understand the behavior of young children and hearing-impaired infants and youths as well as parents' coping behaviors. These are complex internal and external forces that reciprocally influence child development. There are no easy answers to the educational task. Teachers must be well prepared in order to seek the wisest solutions for each child and his family. To be less than prepared is to jeopardize the child's growth and development through parent intervention.

Planning and Teaching

To this point we have discussed *what* is to be taught, to *whom*, *when*, and *why*. Although we have alluded to the *where* it is to be taught and *how* it is to be planned, we have treated neither in detail.

When we mention curriculum, we may have opened Pandora's box because curriculum has been defined as: "Anything that affects the child within school," to "a program or range of studies leading to a specific goal." It assumes one proceeds through well-planned detailed objectives. To be an engineer, one must follow a set curriculum leading to an electrical, mechanical, or civil engineering degree. Most high schools have a set curriculum for students planning to enter college, another for those planning to go into the work force upon graduating. Elementary schools talk about a basic curriculum which includes reading, writing, and arithmetic. These curricula often do not vary a great deal from year to year.

For the preschool hearing-impaired child, the curriculum is frequently determined by the staff and followed for every class, year after year. A child is evaluated and placed at what is considered the appropriate place in *the* curriculum based on his performance. The school's pre-determined curriculum objectives are those that the teacher will give for all the children enrolled in the class. While this curriculum may appear on any child's individual plan, it nevertheless also might describe the goals for the entire class.

This same state of educational enterprise exists for the handicapped child in far too many programs today. However, some individualization is entering the system. This, as stated earlier, was mandated by P. L. 94-142 enacted in 1975, requiring that an IEP (Individual Educational Plan) be developed for each and every handicapped child in public educational programs. The IEP then became the child's personal curriculum. Rather than starting with a pre-determined curriculum into which a teacher was required to place a child, the teacher *starts with the child* and tailors the plan for that particular child.

Similarly, programs for parent-child education usually had a set plan for educating parents about deafness and having them teach pre-determined vocabulary or chart responses to sounds, etc. Historically, schools have recognized individual differences among children but not among parents. The same program that perceived each child as unique, often treated parents as if they were all alike. They were viewed as a monolithic group who needed only information and a set of lessons. Parents then were managed as a group, addressed as a group, lectured to in a group, and the hope was that group psychology would suffice. Parents' unique coping capabilities, their particular needs, and their individual abilities were all too frequently ignored. As the evidence cited by Bronfenbrenner (1976) stated, parents need even more one-to-one learning experiences than do children.

The variables of any group are multiplied when the capriciousness of children is added. Children vary in age, intellect, motor skills, size, talent, interests, and emotions. If they are hearing impaired, they present a number of other variables such as degree and type of hearing loss, age of onset of hearing impairment, cause of deafness, amplification, length of time the hearing aid has been worn, and the presence of other handicapping conditions. For the amount of learning children must do to acquire communicative behavior, it is readily apparent that there are insufficient hours in a day, in a week, or even in the 40 weeks of a school year. Parents must always assume the fundamental role of being their child's teacher, but this is not an intuitive process. They need help.

In order to help parents effectively, educators need to be aware that parents can be even more complex than children. All parents do not have the same abilities or resources. They are not homogeneous. For some parents, finding a way to get food for the next meal is their primary concern. For them, having a child with a hearing loss is not the most important problem in their lives. For others, the struggle up the corporate ladder has priority. For some, hearing loss is such a difficult concept that they can be petrified into inactivity. Emotional reactions impede many. Still others come to the task equipped with an unbelievable sense of dedication. Some are "super mothers" needing little or no assistance, while others want help for each and every step.

Parents are at various stages of understanding of children. They may not understand themselves nor their own needs. They may be first-time parents and know little or nothing about parenting, or they may be fifth-time parents, but know nothing about deafness. Parents have tremendous differences. No parent-child dyad (duo) is like any other; each is unique.

In spite of the individual differences, the intervention program must take the "whole child" and the "whole parent" and shape them into a communicating, interacting twosome. This is the challenging task of intervention. The needs of the child and the needs of the parent must be met.

This task can be extremely difficult for teachers. It is especially hard if the teachers were educated to teach in child-oriented programs. But change they must, as the result of Public Law 99-457 which is to be implemented by 1991. This law mandates a family-focused rather than a child-centered approach to early education. While child achievement is the goal, parent involvement is the route.

Family involvement is now a critical part of early intervention wherever it takes place. In a school it might be in the Home Economics room or an adapted classroom. In a clinic it could be a special office and in a hospital any spot near the audiologic center. However, one of the authors found a home demonstration center to be effective for parent training (Simmons-Martin, 1981). With the *where* flexible today, the *how* remains to be addressed.

If the question, "How do you teach parents and their deaf children?" were asked, many teachers and administrators would reply, "We use such and such curriculum." The "powers" with much or with limited experience have set down the steps thought to be necessary for a deaf child to learn to talk. These steps usually center on the child with parents simply following in lock-step the orders specified in that static curriculum. Possibly, it was to prevent the continuation of such practices that the legislators supported and passed P. L. 99-457.

Instead of stereotyped lessons for each child and his parents, the focus has shifted. A rigid curriculum is no more. The process is individualized for each family.

If intervention programs are to implement the new mandate, they must assess not only the child, but the parents. Professionals need to find out the family's needs and capabilities. They have to be alert to aspects of family functioning as it relates to the child in the intervention program. The time for recognizing and responding to individual differences among families has come.

Public Law 99-457 mandates that staff working with handi-capped infants develop a written Individualized Family Service Plan (IFSP). The multidisciplinary team assists in the development of the plan with the parents participating. Family strengths and needs related to the improvement of the child's potential are listed along with a statement of the major outcomes.

Some precedences had been set in 1975 by Public Law 94-142 which mandated that special educators prepare an Individualized Educational Plan (IEP) for each handicapped child. The plan had to include the student's present level of educational performance, annual goals, and short term objectives. It had to indicate what special education was necessary and what related goals were needed. The IEP had to include the beginning date and the anticipated duration of services as well as the annual procedures which would be used to determine whether the objectives had, in fact, been met. A similar plan for preparation and execution of an Individualized Family Service Program is an attempt to insure that early intervention programs are planned and individualized for each family.

This radical change in professional responsibilities calls for training of staffs that can assess family needs and evaluate family functioning. The assessments then provide direction for specifying family goals. The intervener is required to discuss the needs with the family members and jointly decide their priorities for service. As expected, the IFSP goals, like those in the IEP, must be stated in operational terms.

Individual Curriculum Development

Though educators know the advantages of an individualized program are many, parents will need to be taken through the process of planning a *personal curriculum*. This is a new and perhaps overwhelming experience for them. Constant guidance is necessary.

Bailey and his colleagues (1988) proposed a model for planning and evaluating individualized family services for early intervention. His model, Family Focused Intervention, specifies six steps: (1) assess comprehensively family needs and strengths; (2) hypothesize child/family goals based on the assessment; (3) interview parents to discuss needs and determine mutually acceptable goals; (4) review goals set in step two; (5) describe services provided to achieve goals; and (6) provide for periodic assessment.

Determining current levels of development

Abraham and Stoker (1988) stated that there has been no directed effort to establish a data base regarding language assessment practices actually used with hearing-impaired children. The primary difficulty is, as they see it, related to the test instruments themselves. Most of those in use were standardized on hearing populations, and no norms have been given for the hearing-impaired child. The article by Abraham and Stoker (1988) lists the eleven to thirteen tests available and used with the deaf population. While expressive language and form can be tested, nothing is available to assess language **use.** Their conclusion following the study was that training institutions should offer programming in specific assessment techniques, procedures, and instruments for use with hearing-impaired children.

Based on the information gathered from available and valid formal testing and informal assessments, the teacher of the deaf can determine the present level of educational achievement for the child both in approximate age ranges, i.e., twelve-month level, eighteen-month level, as well as a listing of mastered skills. The hearing loss, the aided audiogram, and other pertinent information on level of hearing and responses to sound and speech will need to be obtained from the audiologists.

The psychologist will conduct an evaluation of the child's overall developmental functioning. These reports would be the result of evaluations at the Center as well as those provided by other agencies. All of this information on the child's current level of functioning will be presented by the multidisciplinary team at a staffing with the parents. At that time, "a best estimate" of the child's current functioning is reviewed as a basis for jointly setting goals for the child.

Assessing needs and abilities of parents

Since formal family involvement is relatively new, few scales of parent's functioning ability are available. The assessment battery described in Bailey and Simeonsson (1988) addressed child characteristics likely to affect family functioning, critical events, parent-child interactions, and family needs. Bromwick (1981) developed a scale for evaluating mother-child interactions. Though the measures reported have not been used with parents of hearing-impaired children, nevertheless, these two scales do assess some helpful generalized parent behavior.

In the meanwhile, procedures for planning must include many observations of parent and child in a natural setting and in contrived situations. Much conversation and discussion with interview-type questioning will help in making some substantive observations regarding such things as parent's:
- awareness of child's communication attempts;
- response to child's communication attempts;
- frequency and quality of attempts to initiate communication with child;
- ease or discomfort with hearing aid;
- awareness of normal child development;
- understanding of the type and degree of hearing loss;
- understanding of their child's communication abilities;

- behavior management strategies;
- questions and concerns.

As was found in the Missouri study conducted by Burton White, first-time parents did not know what they needed to know. Never having been parents before, they did not know what skills were needed to "parent" an infant, a toddler, or a preschooler. Too often, the professionals overlook the fact that many parents are not "super parents" initially. They nevertheless have the intuitive need to be superior. These needs, too, must be given much consideration.

Assessments of parent needs have to be made over time and can be made only after mutual respect is built between the intervention staff and parents. The intervener must acknowledge the parents' expressed needs, and with discussion develop objectives appropriate to their accomplishment. She will also need to know when specific information or strategies should be programmed and be able to discuss the rationale behind the given objectives.

Preparing the IFSP

The staff summarizes the auditory, physical, psychological, and linguistic information and shares it with the family. It must be stressed that the information is based on facts not *interpretations* of what *might* be. The goals that grow out of the assessments must be set for a reasonable period of time. In the case of a very young child, the time probably should be a matter of a few weeks, whereas, for an older child it might be a few months.

Judgment must be used in discussing the information, especially for a family that is perceived as being vulnerable. A family that is still in the stage of trauma from the handicapping diagnosis can readily be overwhelmed. So can the first-time parent who is very unsure about her parenting role.

Caution must be used to see that the handicapping condition does not outweigh the need for a *strong parenting environment*. Parents must be first-rate parents, not second-rate teachers! Therefore, the IFSP must give "equal time" to the support and guidance of parents.

Sometimes the family's perception of assets and needs differs from those identified by the professionals. The staff may perceive that the family has different needs from those the family may identify. In these cases, the staff must respect the family's priorities and acknowledge the need for development of objectives that will best direct them. Or the staff may discuss certain goals and objectives and suggest postponement until the time is appropriate, sharing with the parents the rationale for the delay. Parents need assurance that it is only that — a postponement, not elimination.

Formulating objectives

The more clearly the objectives are written, the easier it will be for all to implement them and document their mastery. Several components should be included in the writing of an objective to make it clear: What the child or parent will do in what situation, with what materials, presented by whom, with what percentage of accuracy, how often, and by what date. For example, if the intervener wants the child to wear his hearing aid all waking hours, the objective might state: "Timmy will wear his hearing aid during all waking hours by October 30." If the intervener wants the child to understand simple sentences, the objective must be specific: "Timmy will recognize four out of five experience-based sentences in a closed set by October 30."

It is important for the educator to be accountable for the objectives. If the objectives are written clearly and specifically, the teacher and the parents will both understand what is expected of the child and of themselves. Furthermore, it will enable the intervener to document progress and achievement in an organized fashion and on a regular basis.

It is assumed that the staff will work to establish the family's trust. They give evidence of being knowledgeable about *parent* education and familiar with the necessary environment for language development.

Helping the parents interpret the objectives

Even though the parents may have attended the curriculum planning conference and heard all the objectives read aloud and explained, they may still need to have further explanations. First, they need to understand the order of the objectives. Second, they need to have the specific short-term objectives listed for them along with two or three examples of natural home activities they can do to support these objectives. These should be updated with the parents every two to three months as the child makes progress and accomplishes the objectives. As soon as mastery of an objective is documented, new ones should be identified.

These objectives must be realistic and clearly written. The careful assessment of family needs and the involvement of parents throughout the process should insure that the goals are attainable.

Paramount to the achievement of child goals and family goals is the need to understand the purpose. Knowing the purpose and the dynamics of their relationship with their child expedites parents' accomplishments.

Implement objectives

Once an appropriate and clear individualized "curriculum" (IEP or IFSP) has been developed, the intervener's main task is to see that the plan is implemented and documented during every individual session. Many approaches can be used. The authors provide a possible routine for accomplishing the objectives.

Routine Procedures for Parent-Child Sessions

1. Rapport Reestablished

Rapport should be reestablished with parents and child at each session. Parents need to know that the teachers care about them and the things that are happening in their lives.

2. Parent and/or Teacher Activity

The parent may conduct an activity brought from home. (This activity should have been planned and discussed at the previous session.) The teacher should also have an activity planned that can achieve a pre-determined goal in case the parent forgets or expresses too much discomfort with the task.

The parent activity is prefaced with a brief discussion outlining:

- The purpose of the activity.

- The particular language the mother will use.

- That Mother will check the language to be sure it is applicable to the child's thought.

- The points of the activity that will interest the child.

- The events that might be anticipated to happen.

- The strategies Mother will use to conduct the activity.

- The alternative strategies she has in mind.

- The frequency of this activity at home.

- The application of the language and concepts to other familiar situations at home.

3. Evaluation

Following the activity, the parent and teacher should evaluate answering such questions as: How did it go? Was it fun? Did it achieve the goal? Would Mother do anything differently next time?

4. Teacher-Parent Instruction:

There are times when the teacher gives the parent information necessary to the understanding of hearing loss, language development, improvement of listening skills, speech development or child management. At times a more urgent need may supersede planned topics.

Parent questions take precedence over any other activity and must be answered as clearly as possible. Effective communication with the parent is a given. Caution must also be the guide word here: The session must not be cathartic only. If the parents have problems beyond the skills of the intervener, referral must be made for professional counseling.

5. Parent-Home Activities

Parents need suggestions for things to do at home. Some parents want *specific* "assignments." Others want general suggestions. The teacher needs to get to know the parents and find out their wishes. The emphasis in either case is on using normal interactions throughout the day for language intervention.

6. Wrap Up

The intervener should summarize the session and discuss plans for the next session. She could help the parent plan the activity she is to bring the next time, if the parent wants help. If the parent is uncomfortable planning the activity, determine her objective.

7. Charting

The teacher should note any progress or critical observations on her lesson plan, immediately following the session. Furthermore, any issues raised by the parent that require later attention should be noted.

8. Periodic Assessment and Revision of Objectives

Records of achievement should be plotted over time and the results shared with the family. The interval of the child's birthday and six months thereafter make convenient reporting periods. Objectives may need to be revised to fit with possible changes in family or child.

Summary

The Federal mandate for the Individualized Family Service Plan (IFSP) in early intervention is consistent with the philosophy of the authors of this text. Services for hearing-impaired infants and toddlers must be family centered. The intent of a parent program is not to tell parents how they "ought" to be. Rather, it is to guide them in discovering how they can use their *own* potential to create a home environment which furthers the child's whole development and which is also satisfying to them as parents.

The professional who is to educate the parents must have specific preparation for working with adults (the parents) and understanding infant growth and behavior. Parents need to know what programs to seek for the best help for themselves and their child. There is no *Consumers Guide for Intervention Programs* as there is for cars, appliances, etc. Parents must shop for the center that reflects their own philosophical orientation. This chapter has outlined some of the criteria for their selections.

Chapter 7

Then There Is Language

Critical to the discussion of language is the description of what it is that the child has to learn. Since it is contrary to the philosophy presented in this text to dissect the language into segments, we have waited until this point to fragment the process. Learning language is a very complex process rather than a simple linear learning procedure. Because language is made up of so many interacting segments, we call it GLOBAL, indicating the wholeness of language rather than its parts. Because so much of the meaning in language is auditory, this total learning process has been called AUDITORY-GLOBAL. The basis of the process is THOUGHT, which is, of course, MEANING.

Even though the "whole is greater than the parts," there is need to illustrate some of the parts. These elements of the whole are phonemes, morphemes, syntax, and semantics. The process is the matching of the interaction of the elements with *thought* to express or receive *meaning*.

What is particularly amazing is that language behavior is achieved in a relatively brief period in early childhood. By the age of five, hearing children have adequate language ability to sustain them throughout their adult life.

Other than parental input, the actual procedures by which children learn their "mother tongue" are, in many respects, a mystery. The even greater mystery is how, through experiences in which the children are presented scanty and even unsystematic data, they are able to acquire such complexity as a three-year-old demonstrates. By that age, a hearing child exhibits language behavior that is functional and by five years of age, he is a skilled speaker. His syntax is complete except for dependent clauses in complex sentences and passive voice. His vocabulary includes over two thousand words including function words and idioms. His phonologic skills of intonation, phrasing, and stress are well established. While not perfected, his articulation is adequate and effectual.

The hearing child acquires this behavior by being engaged in full-time listening. He is presented with a tremendous variety of utterances, not sequenced according to any outline, not ordered by any curriculum, not programmed in any stereotyped way. Apparently, the system the hearing child uses is induction. The age of the child negates any notion that instruction was the procedure used. He must induce the rules of the code.

Citing the fact that children go from knowing nothing to mastering a language in three or four years has led some people to call all children linguistic geniuses. Hearing-impaired children can also be linguistic geniuses if they receive the natural program similar to that which hearing children receive.

Contrary to the numerous reports on the poor language use of hearing-impaired subjects, it has been found that given the opportunity, deaf children can develop as do their hearing peers. They may develop more slowly, but achieve language competence, they can!

It is the opinion of the authors that traditional deductive teaching approaches do not yield adequate results. This fact is compounded by the fallacy that speech, language, and auditory development are separate subjects. Often they are considered so separate that they are taught at periods set apart from each other, with altogether different material, and often by a different teacher. Another factor is that in this age of quantification, people rely heavily upon measurable items such as vocabulary and syntax which can be tabulated. To suggest that such complex behavior as language can be measured by simplistic means is naive. Yet, such requirements are made by the public laws governing education.

It was this concern with numbers of words, numbers of modifiers, mean length of utterances, numbers of phonemes articulated, and other atomistic, artifically separate language units, that led to the writing of this text. Furthermore, the findings relative to traditional teaching systems motivated the authors to challenge the approaches used to instruct deaf children over the past two decades.

The authors' rationale is that language is a code which children learn at a very early age, progressing from large items (intonation), to the particular (the phoneme), over a relatively short period. Rather than starting with language, hearing-impaired children, like their hearing peers, learn their first language by determining, independent of the words, the *meaning of the message*. They discover the intention of the speaker, and by working out the relation between meaning and the utterance, children induce the principles of language. To put it another way, *the "linguistically young" child uses meaning as a clue to language — **not** language as a clue to meaning.*

Stressing meaning as critical to language learning does not infer that language and thought are separate entities. Whether language is different from thought or inextricably bound to it, we leave for the researchers to determine. It is clear, however, that language abilities closely accompany, parallel, or interweave with the development of mental abilities.

Language

Language serves to assist memory and communicate meaning, to express feeling, to state intentions, and to influence the actions of others. It is an auditory-vocal process essential to human development which children learn without specific training and without special reward. This points to an important principle. The child does not learn merely to speak or to understand words or to build up a stock of words. Rather, he learns a whole mode of oral behavior, the linguistic, which is prior to any particular symbolic act in which he may engage.

Function

The function of all speech is social in origin. It is for communication and social contact. The child's primary use of language is to describe his world and manipulate people. It has been said that throughout his language development, the child learns what verbal or general responses will get what he wants or let others know what he dislikes. He learns what responses, on the part of others, are the cues for what he wants or does not want. The *FUNCTION* will be decided for him by the way his language "pays off" — the way he moves people to do his bidding. This is the role of *FUNCTION*, the "why" he speaks. He learns that he can manipulate his environment through verbal symbols. He obtains food, drink, and, most importantly, attention. A specific response is his first control over his environment. At first, the responses involved are very gross or global, but gradually they become differentiated and structured.

Content

Content is the referrent for language. It is the meaning conveyed by speech, the context, concepts, percepts, ideas, wants, problems, and feeling, to mention a few.

Development of content is a process of acquiring increasingly complex concepts, perceptions, and cognitive patterns through interaction with the environment. The content will vary from child to child because home environments and family interests vary. The content of the young child is very much the here and now. As his language matures, it can become more vicarious. However, when experience is scanty, that kind of language is not readily acquired. Thus, experiences for the child should be multiple.

There is a very subtle line of separation between the *Function* of language, the "how" or "why" one uses language, and the *Content* which is the "what" one says. Both function and content are held together by a third interlocking facet — the *Form* of language.

Form

Form is the system of transmission and reception of meaning. Ideas emanate from the mind of the speaker and are coded so as to be transmitted to the mind of the listener. *Form* incorporates *phonological, syntactical, morphological, and semantic* components. These components interlock just as Function, Content, and Form do. Rules govern the combinations within the units and the units with the other components. The rules are systematic and understood by all speakers of the same language. While the code is rule-based, the principles have been induced by the child as young as three or four years.

Form is a system of arbitrary components and rules for putting them together; arbitrary because syntax and semantics are constantly undergoing change in the English language. For example, nouns become adjectives as "parent" to "parenting" and "time" to "time-wise." Prepositions become conjunctions as in "Winstons taste good *like* a cigarette should." Even grammar is changed. "It is I" no longer is necessary and "It is me" is acceptable. The most stable unit is *phonology*, and it is the largest component of the code. This and the other three components — morphology, syntax, and semantics — will be discussed briefly.

Phonology

The features of phonology are phonation and phonemes. Phonation is the language's vocal system, and the first component to be learned or acquired. It is, in fact, the fundamental linguistic feature.

Phonation

Phonation was the feature talked about earlier in this text where the authors stressed the urgent need for parents to reinforce the child's phonations, each in a different way. The cry would get dry diapers, the whine would get the child picked up, and the coo might get him some play. These early sounds are the first audible features to emerge, and as such they are extremely important.

Phonation may be prosodic or melodic. The former has more function in code learning. In the beginning the meaning is usually affective or expressing a need or concern. Melody is not necessarily linguistic but has more to do with the quality of the utterance and interpersonal feelings.

Prosody. The prosodic features of language include intonation, rhythm, accent, and stress. *How* a thought is said is probably more important than what words were used to express the thought. The nuances of speech convey the speaker's meaning more than the specific speech symbols.

For example, nonsense syllables such as "du du du du" can express a thought and be interpreted even if the content is unclear. One of the authors (Simmons-Martins, 1972) described this system when giving her rationale for the auditory-global approach. She suggested that if a topic were the President, for example, the listener could obtain sufficient evidence from the speaker's prosody to establish the latter's political preference. "Dudududu" said in a monotone would reveal the speaker's apathy. On the other hand, if the same nonsense syllables were uttered with gusto, the listener would know immediately how the speaker voted.

Intonation. Interpretation of meaning is dependent upon the speaker's use of prosody, not the words. For example, the utterance might be "Isn't Tom great?" It is possible that it is complimentary, but it could also be sarcastic and uncomplimentary. The intonation the speaker uses clarifies the intended meaning.

Sentences and phrases are marked with declarative, exclamatory, and question intonations, and their intonation appears in the babble or jargon of six- and nine-month old babies. The hearing infant shows adult-like intonation patterns and is able to imitate adult intonation patterns long before he attempts the phonemes of English.

While children use intonation patterns in their vocalizations, they also seem to understand the meanings of emotive language as different from scolding sounds. When given positive prosody as "the pretty girl" or "a big boy," children wiggle, smile, and seem pleased. The same words given with negative or scolding patterns elicit crying or fretting.

Hearing-impaired children, like their hearing peers, need this opportunity to gain meaning and sentence intonation at the pre-linguistic level. This is the essential beginning of auditory training. "Love talk" and vocal play by the parent are necessary first steps. As the child moves on into school, the teacher needs to provide definite opportunities for continuing this learning.

Contrast, for example, the material observed in two separate nursery classes with deaf children. In one class there was a chart as follows:

> We went to the zoo.
> Mary saw a tiger.
> Susie saw a monkey.
> Jimmy saw a lion.

In the other class, the same experience was used with the following language:

> The class went to the zoo.
> Jane petted a baby zebra.
> It jumped away!
>
> Nancy watched the monkeys.
> Oh, she was happy.
>
> Brian liked the giraffe.
> It was so tall.

Not only is the intonation different, but the rhythm of each sentence varies. Some sentences are short, others long. Some have exclamatory intonation, others express happiness or surprise. Auditory training should begin with these meaning-bearing intonation units, not drums, whistles, or other noisemakers. Language is the purpose of listening; therefore, language should be the tool of auditory training.

Rhythm. The number of speech units spoken in a given time is important to speech intelligibility. This has more bearing on the quality of speech than the precision of the phonemes uttered. The utterances of hearing children, even those with articulatory problems, are often more intelligible than precisely spoken ones of deaf children. While their articulation may be excellent, their speech frequently lacks rhythm and proper timing.

Because attention often is focused on individual sounds and words, children with a hearing impairment do not get practice on synchronized breathing and speaking. Because of the atomistic (sound by sound, word by word) approach, their speech is slow, distorting the time in which the message is delivered. The prosody is destroyed, and the consequence is unintelligible speech.

The code dictates the number of sounds to be produced in a given interval of time. Vowels, for example, take twice as long to articulate as consonants, which average .15 seconds. If emphasis is put on units of meaning and the child is encouraged to imitate the utterances which observe the principle of rhythmic language, hearing-impaired children do not need to take three or four times longer than a child who hears to express the same material. Deaf children *can* observe the rhythm of speech producing utterances within the *normal* time. They can do it when their auditory training has been directed to *linguistically relevant* material based upon experience, and their attention directed to the meaning, not the sounds.

Accent. Accent is one of the arbitrary rules which help distinguish one class of words from another, i.e.:

réf use	re *fúse*
súb ject	sub *ject*
cón trast	con *trást*
pró duce	pro *dúce*

Mispronunciation and incorrect accenting influence intelligibility of speech. The message being delivered to the listener may be confusing if the speaker states that, "Someone re*fúsed* to put the *réf*use out."

Accent is that part of "Form" which interlocks more with semantics than with syntax. Again, attention to single words out of context muddies up the whole phonologic component of inflection and negatively affects speech intelligibility.

Stress. While accent has more to do with vocabulary, stress tends to be phonemic. Stress, which is the loudness or softness of speech at four levels, communicates specific meaning. Some examples using primary stress patterns are:

> *Whý* is he going to Paris?
> (What is his reason?)

Why is he going to *Páris?*
(and not some other city?)

Why is *hé* going to Paris?
(and not someone else?)

Stress can be used to communicate excitement, fatigue, disappointment, pleasure, contentment, sadness. These meanings transmitted phonologically could be derived from a single word, "Oh!" or even two words, "Oh, my!"

Perception of stress patterns assists the child in achieving better rhythm and prosody in his speech production. Therefore, we encourage the child's imitation of the adult model of utterances, not as parroting, but rather as training. The match of stress, accent, rhythm, and prosody to the language related to his experience gives the hearing-impaired child the correct data for processing through his auditory-vocal-mental process.

Phonologic features of prosody, rhythm, and stress cannot be taught out of context. Since every utterance a child makes is unique, the suprasegmental features mentioned above will differ. Rules cannot be delineated for each feature. The child must come to induce the rules as he experiences them in real-life language. The adult who models for the hearing-impaired child must provide sufficient data whereby he can assimilate the principle as it relates to meaningful language.

Phonemes

The most basic unit in the spoken language system is the phoneme. While in English there are only forty-six phonemes,[3] an infinite number of sentences can be composed from them. Hence, too often these are seen as tangible aspects of language which can be presented as entities. This is regrettable. These are rules which must be induced; for example, the forty-six phonemes are grouped into consonants and vowels. These in turn are organized into syllables but in a very definite and systematic way. Each syllable must have one and only one vowel sound; though it may have one or more consonants before the vowel and one or more after the vowel.

Vowels are more powerful acoustically and are likely to be perceived and discriminated by hearing-impaired individuals. The energy of the vowels extends down to frequencies as low as 250 Hz., not so the consonants. Fortunately, deaf children can perceive

[3] Phonemes or distinctive speech sounds, consonants or vowels, diphtongs, etc.

most of the consonants when they lip-read as well as listen, even though some may never hear them as sounds.

Through imitation, many of the phonemes develop naturally. For those, no drill need ever be given, and for those that may need attention, we recommend delaying work until the children know the linguistic structure for what they want to say. While phonation and prosody are the first vocal efforts of a child, phonemic acquisition is the last act of Form learning.

There is in all children a latency connected with phonemic understanding; deaf children are no different. The actual development of the phonemes by hearing-impaired children follows much the same order as for hearing children. Vowels precede consonants. Visible consonants, "h," "m," "p," "th," "sh" tend to be learned fairly easily.

Unfortunately, there are still too many people "working" on single phonemes. First of all, the child gets a distorted view of the production. The model's mouth is usually opened wide with accompanying excessive jaw movement. Secondly, the sound is never given the amount of time in connected discourse that it receives singly. Furthermore, the production of the sound differs when it is given initially, medially, and finally. The consonant "p" in isolation is quite different from "p" in "pan," "pat," "pick," and much different from the same sound in final position as in "up," "hop," and "mop." Drilling on words abuses the principle that language conveys meaning. Utterances are given in rhythm in a definite time envelope to fit the meaning. This information is more important for the deaf child than direction on manner of production. Only after the child has control over *language use* should attention be given to the parts. If imitation in context fails at that stage, then and only then should the phoneme production be repaired. When that is done, the item should be put back into context to ensure the proper time-envelope factor.

Morphology

Morphology is a difficult category to classify. It is conceivable that it could be considered an integral part of phonology, syntax, and semantics. Each morpheme has phonologic distinctive features, as well as semantic and syntactic properties.

Morpheme is a unit for grammatical analysis, yet is the smallest element in language to which meaning can be assigned. For example -s can mean several or plural as in boys; possession as in Tom's; or third person doing the task regularly as in Tom runs. Morphemes deal with forms and grammatical inflections of words. As words are modified to show tense, number, case and person morphemes take on importance. The most familiar and most comprehensive morphemic categories in English are *roots* and affixes.

walk	-s	box	-es
follow	-ed	rug	-s
sing	-ing	boy	-'s

Affixes may be either prefixes or suffixes:

Morpheme	*Root*	*Root & Affix*
-ly	glad	gladly
-ness	kind	kindness
-ing	run	running
-er	teach	teacher
un-	happy	unhappy
dis-	satisfied	dissatisfied

A simple change of a morpheme can change the meaning of a sentence:

The principal ask*s* to resign.

The principal was ask*ed* to resign (by the board).

There is abundant evidence to support the notion that children learn these forms first by imitating the various inflected forms heard as they occur in sentences and phrases spoken by mature speakers. Sometime during his third linguistic year, the child may be heard experimenting with false anological forms like "bringed." It was a red letter day for the authors when a five-year-old deaf boy volunteered "At night it's moony," after a discussion about "sunny." Another child had contributed, "Our seed grow*ed* because we tak*ed* care of them." These children, though making errors, were inducting the language rules — a great achievement.

The ability to produce the inflections of the regular words precedes by a year or more the use of affixes on irregular words. While the past tense regular verbs and regular plurals of nouns proceed smoothly, the "runned," "breaked," and "drinked" as well as "mouses," "mans," and "foots" continue for a time. This induction of rules leads linguists to conclude that morphological devices are a luxury of fully-developed language. A small child can get along quite well without them for a long time.

Syntax

In addition to phonologic and morphologic components, language uses structure to convey meaning. Structure principles are Word Order and Functors.

Word Order. Words can have lexical meaning as discrete items, but when put into context the interpretation varies. It is the interrelation of the words that influences the meaning.

The same three words, "bit," "dog," and "boy," can produce quite opposite meanings:

> The dog bit the boy.
> The boy bit the dog.

Similarly:

> The man killed the lion.
> The lion killed the man.

- Addition of the morphemes changes the meanings even more:
  > The men killed the lion.
  > (It took several to conquer one lion.)
  >
  > The lion*s* killed the man.
  > (The visual image is different.)
- Words have certain restraints, i.e., parts of speech which influence word order:
  > Tom *rakes* the *leaves* in the yard.
  > Tom *leaves* the *rake* in the yard.
- Some words require adjustment to the rest of the sentence:
  > The banks overflowed with customers.
  > The banks overflowed with muddy slush.
- The syntactic pattern will clarify some meanings:
  > Is that dog running in the yard?
  > Is that dog running in the yard, a poodle?
- Word order includes phrase order also:
  > I threw a kiss to my mother from the train.
  > I threw my mother from the train a kiss.

Phrase structure in preschool teaching needs to be programmed:

The experience,	"First we squeezed the lemons. Then we made lemonade."
Can be recorded:	"After we squeezed the lemons, we made lemonade."
More difficult would be:	"Before we made lemonade, we squeezed lemons."

One of the problems teachers encounter is teaching children sentence forms without making the form of the sentence the principle concern. If deaf children are taught to have complete integrity about expressing their *own* ideas, then the proper relation between form and idea can be established. Children then learn they need syntactic form to express their ideas. Hearing children can do this by four years of age. They work out the relationship unbeknownst to themselves. They need no artificial crutches. They apparently learn the structure or syntax by hearing and assimilating countless repetitions of the basic language patterns.

Deaf children are said to have more difficulty interpreting linguistic meanings that derive from formal or structural patterns of language than from word meanings. Therein lies a strong reason why children must not be taught or drilled on single words. The models they receive like those hearing children hear *must observe the principles of linguistic form* — the RULES OF THE CODE (the grammatical rules of their mother tongue).

Linguistic rules dictate that certain words can only be combined with others. For example, an adjective, "pretty," can mark a noun, i.e., "girl," ("pretty girl"), but it cannot mark a verb, i.e., "eat," not "pretty eats." A noun, "girl," can be combined with a verb, "eats," but not with an adverb, "slowly." These rules allow the user to differentiate strings of words as grammatical or nongrammatical:

"The green grass sleeps silently." is grammatic; whereas,
"Sleep grass green the silently." is ungrammatic.

Not only can a string of words be recognized as a sentence, but questions can be answered regarding the content, nonsensical as it may be. If a six-year-old hearing child is told, "The rinky boof bliffed his blop," he could answer questions about it as follows:

Who bliffed?	The rinky boof.
What did boof bliff?	His blop.
What kind of boof was he?	Rinky.
What did boof possess?	Blop.

Knowing the principles of the sentence code means, among other things, that the child can form new combinations of words, new combinations of patterns. Nearly every sentence is unique; nearly every sentence is novel; nearly every sentence is a creation. Parents and teachers need to supply the data whereby children can induce the principles of syntactic structure and create their own. He, too, must become able to compose an infinite number of sentences, each having unique meaning.

A child is capable of understanding more complicated structures than he can use; therefore, caution must be exerted to prevent "rubber-stamping." (Simmons, A., 1971) "Rubber-stamping" is coding back to the child what he is capable of using. When he can use, "The boy has a ball. He has a bat." code back to him, "The lucky boy has a ball and a bat." Similarly, when he can say, "Mary has a balloon. It is red." code back, "Mary has a red balloon." And later, "Mary has a big balloon which is red."

Functors. While word order signals meaning comprised of the interaction of one word with each of the others in a sentence, structure words or functors, sometimes called function words, convey precise meaning. For example: "man," "gave," "boy," "money," have lexical meaning in the sentence, "No *man* would *give* that *boy* any *money*." The meaning of that sentence varies from another using the same content words in, "The *man gave* the *boy* some *money*." In the first sentence, the difference in meaning is caused by the functors "no," "would," "that," and "any." The determiners "the" and "some" in the second sentence indicate that it was only one man and one boy, but they were particular people indicated by "the" which indicates an earlier referent. The amount of money is indefinite.

Note sentences such as:

Take the medicine *in an* hour.

Take the medicine *on the* hour.

The functors "in," "an," "on," and "the" demand entirely different action. In the first instance, it may mean only one dose of medicine per day; whereas, in the second case, it could mean twenty-four doses a day.

There are less than two hundred functors in the English language, but these are used and reused many times. If one were to count out one hundred words in any paragraph, he would find at least thirty to thirty-five percent of the words were functors. As examples:

Auxiliaries: can, did, will, may, could

Conjunctions: and, as, but, if, so

Determiners: a, and, the, some, many

Intensifiers: very, most, last, only

While lexical[4] words have meaning, the functors bind them into significantly different meanings depending upon their use. For example:

Any boy wants *a* car.

No boy wants *that* car.

That boy wants *two* cars.

Some boys *do not* want *a* new car.

The same content or lexical words can have different purposes when bound together with certain auxiliaries:

Books that *can* be read.

Books that *should* be read.

Books that *might* be read.

Books that *may* be read.

Books that *must* be read.

In the above examples, word order and lexical words are

---

[4] Words that have meaning when standing alone, i.e. dog, book, etc.

identical, but only one sentence makes the reading of a selected bibliography mandatory. In no way can language be considered simply a task of learning lexical or content words. It is how the words are combined and bound together that is important.

If teachers give any attention to functors, it is usually the prepositions that get singled out for practice. Unfortunately in the classroom, there might be a box and the usual items around the room. The exercise will involve putting something such as an eraser:

> in the box
> in the drawer
> in the closet

In that classroom you would rarely hear "in a pocket," "in a shoe," or "in the teacher's purse." Prepositions of place are important, but so are those of time or manner, as:

> in a minute
> in a flash
> in a hurry
> in the story
> in my dreams

The typical lesson might shift to either "on" or "under" and, again, it would be of place: "on the box," "on the desk," "on the book." The other uses of that preposition are rarely, if ever, considered, i.e.:

> on my birthday
> on television
> on the hour
> on the menu
> on cloud nine
> on fire
> etc., etc.

If one restricts the number of prepositions to only nine (at, by, for, from, in, of, on, to, with), there are over three hundred different meanings involved. This doesn't even begin to take into account the idiomatic uses as a cartoon recently illustrated. In answer to what the character was going to do on his vacation, he replied:

> Fool *around*,
> hang *around*,
> and goof *off*.

Occasionally, these pesky prepositions can be used out of phrases and mean even something different as:

> "on and off" — intermittently
> "off and on" — occasionally

Then there is:

up and down
in and out
over and under

Functors make up only a small percentage of words, but they comprise a very high percentage of words uttered. If one were to measure only one item of a child's utterance to determine his maturity, the evaluator would be wise to find the number of functors used by the child.

Contrast, for example, the utterances of a deaf twelve-year old who had been taught in a good traditional system. The stimulus was a four picture sequence:

A boy went fishing.
The boy took a fish.
Two turtles jumped in the water.
The boy jumped in the water.
The boy put a fish in the water.
The turtles ate the fish.

On the other hand, a hearing child the same age said:

Two turtles jumped into the water, and so did the boy.
After that he caught a fish and threw it back.
It was that fish which the turtles ate.

Words in the linguistic categories of connectors, intensifiers, determiners as well as auxiliaries and prepositions, have no meaning by themselves. Because of this they force the use of language in its total sentence form or at least total phrase structure.

When the child distinguishes "a" from "the" as in "Get *a* cookie." and "Get *the* ball." he must be given the opportunity to use other function words such as "another", "some," "one," as in, "Can you get *another* cookie?" "You may get *some* cookies." or "You may have *one* cookie." When these simple sentences are *comprehended*, more advanced structure should be introduced, e.g., "If you wash your hands, you may have a cookie." The concern is not that the child *uses* "wash," "hands," "cookie," but rather that he is exposed to *if, may, and, a.* At a later time, he will have the background to use these in original sentences.

Deaf children taught by the usual traditional approach have difficulty interpreting structural meanings. They consistently score higher on lexical items rather than structural ones. Furthermore, they use fewer types of functors or omit them altogether.

Young hearing children also leave out the functors giving telegraphic characteristics. But it should be noted that the missing words are unstressed in adult speech, and all are phonetically obscure. To discriminate functors in the flow of adult speech presumably is also difficult for the hearing child, and as a result they do not appear in the child's own speech until he is about four years old or older. Nevertheless, the parent of the hearing child is talking to him at a level that is about a year above his speaking (language) age. To talk at the child's level is merely "rubber stamping" his use and providing him no data from which he can induce principles and grow. Parents and teachers of hearing-impaired children must not "rubber stamp" either, if linguistic rules are to be developed. Because of the importance of functors to the meaning of utterances, deprivation of their use in context would permit very impoverished language or possibly no language at all.

From the first two-word sentence-like utterance, i.e., "Baby cookie," "Mommy shoe." to the very complicated structures that three- and four-year old hearing children use, there is a very fast and amazing development that is completed at the preschool age. Most syntactic sentence structures, most morphological word changes, and most functors are mastered by the hearing child's fifth birthday. From then on the emphasis lies on the expansion of vocabulary, greater use of abstraction, metaphoric usage, and compound structures. By then, adults begin to use more direct explanation. Up to that stage, the inductive way, whereby conclusions or usage is inferred from particular examples, has been the child's primary learning device. Only at the point that the child has *control* over language should the deductive schema (whereby he learns from rules), be used as a class procedure. Deductive procedures are usually employed in upper grades as standard teaching strategy. Note, however, that the child must have a functioning linguistic system quite in place and functioning before deduction is used. A young child's language can be gravely inhibited by formal rules taught for deductive learning. Young hearing children learn inductively. So do deaf children if given the opportunity.

Semantics

The dictionary description of the word *semantics* is significant at this point. Semantics is the science of meanings, as contrasted with phonetics which is the science of sounds. It is the particular kinds of meanings with which this section is concerned. Volumes are available on the topic of semantics; thus only a brief introduction will be given to demonstrate the amount of complexity in vocabulary alone.

Words are meaningful units for analysis. They may be divided into two groups, lexical or referential, and functional or syntactical. The latter class — Functors — were discussed above.

Lexical classes are few in number, but have many members. In English the classes are nouns, verbs, adjectives, adverbs, and pronouns. Children, however, do not learn vocabulary as members of a class of words. They come to discover that everything has a name, not only objects and people, but qualities, activities, relations, and such. Furthermore, they find that one item can have more than one name: as "daddy" who is *daddy*, also a *man* and a *boy*, who may be *sweet* or *angry*, *sleeping* or *driving*. Then he learns that daddy is a man, but Uncle Joe is a man also, so is the gentleman next door, and the postman, and Grandpa. He induces this before he combines the words to form larger units, phrases, and sentences.

Contrary to the common notion that learning the vocabulary of his language is the simplest task that confronts the child, it is one that requires a very high level of conceptualization. While it may appear that all a child has to do is relate objects with their names, such is not the case. Nevertheless, that might be the reason there are programs which we call "The Ball, Fish, and Shoe" school of thought. These three words are often in the first lessons of those programs. The labels get associated with the objects. In the case of "fish," it is usually a plastic one, and then pictures replace the actual objects and are used for the drill. Such an approach is not only non-linguistic, but conceptually non-challenging.

Nouns

Consider just the word "ball" for example. The toddler knows a great deal about the big ball people use in play with him. He knows it rolls to and away from him. He knows it is round and bouncy. He knows he can hold it, but not eat it. He knows it smells different from his teddy bear. He knows it can be red or blue or many colors. It is not cuddly, but it can be small or very big. It can be played with but not worn. It can be used within the house or outdoors. All of these perceptions need to be experienced for the concept of "*ball*" to be meaningful to him. He will recognize the word "*ball*" as having these attributes long before he utters the sound himself. If he does not have the experience, he is not likely to know the real meaning of the word.

Consider the concepts connected with another noun, i.e., *soap*:
One can

bathe with it	clean the car with it
wash the hands with it	wash the dog with it
rub it on a cloth	make bubbles with it
buy it	unwrap it
wash dishes with it	soap windows with it
carve something from it	pour it if it is liquid soap

A variety of concepts can be associated with *soap*:

It can be solid, liquid or granular.
Soaps come in many shapes.
It is not edible.
It is not heavy.
Some soap floats.
Solid soap cakes can be counted.
Liquid soap takes different functors.

a cup of
some
a dash.

A child gathers this knowledge through interaction with his social and physical environment. He learns as he experiences the concepts and the adults discuss the content.

Count and Mass. Ball is a count noun, and that principle needs to be understood because its modifiers differ from those used with mass nouns such as soap.

a ball	some soap
three balls	a cup of liquid soap
a big ball	a large amount of soap

Count nouns use regular or irregular plural endings:

ball, balls	box, boxes

Mass nouns have no plural form, but the determiner (modifier) changes:

water — *a lot of* water   milk — *a gallon* of milk

Categories. By six years of age, a hearing child is able to recognize that:

dogs, cats, and horses are all animals.
chairs, tables, and beds are all furniture.

By that age, he should be able to tell how a peach and a pear are alike and respond to questions such as:

Can you name the animal that says "meow?"
Which animal likes milk?
How are a cat and a dog alike?

While most deaf children can categorize pictures easily, they have difficulty doing the same thing with words without pictures. This is all the more reason why children need verbal exchange and opportunities to discuss, compare, group, and categorize things and ideas.

Synonyms. If the adult "rubber stamps" the language the hearing-impaired child is using, the child will rarely get the synonyms of the vocabulary he knows. The deaf children in a comparison study (Simmons, A. A., 1965) used only the word *boy* to denote a young male person; whereas, the hearing children also used, in addition to "the boy":

lad	he
chap	kid
fellow	guy

To be sure, these will not be taught in a deductive type of lesson (deducing particular examples from general principles) until the child is beyond seven years or so. However, he must be given the opportunity to induce (derive the general principle from the particular example) the meaning very early. *Once one word is comprehended*, the adult should start using synonyms (words meaning the same) and even antonyms (words meaning the opposite) in real situations.

Verbs

Verbs denote some kind of occurrence, action, or mode of being, i.e., "close" can denote action as in, "Close your eyes" or:

Close the door.
Close your mouth.
Close the drawer.
Close the box, etc.

"Brush" denotes action as in, "Brush your hair" or:

Brush the dog.
Brush your teeth.
Brush the snow off.
Brush the scraps off the table.

Verbs must occur in sentences in order for the child to induce that it is the action. There is also an actor and something happens.

Intransitive verbs require no objects.

The airplane *flew* by.
The bird *sang*.
The boy *walked*.

Transitive verbs, on the other hand, require objects.

Mother *made* a cake.

Susie *drank* her milk.
The bird *laid* an egg.

One class of deaf children that one of the authors visited presented an extreme example of being taught distorted language. The teacher handed out pictures of people which she labeled as *walk*, *run*, *jump*, and *skate*. Since the teacher said so, that must have been action, but it was not obvious in the picture. The actions were only a part of the busy picture. The teacher then had the children pull a picture and she asked:

Who has walk?
Who has skate?

The responses were to be, "I do." or "I do not." If she had to drill in this fashion, she should have at least said: "Who has the *picture* of people walking?" which would have provided appropriate concepts.

What principles can children induce from "Who has walk?" If it is the question "Who has walked to the store?" the form of the verb is walk*ed*. If the teacher wants the picture of someone walking that should be the question, "Who has the picture of someone walking?" In the first case, the word "has" is an auxilary or a functor. In the second case, it is the verb "to have" which indicates possession. One possesses objects or ideas, not action. In other words, possession would be of *nouns*. Therefore, programming "Who has jump?" teaches two errors and programs the child for confusion. Fortunately, hearing children do not receive incorrect rules. They may get incorrect grammar, but the basic principles of the language code are not broken. It is the hope of the authors of this text that hearing-impaired children do not receive mutilated language code. The plea is that one consider language, not as made up of items, but made up of *thoughts* which are spoken in a natural and appropriate code.

Pronouns. Pronouns are possibly the most abstract labels that children have to learn, yet hearing children accomplish the task at a fairly early level. "Me," "my," and "mine" follow the principles of all learning. What is personal is learned first, so these pronouns are among a child's first words.

Number, person, and gender dictate the pronoun to be used. So does the syntax. Nominative and objective forms differ for each of the items above. For example:

I   can only be used in the nominative form.
Objective form is *me*.
I can be used by Mary or Jim to refer to themselves.

She	is also nominative. It can refer to Mary if it is used by another speaker.
He	is the masculine nominative which can refer to John if someone talks about him.
Me	can refer to either Mary or John if they use it, but
Her	can only refer to a female, and
Him	is the objective form for a male.
They	may refer to both Mary and John, and
We	may be used by Mary and John if they are speaking.
My	can be used by Mary or John to refer to their possessions.

> *My* ball.
> *My* dog.

Mine	refers to possession, but does not delineate what.

> It is *mine*.
> That is *mine*.

Our	is the possessive plural.

> Ah, *our* house!
> It is *ours*.

Their	is the plural for both genders, and
Theirs	adds the morpheme "s" as does our*s*

> That is their*s*.

You	can refer to either Mary or John singularly or to both of them. Similarly,
Your	is possessive, and
Yours	is like "theirs" and "ours."
It	is the pronoun for inanimate objects.

The above are *personal* pronouns; there are also relative pronouns of "who," "whom," and "which" which have a dual role. One, they introduce questions, but they are also functors called connectors.

Multiple meanings

Another idiosyncrasy of English is that so many words have many meanings. One of the authors became concerned about this while teaching arithmetic. When the children had the problem: "Tom could run a mile in a *quarter of* an hour, how long would it take him to run five miles?" One of the boys in the class asked, "Why did they pay Tom?" Being confused, the teacher asked where he got *paid*? Rick responded that "a quarter" was twenty-five cents. Whereupon, that teacher taught "quarter of" as the fractional part, and the class got "quarter of a yard," "quarter of a foot," etc., until Rick finally said, "Oh, that is why twenty-five cents is called a quarter." At that point, the math problem was then developed.

But following that instance, there was a problem in which, "*Bill* paid his *bill* with a five-dollar *bill*." That led to the study of multiple meanings in first and second grade arithmetic books (Simmons-Martin, A. 1949). In researching the topic, it was found that these confusions were of concern to teachers of hearing children also. How much more practice would hearing-impaired children require!

The first investigation concerned with this problem studied primary level dictionaries. Instead of the five hundred seventy words which the authors of the reading textbooks presented, there were seventy thousand different meanings. The word "run" alone had eight hundred different meanings.

One of the examples from the arithmetic books was the word *figure*. It was used in the second grade book as a noun, a verb, and an adjective.

Noun: Look at the *figure* on page three.
Draw a *figure* of Santa Claus.
Which *figure* is a triangle?
Write your *figures* carefully.
One *figure* in the chart represents twenty boys.

Verb: *Figure* your answer in the margin.
Can you *figure* out the mystery?
"It *figures*!" said Tim.

Adjective: She bought two yards of *figured* material.

This experience of finding that hearing children encounter the same word used differently very early, lead the authors to completely reject the "Ball, Fish, and Shoe" philosophy of teaching deaf children. Such a limited approach does not prepare these children for the variety of meanings to be met in all subject areas.

Idioms

Like multiple meanings, idioms present similar problems:

Catch a plane.	Catch a cold.
Catch his eye.	Catch the waiter's attention.

Sally's friend left a doll for her. When Sally returned she was told that the friend had "to catch a plane." Sally became very cross, arguing at her language level that "you could catch a ball, yes. A plane was too big!"

Our language is replete with idioms.

Throw a kiss.
Throw his arms around her neck.
Throw a curve.

Or:

Which way does your street *run*?
She has a *run* in her new hose.
Run on back.

Unless the child has experiences which are labeled in conjunction with the experience, he can have insufferable problems with words which are taught as single entities.

Conclusion

While this partial analysis of language does not go into great detail, the sample needed to be presented to show the basis of the "global approach." Language cannot be taught in any compartmentalized form. For language to be meaningful, it must include all the necessary meaning-bearing items in the system of spoken language used in our society. The child speaks *thoughts*, and he needs the words to express *those thoughts*. In order to be understood, he must use the same code as the listener. The child must observe the same rules of phonology, syntax, morphology, and semantics as the listener. Listening and speaking use the same code.

Code Learning

Speakers of the same language use a code to relay messages from one to another. Language code, like any code, uses symbols to transmit the message. Morse code uses dots and dashes. English code uses sounds, words, phrases, and word order. Rules govern the combination of the units within the code. The rules are systematic and influence the smallest to the largest elements. There are rules to express meaning; there are rules for speaking phonemes; there are rules for combining nouns and verbs; there are words to use that convey meaning between words; there are a limited number of functors that are used with a great deal of frequency.

Even though the code is rule based and systematic, it is learned by age five years if the child has intact hearing. It should not be much later for the hearing-impaired child: if his parents provide the same information as the parents of the hearing child do, if he has received a hearing aid(s), if the parents have good parenting skills.

Because language follows a set of rules relating to sounds, morphemes, words, and word order, every user of the code employs the very same rules. Because the listener knows the rules, he can predict the words that are likely to be used by the speaker. This *prediction* ability is built upon familiarity with linguistic strings. Prediction is like guessing: given a specific situation; from a series of sounds, words and sentences can be predicted. For the deaf child to gain this familiarity, he needs thousands of hours of code use in meaningful situations.

"Information Theory"

For many years, the telephone company capitalized on the predictability of language. Even though their transmitters at that time were not able to send signals with true fidelity, the company knew the listeners would be able to understand the messages being delivered to their ears. That was because the listener had the ability to guess, to predict what is actually being said in less than ideal listening conditions.

Unbeknownst to the user, "Information Theory" is constantly being applied. The pilot in the cockpit of a plane probably uses predictability more often than the average listener. Because he anticipates the language, the pilot is able to understand the message that the tower sends even though the message may be garbled due to engine noises. "Information Theory" aids in this comprehension. Similarly, people may catch only a word or two delivered over a public address system in a noisy place. Yet, they interpret it because they know the code and can predict what was said.

Code-learning should be of the utmost concern in helping the hearing-impaired child learn to speak. Since sounds, words, follow each other in accordance with the structure of the language, the listener, familiar with the code, will be able to anticipate at any point in the sequence what elements are most likely to come next. His ability, it must be stressed, is entirely dependent upon his experience with communication. This knowledge of the language code is so important it carries much more weight than the individual sounds of speech themselves.

If the child applies the knowledge of the code to information, even though imperfectly received, he should be able to supply those missing linguistic elements. In a lesson, he might hear:

u bi baw ol dow u ee

If he knows the code, he can fill in:

The big ball rolled down the street.

The strength of our knowledge of possible speech sequences helps us fill in any gaps in a stream of words we hear. For example, an English nursery rhyme can be understood with one-third of the letters missing:

M*R* H*D * L*TTL* L*MB
H** FL**CE *A* WH*** *S SN**

The great importance of knowing the code and being able to guess what is said or is to be said can be demonstrated with another example from Denes and Pinson (1968). The experimenters chose a sentence and without giving any hint as to its nature, asked the subject to guess the sequences of sounds that made up the sentence. In the sentence, "Speech is an important human activity!" three-fourths of the letters were guessed correctly on the *first* try. The person who was doing the guessing had no preliminary information of what the sentence was about or how it was constructed; he just guessed. It took six guesses to get the first sound, but only one guess thereafter, up to the word "human." The first letter of that word took twenty guesses. Human was not anticipated as important to speech so the subjects had to take more guesses.

611111 11 11 111111111 205541 69112111
Speech is an important human activity

The listener with normal hearing is guessing a good deal of the time, and when reception becomes difficult because of noise, the proportion of guessing increases. Significantly, the hearing listener has the pattern of speech to which to match the received signals or pieces of language code.

What is important for the hearing-impaired listener is the demonstration of how much can be "guessed" in the absence of a large portion of the message. Code interpretation that is possible with a small amount of residual hearing, and with proper amplification, is appreciable. In order to accumulate the knowledge of the linguistic code, however, the hearing-impaired child needs *as much — not less —* listening to the code as does the normally hearing child.

Hearing-impaired children must be trained so that they, too, can take an imperfect message, apply "Information Theory" and thereby receive the correct message. Hence, we are insistent that children receive natural sentences, appropriate to the situation in which sounds, words, and phrases follow the code rules.

That language code knowledge is more important than word knowledge has been successfully demonstrated with hearing-impaired children by Whetnall and Fry (1964). Fry, a linguist, showed that deaf children learn the code system when given the opportunity. He concluded that once a hearing-impaired child learned the code system, he could guess as efficiently as a hearing child. The deaf child, however, needed more speech, more amplified speech to which he could listen. He also needed more opportunity to practice it. Sufficient code information is available in everyday speech. Deaf children must be given enough information to apply "Information Theory" to the task of communicating in order to become competent in the English language.

"Information Theory" is not in itself a panacea for the intricate task of developing language competence, because if it were, the old procedures of incessant talking to the child would have been successful. Instead, *it is what is in the child's mind* that must be combined with the language code. His thoughts, his ideas, need the code. It is the cognitive organization of experiences in language, not the words, which builds the statistical information necessary for prediction. The semantic information is available only insofar as the language code system is known.

Children do not need to analyze or understand fully the internal structures of utterances as long as they understand and can exploit the *functional* communication value of utterances. When language functions for him, the child induces bit by bit the complex set of behaviors involved in the language process.

Communication is accomplished through the use of language. Communication is possible because both sender and receiver understand the "language code". Because communicators understand the "language code", the receiver can predict the units of the message even though he actually hears only parts of it. Therefore, it is critical that the deaf child learns the code in its global entirety and attends to it auditorially. The process — called "Auditory-Global" — is the rationale on which this text is based.

Chapter 8

Preschool

Despite his handicap, the hearing-impaired child has great ability for learning, but like his hearing peers, he requires education to realize that potential. The overall expectations for the deaf child — educational, cognitive, and social — govern the goals. These, in turn, dictate how the child is to be educated.

The only valid basis for education is the *child*, beginning where he is and taking him as far as he can go. This does not mean as far as someone arbitrarily determines he should go. Such a determination is frequently made when programs are remedial rather than developmental. For the latter, the goals are unlimited. When teachers teach the *children* not the curriculum, children demonstrate their unlimited potential.

When teachers (and parents) pick up on a child's cues and curiosity, they are helping the child achieve greater heights of learning. When adults reinforce the child's growing interests by using appropriate language to expand the experience, they are setting the right direction for assisting the child to develop cognitively.

The learning process must center around children and their needs. The deaf child, like all children, needs to be loved, to be secure, to play, to feel that he belongs, to interact with other children and with adults, to learn to make decisions, to develop initiative. In short, he needs to be allowed to develop a good self-image which is basic to active learning. Fundamental to this is maximum use of residual hearing which enhances his feeling of participation and improves his communication ability.

The child learns best when there is continuous, affectionate interaction between him and his teacher. The teacher needs to combine genuine friendliness, acceptance, warmth, and interest with deep concern for children. In a classroom where there is mutual trust and respect, the teacher is sensitive to the child's opinions and feelings. Teachers cannot *cause* learning to occur. They can only establish the optimal conditions in which learning is most likely to take place.

The child develops through personal action upon, interaction with, and reaction to objects, events, people, and ideas. The child is an explorer, a scientist, an inquirer, and an artist who pursues, constructs, and organizes his environment. Intelligence is the adaptation of the child to the physical, social, and intellectual world. Although it is not possible to speed up a child's rate of development through instruction or drill, teachers must be ready to act on the child's cues and spontaneously enrich his environment in order to accelerate his learning.

In organizing materials for his education, it is necessary that the focus be upon the multiple purposes of learning the content, of learning to think, of acquiring attitudes, and of developing skills. All of these are embedded in language which is the cornerstone of knowledge. While language is exceedingly and distressingly complex, it and the content are not mutually exclusive. In fact, content and language are inextricably interrelated.

The language teaching for hearing-impaired children herein discussed differs from that traditionally outlined for their education. Along with ideas, teachers need to stress the linguistic code observing all of the principles of form and function, thereby allowing the children ample opportunity to develop inductively (i.e. from particular examples to general principles) the rules inherent in language. Language can then emerge as the main system of representation.

The setting for the hearing-impaired child is that of a typical nursery or preschool, equipped, however, with unusual attention to audition — the room treated with acoustic tile, rugs, and if possible with draperies. The critical factor, however, is *not* the physical classroom; it is *not* the equipment; but it is the *teacher*. The teacher must have the appropriate educational background plus the additional dimension of dedication; dedication to the concept that deaf children can learn normally and at an early age.

The teacher should know and understand young children and therefore young children who incidently have a hearing loss. The techniques she employs in the classroom should demonstrate a grounding in audition and linguistics as well as child development.

Auditory-Global

The approach described herein has been called "auditory-global" by the authors. It is broad but also comprehensive. The concern is with the total child, his hearing ability, his developmental age, his interests, his cognitive experiences, and his social functioning. The content of the auditory stimuli is the *global* language, not discrete sounds or words. Language is not parceled into separate entities. Instead, the connected spoken language which is appropriate to the situation contains all the suitable nuances of speech, the rhythmic structure, the intonation, and the stress as well as the connected phonemes; always spoken at the natural rate of utterance.

In each communication situation the teacher should attempt to provide for language *understanding*, ensuring that the child receives language form through many, varied, and clear samples. In order for the hearing-impaired child to build up a knowledge of the structure of language, he must hear a great deal of speech. In fact, the quantity of speech that is connected language should be greater than that heard by normally hearing children. Therefore, since the goal is for the child to develop an ability to predict the events in language — the phoneme or speech sound, the word, the morpheme (or inflected grammatical affix or root), word order, the next sentence or phrase — the code information must be processed through the auditory and vocal systems of hearing and speech. By providing the natural linguistic code, the teacher programs the information of language, combined with meaning, giving the hearing-impaired child opportunities to induce the rules of grammar from specific examples.

The thought, ideas, and concepts can be made meaningful by *first-hand experiences* through nursery and the primary levels. The educational program should be oriented appropriately to contrived and spontaneous experiences. Accompanying and following such experiences, they are described in language. When a teacher is presenting the concepts of dissolving and chilling, she may use:

After Mark poured the water into the pan, Lisa stirred it.
Brian put the jello in the refrigerator to chill.

These and other related sentences also become the stimuli for auditory training during which the child repeats the structure, imitating the intonation and timing of the teacher.

The young child needs a stimulus for his verbal responses. Verbal stimulation takes place throughout the day. Language has to be modeled during contrived experiences or incidental happenings while attaching language to the child's ideas. This is important, too, when the teacher is asking the child to respond to the many verbal directions given throughout the day. The language used and expected is appropriate to the child's understanding while at the same time, his existing expressive language is being expanded.

This interaction of idea and language is related to the real world or more importantly to the child's real world. It may be related to science, e.g., planting seeds, using magnets, floating wood, or art activities. It can be the language of snack time or games. The teacher may give the children language for social interaction, or she might be just chatting with them. *The important thing about this interaction is that it is not a monologue on the teacher's part.* Rather, it is a *teacher-child interaction* which is *based on concrete experiences* and thus has meaning for the child.

In all of these experiences, the teacher, while guiding the children in the fun and fascination of noticing what things are really like, can introduce, present, and drill upon language related to the concepts. For example, to acquire concepts of evaporation, the teacher could contrive such experiences as:

Washing clothes:	Genny washed the doll's dress. Jennifer hung it up. After a while, it was dry.
Finger painting:	Tom painted with red paint. He hung his picture up. It dried by noon.
Puddle dry-up:	This morning there was a big puddle by the door. By noon the puddle was dry. The water had evaporated.
Ice chips melt and evaporate:	Susie dropped her snow cone. Mark swept some of it up. The rest dried.
Water in the aquarium:	Jim forgot to water the fish. The water in the aquarium is low.

Other experiences for the related concepts might include boiling water, shedding rain from rain gear, freezing water for popsicles. A wide variety of situations assist the concept acquisition and the language understanding. With a breadth of experiences he can learn that he can express the same concept in a variety of ways.

Only one experience repeated with the same language, no matter how often, does not develop concepts.

It is mandatory that the teacher knows what a four-year old likes to do and what a five-year-old likes to play with. However, she must also know about cognitive processing. Concepts develop from multiple percepts. In the case of evaporation, children need to know about pouring, spilling, wetness, and dryness. The teacher calls to the child's attention the important elements by labeling them and showing their attributes. This attention assures the meaning level of awareness.

To be sure, the teacher has influence on what interests a child. While the content of a child's lesson might be, "John has on new shoes." or "Tom threw a ball," his interest will be quite different from the child whose lessons are centered on making a garden, feeding the birds, flying a kite, digging for worms for a fishing trip, working a pulley, using a magnet, climbing on a fire truck, or shopping at stores. The latter child is gaining a variety of information about the world in which he lives. In addition, he is learning the language necessary for understanding and expressing these concepts.

There is no precise sequencing of what the child has to learn. He should be offered a tempting smorgasbord, not a carefully prescribed diet. He needs exposure to sentences in the context of conversations that are meaningful and personally important enough to command attention. He needs to be talked with about topics of interest in the context of his ongoing work and play. This is the "global" approach to the total child. To be sure, he needs very specific kinds of help — help with meanings created by combinations of functors and content words; help with pronunciation; help with proper syntax — but most of all help with *communicating information through language*.

The important catalyst is not the language, however, but the child's experience and verbal interaction with his environment. Children need experiences which in turn need labels, but it is the *thought* in the child's mind that needs language form. Without *the meaning* being in the child's mind, words can be piled higher and higher, but no real language *behavior* will result.

Strategies

Teachers cannot merely wait for learning to occur; they must create optimal conditions in which learning is most likely to happen. There are some important strategies which need to be incorporated into the process. The strategies which help meet the challenge of providing the optimal language learning environment are:

- Tuning in
- Reinforcement
- Imitations
- Verbal stimulation
- Expansion
- Modeling
- Provision for rule induction
- Auditory practice

Tuning in

When the teacher "tunes in" to the child, she should try to determine from both verbal and non-verbal cues what it is that the child wishes to say. She then matches the appropriate language to the *child's thought*. She must anticipate the language from the child's point of view. In other words, she gives the child the model for what *he* wants to say in that situation, not what another classmate is capable of saying. The sentences she models at first are usually short and simple. Basing language instruction on ideas the child originates makes the exchange meaningful.

Like the "super mom," the teacher must learn to "tune in" to the preschooler. She must learn to find out what the child is trying to tell her, to listen, and to assist him in learning to make his decisions. He cannot do this in an atmosphere of failure. Instead, the teacher creates a climate where the child is willing to take risks. He is willing because her previous reinforcements were pleasurable. This helps the child develop the willingness to try, so important to any learning.

Reinforcement

Many opportunities need to be provided for successful experiences which help develop the child's self-confidence and positive self-image. Success needs to be followed by positive reinforcement rather than testing the child to show him what he cannot do. Instead of telling the child how often he is wrong, the teacher should tell him how correct he is and show how pleased she is with his efforts. The child should *not* hear *NO* very often, and then, only when he is in physical danger. Failure and subsequent frustration have no place in the language-oriented preschool.

Some behavior from the environment or some reaction within the child must reinforce language behavior. The child's own internal responses or the behavior of other people will be reinforcing if the responses or the behavior increase the probability that the child's behavior will occur again in circumstances similar to those in which it was reinforced. For example, if the child is hungry and says, "oo-ee," and is reinforced by getting a cookie, the likelihood that he will say, "oo-ee," the next time he is hungry is increased. The critical skill for the teacher in any operant conditioning situation, is the reinforcement — both how and what to reinforce.

An inherent problem in language reinforcement is whether one reinforces content, function, or production of language. If a child gets reinforced for "Why me do?" by a response "Because we have an appointment," what happens to form and production? Parents, however, correct children on *what* the child has to say, not the structure nor the pronunciation he uses. Instead of responding to the vocabulary, grammar, or articulation, the mother responds to the truth value of the proposition the child intended to express. In general, the parents fit propositions to the child's utterances, however incomplete or distorted, and then reinforces if there is correspondence between the proposition and reality. The form of reinforcement needs not be a concrete item such as an M & M, but rather an intangible one such as a pat or a smile. The most important reinforcement to a child is achieving the item or recognition because the contingency was met.

If the child can achieve things as a result of talking, the use of speech is learned. A constant rule is that the child accomplishes things because he talked. He may get the scissors because he said, after the teacher's model, "I eed the issors." At another time, it might be paper, paste, milk, cookie, etc. Perhaps the adult is really reinforcing the *function* first, the *content* later and *finally* the correct *form*. So as he progresses, this behavior is shaped accordingly. However, the teacher must encourage whatever the child does correctly at the *time* he does it.

Just recently, a teacher was rewarding, and rightly so, a six-year old for saying, "Our seeds growed because we taked care of them." That child had a morphological rule of forming tenses under control. He had mastered the use of " — -ed" to signify the past tense. Since the concept of tense has been inductively learned, the teacher's task is smooth. That child had observed a language principle and as with hearing children, he, too, was testing his linguistic data. Of course, the teacher gave him the corrected model to imitate, but his attempts were warmly received. In fact, the corrected model was so well handled that the handling itself became motivation to try harder.

Imitations

The role of imitation in language learning has been a very controversial issue among linguists. There is considerable evidence that imitation may not play a very important role in the actual acquisition of syntax or vocabulary. It is generally thought to be more important in articulation development. However, the interaction between the teacher and child resembles the imitation mother and infant performed successfully in the early stages.

Using imitation as a strategy, the child may extract several things from the material given him to imitate. This strategy is especially effective with phonologic acquisition. Intonational patterns are available to the hearing-impaired child. Duration is especially important. As the child imitates, he matches his production to the teacher's time and in this way assimilates the timing of an utterance. Deaf speech tends to be five to six times slower than normal speech. Imitating an utterance in the same time envelope as the teacher's works to accomplish normal rate. Needless to say, just employing the speech organs in imitation gives the child practice not dissimilar to that of young hearing children. The involvement of the kinesthetic and auditory feedback systems has a value which eludes measurement.

The auditory discrimination task of imitating the teacher's sentence chosen from many sentences is readily apparent. Another dimension that seems valuable to language acquisition is that of auditory memory. To be able to imitate sentences which grow increasingly longer and then increase in number certainly must require memory for sequencing.

Imitating the teacher's model is an integral part of speech teaching. It is important for the hearing-impaired child to imitate both models and expansions. From his repetitions, he will get the kinesthetic-auditory feedback to help monitor the language-learning process and thus store structural principles.

These imitations seem to follow a fairly definite sequence. In the early stages of language development, particular emphasis is placed upon the child imitating the time envelope of the teacher's model. This provides the child with necessary articulation practice of vowels and consonants while giving appropriate duration to the phonemes. At first, the imitations resemble the jargon of the hearing child in that the correct intonation and timing are present even though the individual words may not be intelligible. Just any vocalization should not be accepted, but seek the closest approximations that he can make. Gradually, most of the vowels and many of the more visible consonants begin to appear appropriately. As this happens, the child's imitations more closely approximate the sentence patterns. More words and phrases become intelligible. The child should imitate as much of the adult's model as he is capable of producing. The imitations are often very similar to the child's original spontaneous utterances. Once the timing and intonation stages have been mastered, it may be helpful to break the sentences into smaller segments for closer phoneme approximation, but the timing, phrase structure, and intonation should keep their integrity. The sentence is always repeated in its entirety so that it can be stored as a whole thought.

While the observable values can be noted in phonologic growth, some vocabulary acquisition through imitation can be anticipated. When the child sees the situation, experiences the feeling for it and then receives the label, the chances of a label being retained are high. A measurable objective might be the time interval between presentation of new vocabulary in the language of an experience and its spontaneous use by the child.

Verbal stimulation

The young child who is in the early phases of language development is primarily involved in motoric interaction with the environment; the teacher must provide the stimulus for his verbal responses. Verbal stimulation takes place throughout the day. The important thing about this kind of interaction is that it is not just a monologue on the teacher's part, but there is teacher-child interaction which is based on a shared experience and thus has meaning for the children.

In the preschool, the experiences must be selected so that the children will *talk* as much as possible. Children who watch a moth come out of a cocoon, become excited and talk a great deal. Children who see chicks pecking out of their shells want to talk enthusiastically. When the kite gets caught in a tree after experiencing the thrill of getting it up in the air, there is a need to communicate. Here, then, are opportunities for the teacher to take the children's meager linguistic contributions, phrase them into sentences, and put them through the children's sensory receptors. When the children use the expanded language, they get auditory and kinesthetic feedback about something in which they are involved, something for which they comprehend the meaning.

Contrast such experiences with the less exciting, less live, less functional "News" of Johnny doing something (unknown to the class) with someone (unknown to the class) at a place (unknown to the class). Or for that matter, consider the "boredom" of mastering, "Suzie has on a blue dress," or "Jack has an apple in his lunch," or even, "It is rainy." Children are interested in their own experiences.

Fortunately, today the situation has changed. A few years ago in setting after setting, there was *sameness* regardless of location, makeup of class, amount of hearing of the children, age of hearing impairment onset, or use of hearing aids. At that time, there was a set curriculum used throughout the country. "Frozen" would be a more appropriate word than "set." The vocabulary was predetermined and a typical school day in the life of three- to seven-year olds across the nation went much the same way. When and if there was a speech period, pictures were brought out and drill began on "shoe," "fish," and "ball," or was it "ball," "fish," and "shoe"? The brief auditory training period was noisemakers and bells.

There was roll call, calendar work, weather, and news. The latter was written by the teacher, and the children were questioned about "Who," "What," and "What did you do?" There seemed to be a fetish to get *NEWS* from home to school and back to home. Some places even had cassette tape recorders that covered the same route. Other places had notebooks or the teacher had a chat with the person who delivered the child to school. The family and teacher were keeping current on gossip, but what did it mean to the child? No wonder deaf children had difficulty in language behavior when the input he was given was so very vicarious.

One example stands out in the memory of one of the authors. She was at a school where a teacher had had the misfortune that morning to run over a skunk. In no way was the teacher able to get rid of the odor. However, the children's news period consisted of:

Today is Wednesday.
Yesterday was Tuesday.
Tomorrow will be Thursday.
It is sunny.
Johnny bought some bubble gum.
Susie has new shoes.

No, not one word was about "smell," "odor," "skunk," etc. "The children weren't at that level," said the teacher!

Most of the activities with preschool children should be at the sensorimotor level. The older children are able to deal with more vicarious experiences, but not the young preschoolers. Whenever possible, the children need to be actively and physically involved in the activities. It is a "hands on" rather than a "hands off" approach which provides opportunities for the learner to use as many of his senses as possible. The children are able to see, feel, listen to, put together, take apart, or otherwise manipulate the materials, and often even eat the objects involved in a particular learning experience. These kinds of opportunities to explore help to demonstrate the meaning of the words and thus aid in comprehension. Verbal interaction takes place during the experience and appropriate language is processed for the children throughout the activity. The teacher calls the children's attention to the important elements by labeling them and emphasizing their attributes. It is extremely important that the teacher "tunes in" or "listens" to the children in order to foster their curiosity and create opportunities for expressiveness. Children need help to acquire the basic skills of learning which will later enable them to examine, analyze, observe, explore, describe, and organize their own experiences.

The language children are provided is very much in the *here and now*. It is not about other places or even *pictures* of other things. First-hand experiences are the avenues, labeled with sentences appropriate to the children's linguistic ages in number of units, but varied in structure.

If the deaf child starts out behind his hearing peers and is to catch up, he has to progress at a faster than normal rate. One is forced to recognize that time is against the deaf child, and one becomes impatient with any teacher who wastes precious minutes. The hearing-impaired four-year old happily making swiggles at the easel gives the impression that he will be four years old forever. But for the teacher to act as if this were true is disastrous! The "making swiggles" must be the topic of language input.

> John put on a shirt backwards.
> He painted with yellow finger paint.
> Then he used red paint.
> His swiggles looked funny.

Because he experienced the swiggling, John has the *meaning* base of the sentences. This then is real language, not artificial drill.

Expansion

In addition to providing the young child with verbal stimulation, the teacher expands the utterances the child has initiated as his spontaneous language begins to develop. His saying "truck" and gesturing broken, might be expanded to, "Yes, the truck is broken." If he says, "Bobby home," the teacher might respond with, "Bobby is going home." At a more advanced level, a child might say, "After we finish — see book?" and this could be expanded to, "After we finish, can I see the book?" The adult generally retains the child's word order and adds something to it to form a complete sentence. There are many possible expansions that a teacher might provide, and the decision among these is based on extralinguistic cues. Care must be taken not to provide incorrect expansions, especially in the early stages of language development. Nor should every telegraphic utterance be expanded. Parents of hearing children expand only about thirty percent of their children's utterances, perhaps this is all they understand well enough to expand correctly, but they select only about one out of three. The expanded sentence provides acceptance of the child's statement. It also provides the child with a correct model without the discouraging aspects of a direct correction. The child seems to understand that the teacher has understood him and is interested in what he wants to say. When the teacher reads the situation correctly, however, she notes the meaning a child has in mind and provides the proper linguistic form. The percentage of expansions demands sensitivity on the part of the adult.

It is important that the teacher be sensitive to what *the child* wants to say, *never* what the teacher wants to say. As the hearing-impaired child sees words attached to his meanings, he learns a little more about language and how to express *his* ideas.

To assure ourselves that the hearing-impaired child is getting the same information as a hearing child, we ask him to imitate the expansion. In this way, he gets auditory-kinesthetic feedback along with storage in his auditory/visual repository. Just as an example, "Tom hit Bill." The teacher witnessed this and observed Bill's anger mounting as he said something resembling, "No." At that moment, she *expanded* to, "Don't hit me," which Bill imitated. The reinforcer was immediate. Tom, the offender, didn't get attention and Bill got reinforced for imitating the teacher's expansion of *his* thought. It is a circular but meaningful strategy for both language and class behavior.

Modeling

Another strategy which plays a role in syntactic development is modeling. This is making relevant comments or statements about what the child says rather than improving on it, or expanding it. If the child says, "Doggie bark," the person who is expanding would probably say, "Yes, the dog is barking." Whereas, the person who is modeling might say, "It's because there's a cat in the tree." When a child said, "Jimmy wore a jacket to school," the teacher who was modeling said, "Maybe he thought it was cool this morning." A combination of expanding and modeling is used, particularly if the child's utterance is incorrect or a related idea is needed. Expansion limits the conversation to the child's own grammatical elements and ideas. Modeling introduces a greater variety of grammatical elements since it is closely connected with what the child has just said; both seem to play a role in language development.

When the language model is supplied him at the instant a child has the need, language is received and apparently imprinted. Furthermore, the language model must be put through his auditory-vocal system. He needs to derive the critical kinesthetic and auditory feedback considered essential to language learning.

A hearing-impaired child needs an environment which provides him maximum opportunities for exploiting his natural curiosity and fostering his spirit of inquiry. Vivid, vital, and pleasurable experiences are the easiest to remember. They should be selected by virtue of the child's need for learning the concepts and oriented toward daily experience. They may be appropriately contrived, spontaneous or incidental happenings (as the "skunk situation" should have been).

A relatively large proportion of learning time should be spent in modeling, as it were. The teacher formulates the sentences about the experience, about the "show and tell" items, about the storybooks. Importantly, the teacher doesn't stop with input but makes quite certain the child puts the language through his own auditory-vocal system. It is crucial, however, that the child has the concept within him and the language that is modeled for him fits the situation.

There is the great pitfall called "rubber-stamping." Do not model for the child that language for which he is capable of producing himself. If the child is spontaneously using, "I have a ball," give him "I have a big red ball." He needs to be processing language at a level *above* his production stage. The teacher should be continually providing him with language to be stored. He needs to be surrounded with the next level of language, and modeling is an effective strategy.

Provision for rule induction

Language development is characterized by generalizations made from limited input. The skill of generalization may be why language structure develops so fast. If the child waited for enough evidence to justify the generalizations he makes, he would never learn to talk. The tremendous generality of children's first grammar suggests the existence of such a phenomenon throughout language acquisition. Generalization appears early. What requires time and further experience is the modification of these generalizations. Tense endings on irregular verbs and plural endings on nouns such as *ox* or *sheep* are among the many instances that could be cited.

As the experiences are discussed, relived, and put into some permanent form whereby the children can see as well as hear the grammatical markings, rule learning begins. When the event is recalled later, the morphemes, functors, and labels have meaning because they describe a personal encounter. Sometime later, a similar but not identical experience can be shared. Some of the language used in the first experience can be repeated. The language will be familiar to the child though presented in a new, related context. In this way — with multiple experiences — the child can observe the rules implicit in the variety of language samples.

The concept of rule induction raises as many questions as it resolves. Very little is known about what particular events in the environment will help the most in facilitating rule induction. Teaching rules and/or principles, however, have been shown *not to help*. Possibly nothing is more helpful than a chance to practice conversation. Interaction through communication must be ongoing, both at school and at home.

Repeating the language employing the same principles with a certain degree of regularity provides practice. The language is then matched to the experience and to subsequent contrived or spontaneous experiences. When the child overgeneralizes, he receives reinforcement for having discovered the principle, but is then given the correct model very tactfully. For example, Mark, when learning "sunny" and "rainy" in relation to the class' experience, contributed that night was "moony." He was warmly reinforced. Under no circumstance should the improper grammar be corrected without giving understanding and attention to what the child is attempting to say. The process of generalization is a far greater achievement than any possible errors of over-generalization. The encouragement on the part of the teacher is a sensitive one.

Auditory practice

Practice is basic to learning language. While practice takes place in many settings — conversations, response to questions, recalling similar experiences — the critical practice is that related to the auditory perceptions a child develops.

Accompanying and following an experience, a written description is developed, e.g.:

> Jessica and Bobby picked up some snow.
> They brought it inside.
> The snow melted.
> Then we had dirty water.

The sentences are written because the hearing-impaired children may not hear the functors[5] or morphemes[6] but can see "something" in those spaces where they occur. The sentences then become the stimuli for listening experiences. The child is asked to repeat what he heard. This is auditory *training*, not testing, because the child knows the source of information. The stimulus must be familiar, and the child can see it, if necessary. He is then asked to repeat the sentence with appropriate phrasing, intonation, and time.

The length of the sentence may at one time be the unit of discrimination as in the above example. At another time, it may be as small as a word, e.g.:

> Mary washed the doll's *pajamas*.
> Penny washed the doll's *socks*.

Or it may be as large as equally long sentences which have differentiating phonemes[7], e.g.:

> Susie cut the gingerbread man.
> Brian put in the eyes and the nose.

Through imitation, the child stores the memory of syntactic

---

[5] Functors, structure words which have meaning only in context.
[6] Morpheme is a word, root or affix. The smallest meaningful unit of language.
[7] Distinct sound in speech, consonant, vowel or diphthong.

sequencing and use of words. He accumulates data whereby he, too, can induce the rules of the language code.

If the auditory perception has been too faulty, the child may always need assistance from watching the speaker's lips as well as listening. Audition is given priority, but the deaf child is not deprived of his use of vision when needed. The auditory stimulus however, must not be strange to the child. Auditory *training* must never be confused with auditory *testing*. Auditory training for the most part is developed with material the child has had practice imitating.

The purpose in repeating the sentences given through hearing alone is so that the child receives auditory feedback and can match his utterances with those the teacher gives him as a model. Through this auditory feedback system, the child can develop closer precision in speech, particularly as he learns the time-frame — the number of phonemes[8] per second — and the intonation patterns.

The "auditory-global" approach allows the child to attain important acoustic characteristics of spoken language. At the same time, he accumulates information about the probability of language rules including morphemes[9], structure words, and sentence formation. Thus, the child's mind is programmed to utilize the sounds of spoken communication received auditorily.

Activities

It is essential that teachers know *what* they want to teach and *why* they want to teach it before they begin to think of *how* to teach it. Once having established the "what" and "why", the teacher can then develop creative ways for the *how* of the process.

The *how* comes from the environment which provides maximum opportunities for the child to exploit his natural curiosity and foster his spirit of inquiry. The vivid, vital, and pleasurable experiences of a child are the easiest for him to remember. They are also the most meaningful. A preschool program needs to be oriented toward daily experiences, either contrived or spontaneous incidental happenings.

Materials required are often the type that the teacher can provide or make herself. The use of familiar objects is most effective in introducing a skill or a concept for the first time. As the

[8] See footnote 7, preceding page.
[9] See footnote 6, preceding page.

children become more knowledgeable about concepts, they can work with pictures and eventually abstract ideas.

Young children constantly explore the world around them. This exploration helps them gain concepts about the physical world. Satisfying their curiosity is essential for cognitive development and for their comprehension of order and relationships within their environment. While the activities of the younger children are at the sensorimotor level, they need also to be events and phenomena of the child's own environment. This means that the classroom needs areas for exploration, science, art, social studies, numbers, and cooking. However, the learning must not be confined to the enclosed room. Field trips and experiences throughout the school and outside of school can ensure that the children are actively and physically involved in activities that can be developed and expanded with language.

Language-learning is acquired and used in social contexts. Therefore, the program must use communicative language or conversational style of language at all times. The time for formal language can wait for readers and textbooks. In the preschool, children must acquire linguistic competence in basic semantic knowledge and code rules. Communicative competence involves general knowledge of how language use is affected by persons, places, situations, and events. In addition, of course, communicative competence includes knowledge of patterns of sequencing in conversation, forms of address, and standard verbal routines.

The class activities take many forms, such as:

> Language opportunities
> Experiences in science
> Exploring the arts
> Play
> Field trips
> Social Studies experiences
> Pre-math
> Story telling
> Picture description
> Songs
> Scrapbooks
> Snack time

Opportunities for language growth

These are experiences which provide maximum involvement by the children either through physical action or verbal response.

They are then combined to yield language behavior. These activities can range from making loop chains with colored construction paper to surprise boxes. They can include finger painting, scrapbooks, things dragged from home for object and picture description. The common outcome of all the typical preschool activities is that the child has an opportunity to acquire language related to *his thoughts* derived from *his experiences*.

Many children do not initiate communication easily. If left alone, they would probably be silent much of the day. The most important thing a teacher has to do is to get children talking and keep them interested in conversation exchanges. She needs to talk to the children while they are involved in activities. In this way, she can model for them the language for *their* thoughts. This language can later appear on sentence cards and charts for the constant repetitions children need to acquire the code.

Show and tell

The children can be encouraged to participate in this traditional preschool activity. They can bring in special things from home. Then they can be helped to share them with their peers. However, just because a child brings something to class and is excited about it, this is no sign that the other children will be interested. One day Billy came rushing in with his starfish which his grandfather sent him from Florida. It didn't interest the other children at all until the teacher drew from them:

> Mary Beth felt the starfish.
> It was rough.
> Jason counted the points of the starfish.
> Tim lifted the starfish.
> Billy said, "Don't drop it."

The next day, the teacher's task was easier because the Show and Tell included: "Vivian brought chocolate cupcakes for everyone."

Children at this age are ego-centered. They are interested in the language about themselves. It takes teacher talent to see that two or more children can get involved in the "Tell" part of Show and Tell:

> Jason pushed Jim's truck.
> Jim opened Beth's purse.
> Tim showed us his boxing gloves.
> Everyone held Penny's doll.

Communication is more than adult-child interaction. It moves to child-child and back to adult-child-child conversation and finally to conceptualization.

All the preschool activities recommended for hearing children must find their way into the early education classes for the hearing-impaired children. Not only must these children learn concepts of size and shape, "hard" and "soft", "light" and "dark", "hot" and "cold", but they must have them put into appropriate language at every opportunity.

Children can be asked to bring something (hard, big, to eat, etc.) and that material gets processed in the Show and Tell period:

> Jimmy brought something soft to school.
> Barbara guessed it was a kitten.
> Tom thought it was cotton.
> Esther asked if it was kleenex.
> Jimmy showed us marshmallows.
> Everyone had a marshmallow.

The basis of all language must be *concepts* which form the foundation for language growth. However, cognitive growth must be the primary purpose of preschool education. The secondary purpose, of course, is the language that clothes the concepts. Concepts need to be experienced over and over again in different areas of school. Concepts like "hot" and "cold" can be identified in the classroom with drinks of hot chocolate milk or cold lemonade. At playtime — whether it is too hot for a coat or too cold without one. Cooling — when things are cooked and then frozen. At Show and Tell when the popsicles melted. New and old concepts need to be incorporated into all parts of school's activities. Children need to be reminded of the concepts they learned earlier and similar experiences with some language differences need to be used. This is necessary as well as the use of similar language with different concepts.

The list of preschool concepts can be endless. It can include identifying and classifying foods; learning parts of the body, left and right side; learning shapes; learning size; learning "hard" and "soft"; "fast" and "slow"; "light" and "dark"; to mention just a very few. Language can help focus on the activities and in this way, the children can hear more language, connected language, and conversational language. In this way, children can receive sufficient data to apply "information theory".

Sentences from play can be repeated at Show and Tell, utilized in "experience stories", mentioned at "story telling", and occur in "experience stories" or charts. Sentences such as:

> Johnny used both hands to hold on. (body parts)
> Mary hopped on her right foot. (left and right, body parts)
> Peter sorted the red and white buttons quickly. (color differences)
> Martha used triangles for the Jack-O-Lantern. (shape)
> Bill couldn't bite the hard candy. (hard and soft)
> Susie bit the marshmallow. (hard and soft)

Experiences in science

The "experience" is a pre-planned activity. It is a hands-on rather than a hands-off activity. It provides opportunities for the child to learn through his senses as much as possible. The children should be able to see, feel, listen to, put together, take apart, or otherwise manipulate the materials, and even eat the objects that result such as Jello, orange juice, popcorn, and snow ice cream.

The purpose of providing experiences in science is to assist the child in gaining knowledge about the physical world, becoming aware of the properties of objects and basic "laws" such as gravity, and developing skills to understand the simple ideas upon which science is based. The teacher can help the children do things deliberately so that they may learn from the experiences. For example, she can show them how one thing happens because something else happened first. When they are given a push on the swing, a certain back and forth motion follows. If the child pumps, the movement is maintained. If he stops, the motion stops. If a child drops a block, it will fall to the floor. If he does it ten times, he can be certain that the block will fall to the floor every time. Other things are not so predictable. If he drops a ball, it will bounce back up fairly straight. If he drops a football, it may bounce straight up or to the side.

The children should be given experiences they may not completely understand but which will give them the basis for future knowledge. The principle of conservation — matter may change in form and composition, but continue to exist — is not an easy concept, but there are many examples of such transformations. The changing of water into ice is one example; the water is still there but in a different form. Another is the difference in reactions that take place when sugar is put into one glass of water and sand into another. The sugar seems to disappear but is still in the water, as the children can observe by tasting.

The teacher must work to distinguish between experiences which deal with objects and properties of the environment and those which deal with laws and principles which govern the operation of the physical world. It is one thing to help children learn about eggs and seeds, but another to help them grasp the concept of reproduction.

An example was one in which the teacher was concerned with burning, evaporation and freezing. She was also working on a number of language categories, morphemes[10], function words[11], pronouns[12] to name just a few. The two, language and science, are not mutually exclusive; the children were acquiring both as the stories about their experiences show.

> The popcorn burned.
> It got all black.
> No one would eat it then.

> Susie's mittens were all wet.
> She put them on the radiator.
> They dried very quickly.

> It is cold today.
> The water in the puddles froze.
> Tommy tried to skate on them.

The same class had other experiences such as burning toast, drying dishes, and freezing milk. Similar language was the goal, but the labeling, of course, was appropriate to each situation. Burning, evaporating, and freezing occurred in still other situations, again the language was similar.

One may ask, "Which comes first? The concept or the language?" Invariably, it should be the *concept*. It is the concept in the child's *mind* which needs to get clothed in language.

The urgency of the activity being at the child's interest level, and the concept to be developed, along with the goals of conversational language, is a difficult task for many teachers. They, too, often fall into the error of having the children learn about the properties of the objects, not the concepts.

10/Roots, affixes or inflected endings showing number or tense.
11/Words that indicate function or relationship between other words, i.e. prepositions or conjunctions.
12/A word used instead of a noun or noun phrase (personal [he], relative, demonstrative, [this]), definitive, reflexive or adjective [his dog] interogative [whose dog is the black one?].

Student teachers learning to teach the deaf are inclined to emphasize the language to the neglect of the concept. One student teacher planned a lesson in the fall on colors and size of leaves that had fallen to the ground. She planned an experience to the park to gather the leaves. The story she had planned was:

> We walked through the park
> Sally picked up a big red leaf.
> John found a yellow one.
> Some leaves were small.

The lesson plans passed inspection, and the student teacher was all prepared with the chart partially written or printed. On the morning of the planned lesson, it rained heavily. To compensate for the weather, the student teacher gathered wet leaves and put them near the door. As each child came forward, she held the umbrella as he or she picked out a leaf. The student teacher missed the point of the need of children for *reality*. Some things might be retrieved from the outside without getting wet, but not fall leaves! An alternative lesson might well have been on rain. Or it could have been about the children's feelings because they couldn't go on the trip. Or what would happen if they were to go. Even a fantasy trip could be substituted. Flexibility has to be a necessary characteristic for teachers.

Another student teacher wanted to teach the concept of sweeping with the associated language. Her plans indicated that she was going into a big auditorium which the children had never seen. The janitor would have brushed his sweepings into a pile, and the class would simply sweep them up. She completely missed the need for purpose and reality.

She tried again and this next time planned to enter the classroom covered with snow and dump it so the children would have to sweep it up. The concept of snow melting was only one of the many she didn't have. Eventually, the demonstration teacher took pity on her and began a craft activity. Scissors and paper punches were operated busily. When the activity was over, there was, indeed, cause to sweep. That experience story that resulted went as follows:

> We needed a book for our pictures.
> Jeff cut some red paper squares.
> Bill punched holes for the rings.
> Oops! Scraps of paper were all over the floor.
> Jennifer looked for the broom.
> Genny swept up the scraps of paper.

It is important that children have experiences that begin to lead them to new levels of understanding, even though these levels may not be reached until after they leave preschool level. Similarly, the sentence lengths and linguistic sophistication of the charts anticipate the level that the child will be *using* in a few months. If the child is comfortable with short sentences, the teacher should be lengthening sentences with phrases and modifiers, thereby laying the foundation for more advanced structure.

The essential feature of the entire learning process is ensuring that the child has and/or develops thoughts to which the message of the language applies. It is the matching of the language *form* to the *content* which the child must achieve and the teacher make happen.

The second feature of the process is the relation of each language event to other language events, and the child's ongoing store of knowledge which results. Different experiences employing similar language structures can help the child induce the applicable rules of the linguistic code. Similarly, when related experiences present varied language structures, the child can be led to the generalization of the underlying concepts.

The flexibility of experience planning allows the teacher to be able to take advantage of the child's ideas and input and incorporate them into her goals. Caring for gerbils or a bird may appeal to some children. A snail from the garden, a bird's nest some child may have found, some sea shells from a recent trip may provide opportunities for scientific information. Baking cookies, popping corn, or building a snowman can usually trigger interest in all children. Occasionally, it helps to select a theme such as "changes" whereby the teacher might make cinnamon toast and children observe how bread changes to toast, how leaves change, how a sponge changes when in water. Other themes might be "how things feel," "growing things," "air," or even, "the science table."

Exploring the arts

Some of the teacher's best times for teaching will be spontaneous. These times are when the child is totally involved. These can be activities which concern the affective areas of his life — the visual and tactile "arts," story telling, and play.

When compared with cognitively oriented tasks such as science, children's learning in the arts is more difficult to measure and specify. Because of the stress on teaching formal skills, and because goals in such activities as painting, working with play dough, and dancing are not easily articulated and measured, the arts are often relegated to a position of relative unimportance. However, the teacher can have certain objectives in mind as a natural part of the total day. The teacher may want to let one of the children pound the play dough as hard as he can to work off some of his angry feelings; another time, she may use the play dough to teach conservation of quantity. Whatever the activity, the children are provided another opportunity to have language.

> Miss Smith helped us make play dough.
> Doug put in some salt.
> Tom added the flour.
> Susie poured in just a little water.
> Everybody rolled the dough.

Or another time:

> Peter wanted to play with the play dough.
> Susie wanted to use the big crayons.
> Dick decided to help Peter.
> They punched, poked, and squeezed the dough.
> Jane thought they made a puppy.
> No one wanted to stop.

The preschooler may be at the cognitive age at which he recognizes shapes and figures that seem to represent things in their clay modeling, or finger painting. However, let him identify his work. Teachers should not try to read the child's product.

A favorable form of art many children like is collages. These lend themselves very well to language. If the assignment is to leaf through catalogs and find pictures of "shoes," the collage could contain pictures of shoes which have "tops and bottoms" or "buckles, ties, or no clasps at all." There could be pictures of "party shoes, school shoes, play shoes, and gym shoes." There could be "high heels, low heels, and rubber heels." The language can be about the cutting and pasting and whose pictures were used.

Artistic activities which range from painting to mosaics made with egg shells should dot the school week. There can be mural painting as a group activity in which each child is responsible for his own square which he can take home. The activities can include chalk drawings, cutting and pasting, or other uses of art materials. Teachers need to keep in mind, however, that the arts should be child-oriented and deal with the processes, not the products. It is the *process* that needs labeling. Language such as follows needs to be learned:

> Everyone put on a smock.
> It was an old shirt.
> We put it on backwards.
> Mary got paint all over her smock.
> Jim made the blue and green paint go together.
> Lisa spilled the red paint.
> Miss Smith used a sponge and a towel to clean up.

Some people believe that scribbling and drawing experiences are essentially cognitive experiences for the child. They believe that they are an expression of his mental maturity. By just playing around with crayons and paper, paints, clay, or wood, the child is giving expression to his ideas, he is representing his concepts in a concrete, yet creative, manner. Though the activities are their own reward, the child needs the tools to discuss these experiences. Language, then, becomes a necessary goal, not the work of art.

Play and games

Play can take many forms. It can be spontaneous or planned, individual or group, quiet or active. Play should increase the children's time to talk to one another. While it is called "free" play, the teacher has an important role. She still models language for their thoughts and experiences during play.

Outdoor play should be a part of the children's day. Terms like "Help me," "Push me," "Watch me," and "Let me — — ," become necessary conversational language. Here, too, is a good opportunity to model or teach:

About the swing:
> Shana is swinging now.
> Eric can have the swing next.
> Shana is swinging up high.
> Jimmy got off the swing.

About the slide or jungle gym:
> Rodney is climbing up.
> Molly slid down.
> Tracy climbed up and jumped down.
> Susie climbed up and Miss Smith helped her down.

About the sand box:
> Mary's bucket is full.
> Tom is filling his bucket with sand.
> Lisa liked to run the sand through her fingers.

Games requiring imitation and verbal accompaniment can direct energy and also provide an opportunity for language practice. While the purpose of some games is to gain control of gross body movements, they lead to control of the finer movements of muscles necessary in speech and writing. They can, as do all activities, set the stage for language use. Play provides the child the means for practicing and consolidating a great deal of what he knows.

Preschool manuals are full of games which have language directives such as "Put your little foot in. Put your little foot out," or, "Everybody do this just like me!" There are games two-year olds like, games for three-year olds, and for the four- and five-year olds; games which range from "Ring Around the Rosy" to "In a Spider's Web."

There are numerous finger games that use language and rhymes to be acted out. Repetition of the language leads to the children saying the rhymes and directives without the teacher's model. "What was the most fun?" "Did you have fun?" can be part of a discussion about their favorite activity at the quieting down period following such games and finger play.

Guessing games, where the child has to ask the teacher questions about what is hidden in a bag, is not only fun but provides necessary language practice. This beginning of "Twenty Questions," i.e., "Is it something to eat?" "Is it round?" "Is it hard?" leads to the cognitive experience of categorization in addition to question development.

This variety of games, games or curiosity expansion provides, as does everything a teacher does, opportunities for a child to practice his developing language skills. The play of the child is of utmost educational value. Young children require freedom and time to play, indoor and outdoor space to play in, things to play with, and an adult to give them the necessary language at the moment it is needed.

Field trips

The teacher plans for a field trip in much the same way she plans for a language or concept-building experience. She analyzes the cognitive and linguistic needs of the children and decides if a given trip is appropriate and would enhance this development. A trip to the children's zoo might be in order, but one to a horse stable could be inappropriate. A trip to the riverfront would be of little value, but one to the fire station could be good for social studies and would be within a young child's range of interest.

In preparation for the Halloween party, a trip to the pumpkin farm is always fun, and even more so if parents repeat it later. Because of its previous experience, the children would have enough language that both parents and children would enjoy it and be able to talk about it. The teacher needs to "preview" the site of the field trip and see what specific items exist. Then she needs to plan what language can be used. Such a story might be planned:

> Our class went to Miss Brown's farm.
> There were hundreds of pumpkins there.
> Beth picked out a big one.
> Bob liked the long skinny one.
> Brian and Matt carried our big one to the car.
> Lisa dropped her pumpkin.
> What a mess!

An added value in taking the learning beyond the classroom is that children learn that everything can be the source of learning. Furthermore, the children have opportunities to interact with strangers yet have the teacher nearby to model the appropriate responses.

Social studies experiences

A study of the geography aspect of social studies cannot take place entirely within the confines of the school. The children must be able to go on those field trips to experience their larger world. Trips to the shopping centers to see the kinds of stores there, to the grocery store to see the departments, to the teacher's home to see that the teacher lives there, not at school. Well-planned, carefully selected field trips give children real experiences with the wider world, geographical concepts, and appropriate language.

A field trip to the nearest gas station acquaints the child with the smells of oil, tires, and gasoline. And the men at the station do so many interesting things to cars with machines, pumps, lifts, and tools. Other places of interest might be the shoe repair shop, television repair shop, bakeries, laundromats, beauty parlors, hamburger stands, paint stores, Post Office, police station, and library, all of which expose children to concepts needed to understand community life. One class' outstanding field trip was to and through a car wash. Essentially, the teacher was only extending the meaning of "wash," but the learnings far exceeded the limited concept of "wash."

Social studies' trips lend themselves very well to the type of language five- and six-year olds will be meeting in the social studies textbooks as well as science books. These trips can offer opportunities to make the bridge between conversational style and the written style of language. For example, a first-grade text had a story something like:

>Long, long ago, the Earth was different.
>It was very warm.
>There were big swamps.
>There were big forests of strange trees.
>Strange animals lived on the land.
>Some lived in the swamps.

In preparation for that language — expletives, predicate adjectives, functors, indefinite pronouns, and others — a teacher prepared a story about a field trip. The concept she was working on was communities. The language was from the textbook the class was to use the next semester.

Neighborhood Shops

We rode in Miss Smith's car to Forest Avenue.
There were many stores there.
The first shop was a candle shop.
There were many candles there.
There were big fat ones and long skinny ones.
The next shop was a candy shop.
The lady in the candy shop gave us some candy *free*.
The last store we visited was a flower shop.
There were lots of flowers there.
There were roses, carnations, and lillies of the valley.

As the children outgrow the ego-centered stage, there is less need to put their names and their particular activity in the chart. However, until they themselves are using sophisticated language, the language that is presented should be based on experiences. Furthermore, it should be used during the experience. The teacher must model it at the time it occurs. For example, "short, fat" and "long, skinny" were used while in the candle shop. Similarly, the phrase modifying a noun, i.e., "The lady, in the candy shop."

Well-planned, appropriate trips clothed in language can assist the child in both cognitive learning and language use.

Pre-math

Mathematical concepts can be incorporated into every area of the preschool program. The young child learns concepts underlying mathematical operations in many of his daily activities: one-to-one relations occur daily at snack time as in: One cup for Matt, one napkin for Susie, etc.; at play: one trike for Jim, one for Jennifer; at art, at science, and even in the play time: one car for . . .

Numbers are all around. It is *nine* o'clock; *three* children can go to the table; *two* cups of flour are needed; there are *two* children on the slide.

In cooking activities, the children learn sequence and how quantities are related:

Mary put the flour in *first*.
Next, Jane put the sugar in the bowl.
Tom added the baking powder *last*.

Many opportunities to present mathematical concepts are present in both outdoor and indoor play. The smooth stones a child gathers, the acorns he collects, the sticks or cups he needs, the number of children waiting to ride the new bike, all offer meaningful experiences with numbers classification. Basics to future mathematical concepts can be begun when the seeds, acorns, leaves, little cars, stones are sorted, then counted.

Sorting and classifying can be used to assist in the child's learning or recognizing particular attributes. The adult should not guide the children as they sort their materials; whatever classification a child decides on should be accepted. As the children reach the stage where aimless exploration has passed, the teacher may ask why a collection of nuts, bolts, toys, marbles, etc., were sorted in a particular way.

Meaningful counting, rather than rote counting, is imperative. The child must be aware of the fact that he is pairing the term "one" with the first object he is counting. Then groups of two objects are labeled with the term "two." One must caution that numbers be written as words until the child has had sufficient experience to know the meaning of "three," "two," "five," "four," and "one." Numbers are double abstractions and as such must be taught in stages. "Three" represents a quantity of threeness — three balls, three blocks, three cookies, etc. Then the figure 3 represents or stands for the *word* "three." Far, far too often, deaf children get pushed into figures not having had an opportunity to "experience" their meaning. The child must have logical understanding of number concepts rather than rote memory of terminology.

The understanding of mathematical concepts begins and ends

with language. That language provides young children with necessary terms and symbols to communicate and label their experiences. For example, the children will need terms such as:

some	alike	join
a few	as many as	pair
a lot	different	collection
greater than	less than	the same as

They will need comparatives:

big	bigger	biggest
few	fewer	fewest, etc.

Function words of position:

above, below	in front of	up, down
before, after	in back of	here, there, etc.

Terms of weight, speed, linear measure, temperature, and time all are necessary for mathematical understanding. Therefore, the teacher should plan activities to include experiences using that language.

> Jason's kite flew faster than Tod's.
> There were big, round candles and tall, thin ones.
> Shana found more acorns than Susie.
> Tom sat in front of James on the bus.

Story telling

Story telling is a valuable time to extend the children's thinking beyond the "here and now," and to increase their attention span. Books need to be chosen for each class because children vary from year to year. Their interests, their level of comprehension, and their language ability should guide the selection of books for a particular group of children.

Books that relate to what the children are doing in the classroom or the kinds of things that happen in their homes are good to use at the beginning. For those children who are not ready to attend to stories with a great deal of language, picture books may be more appropriate. Teacher or parent awareness of each child's developmental level will dictate the selections to be used.

Children enjoy repeating words and sentences in unison when the story has a refrain. If the book has a simple plot, the children might be asked to tell what happened first, second, and third. Or they might predict what could happen next. Their efforts are to be rewarded through the language. The teacher will probably have to model it for the chidren at first, but eventually they will be able to take turns retelling the story.

Often, children like to act out stories. This gives the teacher another opportunity to model. Discussion of the characters gives opportunities to use the language immediately. Relating the story to themselves helps also. Anticipating "What happens next?" sets up a need for particular language. However, the story telling must always be a pleasurable experience. During story telling many special activities can be used with a book to utilize language. Children can pretend to be one of the characters in the story. They can repeat certain routines that the characters said, i.e.: "I'll huff and I'll puff and I'll blow your house down." The stories of *Three Bears, Three Little Pigs,* and *Three Billy Goats Gruff* are ageless classics, but trips to the library can add current childhood literature.

It is well to have a selection of books available because children should be given opportunities to choose which book they want read or to retell. If the book is new, they need to be told something about it before it is read. Needless to say, the teacher knows the stories so well from her preparation that she can tell them without looking at the pages. Therefore, the book can face the children. This, of course, provides the children the opportunity to relate the language of the teacher with the pictured concepts available to them.

The creativity of the teacher is unlimited in the area of story telling. Books are fun; they expand concepts; they increase language; they provide a basis for vicarious language growth. Most of all, they lay the groundwork for the love of reading so basic to the intellectual growth of every child.

Picture description

Related to story telling from books is story telling from pictures. Pictures of interest to a young child can be discussed. For example, a picture of two barefoot boys fishing by a river on a summer day can lead to such questions as:

> What time of the year is it?
> How do you know?
> Did they go to school?

The teacher can encourage descriptions of the details of the picture by asking other appropriate questions as she shows the pictures. She can also encourage speculation on the child's part about what has happened and what might happen in the "story."

Children can arrange the pictures in sequence if there are several. They can identify the pictures through listening and looking and through listening alone. They can act out the story, draw pictures of the story, or do any of the other activities children enjoy.

Songs

Similar to story telling and picture description is music. The songs should be simple, meaningful, and involve a great deal of body action. Children enjoy repetition of all kinds and will "sing" the same things over and over again.

Choices of songs can relate to other areas of learning, e.g., storytime, Show and Tell, etc., or they can, and probably should, be songs sung by all preschool children. The universality of music helps hearing-impaired children experience a sense of belonging.

Scrapbooks

Some children are not ready to listen to stories; for them scrapbooks might be more appropriate. The earliest picture scrapbooks should contain realistic pictures of familiar objects that the children will want to talk about. It could contain pictures of the child; the child's parents and other family members; his favorite toys and animals; favorite foods; and activities. Needless to say, each child would have to have his own personal book.

Another scrapbook might center on the child's activities of helping in the kitchen, picnicking, going to the store, etc. Or it might be of the child's daily activities, e.g., sleeping, taking a bath, brushing his teeth, etc.

Scrapbooks are a valuable device for teaching language as they are motivators for stimulating talking due to the fact that young children are ego-centered and like to tell about *their* world.

Snack time

"Snack time" is another ideal time for language learning. The child is willing to cooperate to get what he desires. He learns that there is a relation between his need and his vocalization. The goal may be to get a cookie; the vocalization will be "cookie" or, "I want a cookie." The goal can change from "milk" to "more milk" to "I want more milk" to "Please pour me some milk" or "No" to "I don't want any milk" or "All gone" to "The milk is all gone" to "There's no more milk."

Each snack time the class uses cups, napkins, cookies or another treat, and milk. A child can be told to "Go get the cups;" the next day, "Find the napkins in the closet;" "Get the milk on the window sill;" and still another time: "Bring the cups." The reward of accomplishment and/or eating make it all worthwhile to the child.

During snack time the child can learn about questions, too.

> What kind of cookie?
> How many cookies?
> Where is your napkin?
> Do you want more?
> Is that enough?

Snack time also is a good period to learn verbs such as:

get	spill	smell
pass	want	feel
pour	need	like
stir	taste	have

The list of learning activities for young children is endless as evidenced by any preschool textbook or guide. Any of these experiences can become a language exercise or simply a routine drill activity. They become a justifiable contribution to the total preschool program *only* when the teacher utilizes the activity for concept growth and language development. When she directs the activity with the knowledge of how language is acquired as a functional communication system, the children will acquire linguistic competence and expanded conceptual growth.

Techniques

Techniques are devices that teachers can use to help the children receive enough language data so that they may induce the rules of their language. The experiences whereby this is done can be productive and enjoyable. Just as with the very beginning stages, the emphasis is on the positive and none of the activities should ever appear to be drills.

The aim of the "auditory-global" approach is to equip the hearing-impaired child with spoken language which functions for him. In order that the deaf child will be able to predict, just as efficiently as a hearing person, what sounds, words, phrases, patterns, and sentences follow each other, he needs practice — *he must have* much listening practice. He must hear more speech. He must hear more continuous and conversational language. He needs to acquire the statistical knowledge that the hearing child uses when he is exposed to and understands the speech around him.

The deaf child is not learning merely to speak or to understand words, or to build up a stock of words. He is learning a whole mode of linguistic behavior. At first, his learning is very global. The child does not differentiate *form* from *content* from *function*.

Content is relevant with young children when it is related to experiences. The child, as a receiver of language and as a sender, uses form only as a garment to clothe his thoughts. The topic, the content, is his concern, not the form. The primary function of speech is communication, social contact. After adequate exposure to language using the strategies delineated in this chapter, the social speech of the child is divided into egocentric and communicative. Language eventually is used to communicate meaning: to express feelings or disguise them; to state intentions or merely to intimate their nature; to influence or control the discussion of others; to assist memory and facilitate thought.

The task of the preschool is to start the child on his way to being a learner and a participant in society. Strategies have been given, activities described, but some techniques might be helpful. Three that have proved helpful are: 1) Charts; 2) sentence cards; and 3) auditory cards.

Charts

Most charts are based upon the experiences the children have had and furnish the children with functional reference material. They are written by the teacher with "assistance" from the children. They are printed in manuscript as is all writing in the preschool. Chart-size paper should be strong in order to sustain much handling as the children turn the pages frequently. The language is always conversational, not formal style. The charts will be brief at first, but soon grow, as does the children's skills, to as many sentences as can be presented on the sheet, possibly eight or ten or more.

Pictures, either sketched or pasted on the chart, will help the children recall quickly which incident is being described. These charts are in the classroom, each new one on top of the others, creating a progressive display of the children's experiences written in language they learn to comprehend.

The early charts are a sequence of related events and contain the names of the child who experienced the item addressed:

We had a parade.
Alice carried a flag.
Jim beat the drum.

As the child matures in language, the charts can grow longer.

We watched a parade downtown.
Tom liked the clowns.
Jeff saluted the flag.
Mary dropped her popcorn.
Oh, too bad!

They can also grow to more involved, complex language:

The fall parade was on Saturday.
We went to see it with Miss Brown.
There were many people there.
Mary and Jim counted the floats.
Everyone shook hands with the clown.
Many clowns climbed out of a little car in front of us.
It was fun to clap in time with the bands.
Boom! Boom! Boom!

The language that is used is what would be most naturally spoken. The language of the charts is always *global* because how else would the children learn the structure or function words? How else would the children get the information to induce the predictable component of language? In the global form, children receive all of the phonologic[13], morphological[14], functors[15], semantics[16], and syntax[17] information based upon *their* experience. Since children move from meaning to language, the experience story is meaningful and easy for the child to learn.

The task after the chart is prepared is to provide listening practice and enable the children to accumulate linguistic statistical data necessary for induction of language rules. The teacher needs always to work toward the goal of providing the hearing-impaired child sufficient information to apply "Information Theory" in the same way as do hearing five-year-old children.

The charts are a rich source for developing auditory skills. The teacher selects a sentence; the child identifies it and repeats it. A word of caution is very necessary here. Many teachers fall

---

[13] Related to sounds.
[14] Relating to structure of words, roots, affixes, inflected endings etc.
[15] Like function words, indicating function or relation between other words i.e. prepositions and conjunctions.
[16] Meanings of words.
[17] The arrangement and interrelationship of words in phrases and sentences.

into a sing-song habit. This must not be done! The phonologic factors — intonation, prosody, rhythm, and time — are important auditory signals the child must learn. Any unnatural recitation of the sentence distorts the auditory message. The sentences on the chart should be conversational in style and must be "globally" correct (correct as a whole). The imitations required of the child are then complete in all aspects. It is wise to have a variety in length and intonation pattern. This makes the auditory task easy for the child because he can get short versus long, as well as strong versus weak emphasis from the chart story.

The auditory and/or lipreading of the sentences is meaningless for the child who was absent the day of the activity. Those children who participated in the activity and/or were part of the involved group understand the ideas on which the language is based.

Sentence cards

Sentence cards grow out of an experience, contrived or spontaneous. They can come from play, stories, Show and Tell, snack time, e.g.:

Jeff was the leader of the farm game.

Peter told the story of Mr. Bear.

Susie's little doll was sitting on a sled.

Jane brought cupcakes for everyone to eat.

The event should be depicted the way it really happened. These cards can also be used for auditory discrimination, speech practice, and memory storage. The greater the number of sentences the child can store and identify and then tell another person, the greater is his auditory memory.

What role auditory memory plays in speech development is not completely established. However, it is known that children, who can retain the memory of six or seven sentences developed around an experience, do become the more fluent communicators.

It must be remembered that sentence cards are not to teach the children to read, but rather to let them see the printed form of the parts of language which they do not hear, i.e., structure words. Sentence cards serve as a target of what was said and how it was said. This provides models for the child to imitate. To him all such activities must be "like a game" *never* a stilted meaningless drill.

Questions

Questioning is one of the most effective ways to develop children's thinking processes and it cannot be begun too early. Too often teachers use questions only for concrete answers, but these only help recall facts and details. They should move on to probing for sequence and causality. They need questions for drawing inferences, noting contingencies, predicting outcomes, seeing relationships and making judgements.

A perusal of the teacher's manual of any readiness book shows the vast number of questions put to five- and six-year olds. These need to be asked by parents before children enter preschool and thereafter by the teacher. A teacher's manual of Scott, Foresman Company at preprimary grade level yielded such questions as:

What did —— do?

What did —— do next?

What does Tom think —— is?

How do you think —— felt when his bear wasn't on the table?

What did —— want at the beginning of the story?

What might the boys be saying?

How do you think —— found the bear?

How many circles will you make?

How many circles will be little ones?

How many will be big?

What is the middle-size circle for?

What do you do when you are finished?

What happened first?

What happened next?

What happened last?

How do you think Ken could keep the frog inside the aquarium when he gives the frog clean water?

How did Beth catch the frog?

How does —— try to catch the frog?

Did —— help —— make wheat bread?

What did —— answer?

Summary

The basic assumption in the program we have described is that each child reconstructs knowledge through interaction with his social and physical environment. He progresses through stages of development in which his thought-processing qualitatively changes. Therefore, the content of the preschool program must be derived from an understanding of the way children develop and the kinds of experiences which interest each child.

Learning at the preschool level must be active rather than reactive. Through "hands on" opportunities, a child can construct knowledge and seek out information. It is essential, therefore, that the opportunities are *MEANINGFUL* and first-hand. They must challenge the child's developing thought processes, yet not overwhelm him with material beyond his stage of development. The behaviors which the teacher must seek must be those that are essential for the child to develop optimally and function successfully in society.

Part I
References

Abraham, Suzanne, Stoker, Richard, et al. (1988). "Speech Assessment of Hearing-Impaired Children and Youth: Patterns of Test Use." *Language, Speech and Hearing: Services in Schools, 19, 1, 17-27.*

Anderson, Barbara J. (1979). "Parent's Strategies for Achieving Conversational Interactions." in Simmons-Martin & Calvert: *Parent-Infant Intervention: Communication Disorders,* New York: Grune & Stratton.

Bailey, D.B., and Simeonsson, R.J. (1988). *Family Assessment in Early Intervention.* Columbus, OH: Merrill.

Bettelheim, Bruno. (1987). *A Good Enough Parent.* New York: Vintage Books (Random House).

Brazelton, T. Berry. (1987). *What Every Baby Knows.* Addison Wesley.

Bromwick, R. (1981). *Working with Parents and Infants: An Interactional Approach.* Baltimore: University Park Press.

Bronfenbrenner, U. (1974). "Is Early Intervention Effective?" *A Report on Longitudinal Evaluation of Preschool Programs. 2,* Washington, D.C.: Department of Health, Education and Welfare.

Bronfenbrenner, U. (1976). "The Experimental Ecology of Education." *Education Researcher,* May 15, 1976.

Bullowa, M. (1964). "The Acquisition of A Word." *Language and Speech, 6,* (April-June, 1964).

Council on Education of the Deaf, (1975). *Requirements in Teacher Education.* Washington, D.C.: Gallaudet College.

Church, Joseph. (1973). *Understanding Your Child From Birth to Three: A Guide to Your Child's Psychological Development.* New York: Random House.

Clarke-Stewart, A.K. (1973). "Interactions Between Mothers and Their Young Children: Characteristics and Consequences."

Monograph of Society for Research in Child Development. Serial No. 153, **38**, 6-7.

Crystal, David. (1986). *Listen to Your Child, A Parent's Guide to Children's Language.* New York: Penguin Books.

Davis, H. and Silverman, S.R. (1970). *Hearing and Deafness.* New York: Holt, Rinehart, and Winston.

Denes, Peter and Pinson, E.N. (1968). *The Speech Chain.* Murray Hill, NJ: Bell Telephone Laboratories.

Dodson, Fitzhugh. (1970). *How to Parent.* New York: Signet.

Federal Commission on Education. (1988). *Toward Equality— Education of the Deaf Report.* Washington, D.C.: U.S. Government Printing Office.

Gesell, A.L. (1940). *First Five Years of Life.* New York: Harper.

Ginott, A. (1965). *Between Parent and Child: New Solutions to Old Problems.* New York: MacMillan.

Greenstein, Jules M., et al. (1976). *Mother-Infant Communication and Language Acquisition in Deaf Infants.* New York: Lexington School for the Deaf.

Heider, F.K. and Grace M. (1940). "A Comparison of Sentence Structures of Deaf and Hearing Children." *Psychology Monograph. 52, #1 (Whole No. 232).*

Jacoby, Susan. (1988). "Roots of Success Survey." *Family Circle 101, 5* Matoon, IL: Family Circle Inc., a subsidary of the New York Times.

Klinman, Debra and Kohl, Rhiana. (1984). *Fatherhood U.S.A.* New York: Garland Publishing Co.

Koltosova, N.M. (1962). "The Formation of Higher Nervous Activity of the Child." *Psychology Review,* 69, 344-354.

Ling, D. and A. (1978). *Aural Rehabilitation.* Washington, D.C.: A. G. Bell Association.

Maxwell, Barbara. (1988). "Parents as Teachers." *School and Community,* Fall, (36), 10-13.

Pines, M. (1969). "Why Some Three-Year Olds Get A's and Some Get C's." *New York Times Magazine,* July 9, 1969.

Rhodes, M.J. (1972). "From A Parent's Point of View." *The Deaf American.*

Schaefer, E.S. (1972). "Parents as Educators: Evidence from Cross-Sectional Longitudinal and Intervention Research." *Young Children,* 27, 227-239.

Silverman, S. Richard, translator, (1982) **Urbantschitsch, Victor.** *Auditory Training for Deaf Mutism and Acquired Deafness—1895.* Washington, D.C.: A. G. Bell Association.

Simmons-Martin, A. (1976). *A Demonstration Home Approach with*

Hearing-Impaired Children, Professional Approach—Parents of Handicapped Children, ed. Eliz. Webster. Springfield, IL: Charles C Thomas.

Simmons-Martin, A. (1971). "Are We Raising Our Children Orally?" *Volta Review*, Vol. 73, 7, Washington, D.C.: A. G. Bell Association for the Deaf.

Simmons-Martin, A. (1978). "Early Management Procedures for the Hearing-Impaired Child." *Pediatric Audiology*, ed. Frederick Martin. Englewood Cliffs, N.J.: Prentice Hall.

Simmons-Martin, A. (1972). "Facilitating Positive Parent-Child Interaction." *Parent Programs in Child Development Centers: First Chance for Children*. Vol. I, ed. Dave L. Lillie. Chapel Hill: TADS.

Simmons, A. (1949). "Language Problems in Teaching Arithmetic: Multiple Meanings." *Proceedings of Auralism and Oralism*, St. Louis, MO: Larenscop.

Simmons-Martin, A. (1972). "The Oral/Aural Procedure: Theoretical Basis and Rationale." *Volta Review*. Vol. 74, 9. Washington, D.C.: A. G. Bell Association for the Deaf.

Simmons-Martin, A. (1983). "Salient Features of Parent-Infant Programs." *American Annals of the Deaf*, Spring. Washington, D.C.: CEASD and CAID.

Simmons-Martin, A. (1965). "A Student Teacher Learns," *Proceedings of the Convention of American Instructors of the Deaf. Supplement American Annals of the Deaf*. Washington, D.C.: Congress of American Instructors for the Deaf and Convention of Educational Administrators Serving the Deaf.

Simmons, A. A. (1975). "Written and Spoken Language of Deaf and Hearing Children", *Proceedings XIII Congress of International Society of Logopedics and Phoniatry*, I pp. 234-235.

Simmons-Martin, A. and Calvert, D.R. (Eds.) (1979). *Parent-Infant Intervention Communication Disorders*. New York: Grune and Stratton.

Spock, B. (1976). *Baby and Child Care*. New York: Pocketbooks.

Westerhouse, Joni. (1988). "Deaf Education Debate: Signing vs. The Spoken Word." *Medical Record*. Vol. 12, #34. St. Louis, MO: Washington University.

Whetnall, E. and Fry, D.B. (1964). *The Deaf Child*. Springfield, Il: Charles C Thomas.

White, B.L. (1975) *The First Three Years of Life*. New York: Avon.

White, B.L., et al. (1973). *Experience and Environment: Major Influences on the Development of the Young Child*. Englewood Cliffs, N.J.: Prentice Hall.

White, B.L., et al. (1978). "Competence and Experience." in

Uzgiris, I.C. and Weizman (Eds.) *The Structuring of Experience*. New York: Plenum Press.

    Winter, Mildred. (1988). "Parents as First Teachers." *Principal*, *64*, 5 22-24.

PART II
IMPLEMENTATION

Introduction to Part II

Part I of this book presents ideas, suggestions, and methods for establishing a successful program for parent intervention. It is based on the premise that highly trained, skilled, and knowledgeable people are essential in an effective program. Staff competence must have top priority. However, in order to clarify to some degree the objectives we proposed in the earlier section, we have prepared the material in Part II.

As we said in the Preface, the basic idea behind this book is that the most crucial period for language development for a child learning the "mother tongue" is in the early years, even early months. Naturally, the most important teachers are the people who are constantly in the child's environment. This is particularly true if the child is hearing impaired and his language age therefore is not equal to his chronological age.

Parents need a partner who can guide and support them. During the period when the child's language is at the infancy and toddler level, parents need a coach, an implementer or an intervener who will teach *them*. The teacher's role will shift as the child acquires language, but at the onset the teacher *teaches parents*. This is a role quite different from teaching children, as we discussed earlier in the text.

Since we feel strongly that the task of teaching parents differs so greatly from that of teaching in the classroom, we decided to treat it in greater detail in this section. Unlike the traditional approach where parents were told to help the child acquire words, we see language as a much more complex and multi-step process than word-calling. We perceive many levels of parent-child interaction as needed for the foundations of language development.

We have delineated twelve areas needing attention in order for language even to begin to develop. Each of these areas has multiple objectives which could be measured. Rather than have the reader referring back to the chapters within the text where the objectives with the rationale are described, we have condensed them

201

in this section and indicated the pages where they are discussed within each area.

To illustrate how we visualize achieving the objectives, we present a two-column chart. One side describes procedures a teacher *might* use and suggest to parents. The other side tells how the parents could carry out their role with their child in their own environment. These are not "set in concrete" but are ways we have found to get the hearing-impaired child developing competency in language.

At no time do we feel this book is a manual nor is it a cookbook. Rather the ideas and suggestions are only given as examples of the many possibilities for helping parents achieve the objectives. Neither do we consider these ideas to be curriculum. By now, the readers know that our idea of *curriculum* is fluid. It is not something carved in stone for each and every family.

We, purposely, have not sequenced the ideas and suggestions in precise order. Each child and each family unit is *UNIQUE*. Not every activity or recommendation is appropriate for every family nor for every child. The teacher's knowledge of the parent and the child plus her own unique personality, will determine the usefulness of each suggestion. The ones given here are to serve only as stimulii for procedures to implement objectives. We hope these ideas will help orient teaching staff and parents to some techniques whereby the hearing-impaired child learns through meaningful interaction with his parents and teachers.

Some possible objectives that might be considered at this stage are:

- For the parent to be aware of growth and development of other children the same age as her child. **205**
- For the parent to provide appropriate playthings for the child's age. **206**
- For the parent to see that the child is wearing his hearing aid(s) during all his waking hours. **207**
- For the parent to respond promptly to the child's distress calls. **209**
- For the parent to interact with the child. **210**
- For the parent to bring the child to the room or the place where she is working. **212**
- For the parent to watch the child even when otherwise engaged. **213**
- For the parent to anticipate the child's interest. **214**
- For the parent's talk to match the child's thoughts. **215**
- For the parent to respond to the child's gazes, smiles, sounds and gestures. **217**
- For the parent to make frequent eye contact with the child. **219**
- For the parent to smile frequently at the child. **221**
- For the parent to return the child's smile. **222**
- For the parent to frequently demonstrate affection. **223**
- For the parent to use "love talk". **224**
- For the parent to display pleasure in interaction activities. **225**
- For the parent to set limits. **227**
- For the parent to demonstrate consistent authority over time. **229**
- For the parent to respond in a positive way to the child's positive behavior. **231**
- For the parent to handle the child with confidence. **232**

OBJECTIVE: **Parent Will Be Aware Of Growth And Development Of Other Children The Same Age As Her Child.**

How the Teacher Helps	What the Parent Does at Home
Often parents become so involved with the hearing loss and all of its ramifications that they lose sight of their child's overall development. They may need to be reminded that he is a child like any other child.	Suggestions for things parents can do at home to increase awareness of normal growth and development.

How the Teacher Helps

Often parents become so involved with the hearing loss and all of its ramifications that they lose sight of their child's overall development. They may need to be reminded that he is a child like any other child.

- On a monthly basis, the teacher and parent could review the child's overall development by using one of the many commercially available growth charts.

- On-going reading material could be provided to the parents covering child development and child rearing issues of interest to any parent.

- The parent could watch her child at play and the intervener could direct the parent's observation to determine what the child does that makes him like a two-year-old or a three-year-old, i.e., "He's stacking six blocks. That's appropriate behavior for his age."

The hearing-impaired child should be raised like any other child, with all of the benefits, expectations and responsibilities appropriate for his developmental age. Knowledge of normal growth and development will help the parent challenge the hearing-impaired child to reach his fullest potential.

What the Parent Does at Home

Suggestions for things parents can do at home to increase awareness of normal growth and development.

- Parent could subscribe to a monthly magazine for parents dealing with a variety of child development and child rearing issues.

- Parent could read a book such as *The First Three Years of Life* by B. White.

- If parent encounters a question regarding child growth and development either through reading an article, watching a TV program or through direct experience with a child, she should make a note of the question and discuss it with the teacher the next session.

- Parent could observe other children playing at family gatherings, religious school or in the neighborhood and get a "feel" for growth and development of children.

OBJECTIVE: Parent Will Provide Appropriate Playthings For The Child's Age.

How the Teacher Helps	What the Parent Does at Home
Many times the parent's main sources of information regarding the appropriateness of toys and playthings for her child are advertising, knowing the most popular toys in the neighborhood, and reading the age information on toy boxes. The teacher should be a more reliable reference for the parent. • Many of the commercially available growth charts list favorite activities and toys for different age levels. These could be discussed. • Age-appropriate toys could be reviewed prior to shopping for birthdays, Christmas or Hannukah. • Age-appropriate activities also could be discussed along with suggestions for implementing them using materials already available around the house. The provision of appropriate playthings will insure more opportunities for meaningful interaction and language of interest to the child.	• As a related activity, following gift-giving holidays, the parent could examine the child's new toys, observe him playing with them and brainstorm all the language possibilities of these new toys. She could involve father, older siblings or teacher. • Parent can read Brazelton or White on toys. • Parent doesn't have to put out all of the child's toys at once. She can put out a few toys one week and then change the selections in a week or two. This way playthings stay "new" and interesting and language opportunities are varied.

OBJECTIVE: **Parent Will See That The Child Is Wearing His Hearing Aid(s) During All His Waking Hours.**

How the Teacher Helps	What the Parent Does at Home
Most parents of newly identified hearing-impaired children never have had any experience with a hearing aid until the day they bring one home for their child. They don't know how it works, they don't know what it will do for their child and they can't imagine that their child will ever leave it in his ear. Many parents don't know how to put in the hearing aid and approach the task with fear. Parents need help in order to establish consistent hearing-aid use.	• Parent needs to make a special place to keep the hearing aid, extra batteries, battery tester and any other related materials. If Mother is away, any responsible person would know where hearing aids are kept.

• The teacher needs to practice putting in the hearing aid <u>with</u> the parent until she feels more at ease.

• Many fathers, siblings, grandparents and babysitters are slow to learn how to handle the aid. The teacher needs to practice putting in the hearing aid with the father, older siblings, grandparents, friends, babysitters and anyone else available until it becomes second nature.

• The teacher can assist the parent in marking the earmolds and the aids with identifiable markings so it is readily apparent which aid and mold goes in which ear. This helps to reduce adult anxiety.

• The teacher can check the aid together with the parent each time the family comes to the Center.

(continued)

• Parent should post a card clearly indicating:
  – volume setting (for each aid);
  – setting to indicate that aid is on, whether "M" or "O" or whatever;
  – how to tell which aid goes in the right or left ear;
  – any other pertinent information.

• Parent responsible for primary care of the child should ask for help from other family members and friends. Mother may become the only one who knows about the aid and the child's needs. This can become an overwhelming responsibility and prevents hearing-aid usage when Mother is not around.

• Parent needs to establish a routine for checking the hearing aid on a daily basis.

• When the parent is establishing gradually increasing periods of wear each day, she might put some toys in a box that are only to be played with during these times. She also might plan to do something special on another occasion, e.g., blowing bubbles or popping popcorn.

OBJECTIVE: (continued) **Parent Will See That The Child Is Wearing His Hearing Aid(s) During All His Waking Hours. (cont'd)**

How the Teacher Helps	What the Parent Does at Home
• The teacher can assist the parent in establishing a program of daily hearing aid check. • When beginning hearing-aid use, the teacher-counselor could advise the parent to start with a few, short periods of wear each day during which time the child is actively engaged in interesting activities. As quickly as possible these times should be lengthened. • The teacher can advise the parent to be watchful of the child to protect the hearing aid. Another function of watchfulness is for the parent to know the child well enough to anticipate when he is getting anxious about the aid being in place. • The teacher needs to help the parent gain the confidence necessary to adopt the attitude that <u>she</u> is in charge of the hearing aid(s) and <u>she</u> is in charge of <u>when</u> they are to be worn. Consistent hearing aid use will not be established nor continued unless the parent meets with some success for her efforts. It also will not be possible unless putting on the hearing aid is as natural a task as changing a diaper or putting on a pair of pants. This needs to be true for everyone who is regularly involved with the child. Teachers can reinforce parents for this.	• When the child becomes anxious about the aid being in place, the adult needs to intervene and praise the child for wearing his aid(s). The key is to <u>avoid</u> having the child tugging at the aid(s), removing it, throwing it, disassembling it and ultimately getting in trouble when he is wearing it. By anticipating trouble, the hearing aid(s) will be associated with more pleasurable feelings. • When the child removes the hearing aid, the parent should replace the aid just long enough to praise the child for wearing it and then say, "Mommy will take off your hearing aid."

OBJECTIVE: Parent Will Respond Promptly To The Child's Distress Calls.

How the Teacher Helps	What the Parent Does at Home
Parents may be missing opportunities to respond to their child's distress calls simply because they don't recognize these attempts. These distress calls may not be as frequent nor sound the same as other children with whom they have had experience. • The intervener can help the parent become aware when the child is attempting to communicate distress. She could say: "Did you hear that? What do you think Johnny wants? Oh, look, he dropped his rattle. Do you think he wants it back? Why don't you pick it up and hand it to him and see what happens. There. He stopped fussing. I think he WAS trying to tell you something." • After learning to recognize these attempts to communicate, prompt responses can be discussed. The teacher might say: "You know, whenever possible, if you respond to his cries right away like that, he'll begin to know that he got his message across. If these attempts are rewarded, they will increase." Pointing out the child's communication attempts as exciting achievements to be reinforced and rewarded is a more positive approach than tallying the number of opportunities the parent missed. If the learning experience is positive for the parent, the interaction between parent and child will develop more naturally and be more joyful and less stressful for the parent.	Examples of responses to child's distress calls: • When the child is fussing and appears to be unhappy about something, the parent investigates to find that the child has a wet diaper. She may say something like: "Brian's diaper is all wet! Poor baby! You don't like wet diapers. Mommy will take it off. There! That's better!" • When the child has been sitting in his highchair watching Mother work in the kitchen for a few minutes, he begins to fuss and wiggle, leaning over the sides of the highchair. Mother could say: "Do you want down? Mommy will help you. Down-down- down we go!" • When feeding time nears, the child begins to fuss. Mother responds and says: "What a hungry boy! Mommy will fix you something to eat. Look—some cereal. Johnny will eat some cereal."

OBJECTIVE: Parent Will Interact With The Child.

How the Teacher Helps	What the Parent Does at Home

In order for the parent to interact with her hearing-impaired child, it is essential that she be able to recognize her child's attempts to elicit interaction with <u>her</u>.
 	
• It may be helpful for the teacher to provide materials and discussion about nonverbal communication (i.e., body language, gestures, glances, etc.) that <u>all</u> children use to communicate.
 	
• There are wonderful photographs in women's magazines that are advertisements for detergent, baby food, diapers and so on. While the ultimate purpose of these pictures is to sell the item, they also depict children expressing different kinds of needs and inviting interactions. For example, the baby in the saggy disposable diaper is obviously expressing discomfort and wants to be changed. The crying baby with shampoo running in his eyes is telling you that it hurts and he wants someone to take the hurt away. The wide-eyed baby smacking his lips after his first taste of bananas is glowing with pleasure and wants his mother to know it. None of these children are SAYING anything verbally, but they are TELLING the world "whole stories" with their nonverbal communication.
 	
• The teacher could compile a notebook of such pictures and use it as a basis of discussion with the parent:
 	
(continued)
	Examples of situations where the child invites interaction:
	
	• <u>When the child is in the tub splashing and looking as if he is having a good time</u>, Mother says:
	   "Billy likes to take a bath. Can you splash the water?" (Mother takes the child's hand and smacks the water.) "Splash-splash! Splash the water. That's fun!"
	
	• <u>When the parent is changing the child's diaper, he is kicking, waving his arms, cooing and gooing as he looks up at his parent's face.</u> Father says:
	   "Daddy hears you. Are you talking to Daddy? I like to hear you talking. What a big boy!"
	
	• <u>When the child is riding in the stroller he kicks his feet and waves his arms when the stroller stops.</u> Mother might say something like:
	   "Uh-oh, Mommy stopped. Johnny wants to go. Let's go, Johnny."
	
	(continued)

OBJECTIVE: Parent Will Interact With The Child. (cont'd)

How the Teacher Helps	What the Parent Does at Home
"What is that child communicating? If that child were in this room, how would you respond to him? What would you say to him?" For the mother of a hearing-impaired child who seems to be "off in his own little world," the responses and communication overtures from the child may be few and far between. • The teacher may need to show the mother some techniques for improving interactions with her child. • The intervener might suggest that the mother try sitting on the floor quietly beside him and play with what he is doing. She could try imitating his actions, doing something novel and interesting with the objects he has, or developing a repetitive game. • If the mother does these things very casually, without invading the child's "space," the child may eventually begin to show an interest in what his mother is doing. They may slowly then interact more with one another.	Some examples of engaging the child in interaction when he is otherwise occupied: • If the child is playing with <u>small miniature cars,</u> Mother could begin playing with her own miniature cars next to the child. She could begin driving the cars, making "car noises." She could drive the car gently into the child's knee and say, "Beep-beep." If the child likes this she could repeat it and watch for his attempts to invite repetitions. She could make a ramp with books and blocks and drive her cars on the ramp. • If the child is playing with <u>miniature action figures,</u> Mother could begin playing with her own action figures next to the child. She could make her figures walk, jump, fall down, ride in vehicles and so on and watch for her child to indicate interest.

OBJECTIVE: Parent Will Bring The Child To The Room Or Place Where She Is Working.

How the Teacher Helps	What the Parent Does at Home
Since the goal of this text is that the parent becomes the child's first teacher, the parent needs to learn to modify her daily routines to allow for maximum interaction. One modification of routines is to bring the child to the room where Mother is working as much as possible. • The teacher can discuss with the mother times the child can be in the same room with her while she is working. • The instructor can help the mother think of ways to position the child safely so mother and child can mutually observe one another. • As the mother watches the child and begins to spend more time with him, there will be more opportunities for interaction.	• If the child is an infant, the child could be brought to the room where Mother is working and positioned safely in an infant seat, walker, swing or playpen so the mother and child can mutually observe one another while Mother fixes supper, folds the clothes, scrubs the floor and so on. • If the child is a toddler, the mother may need to think of ways to safely confine the child in the same room by the use of baby gates or closed doors. • If the child is a preschooler, it often helps to have his OWN special things to do while his mother is working. For example, the child could "work" in the kitchen with his mother if he has his own drawer there filled with special toys and objects. He could have his own small laundry basket for doll clothes or washcloths when mother is folding the clothes. • As the child gets older, the mother may have a special toy box that only belongs in these "working" rooms to keep the child satisfied. The most obvious and best situation for the child, as he gets older, is to involve him completely in the task at hand. But since his attention span may not last through a full basket of laundry, the toy box could be pulled out.

OBJECTIVE: **Parent Will Watch The Child Even When Otherwise Engaged.**

How the Teacher Helps	What the Parent Does at Home
A teacher and mother can be observed busily engaged in a discussion relating to the child's hearing aid. The child is cooing and gooing and excitedly kicking arms and legs. Neither the parent nor the teacher look at the child. • The teacher needs to set the example of being able to watch the child even when engaged in a discussion. • The teacher can engage the parent in a discussion and watch to see if the parent will stop and note the child's activity. If the parent does not stop and look at the child, the intervener can stop the parent and say something like: "We need to stop and pay attention to Johnny. Nothing I have to say to you is as important as Johnny's attempts to get our attention."	A parent can "connect" with her child in subtle ways through the course of her daily activities. • If Mother is busy preparing dinner and the child is playing with blocks in the adjoining room, she can watch the child out of the corner of her eye and pause in her own activities to interact briefly with the child by: - just saying, "Hi!"; - commenting when she sees the child's interest focusing on something; or - making a mental note of her child's interests so she can expand on them at a later time when she has more time to spend.

OBJECTIVE: Parent Will Anticipate The Child's Interest.

How the Teacher Helps	What the Parent Does at Home

When asked, "What is your child's favorite toy or activity?" many parents will have difficulty answering the question. In order for a parent to anticipate and challenge her child's interests, her awareness may have to be heightened.
 	
• The teacher could ask the mother to watch the child during the week and make a list of <u>his favorite toys, activities, and people.</u> It might be fun for older siblings to make their own list. The teacher may help the mother learn to capitalize on the "favorites" and determine which are good for fostering communication. The teacher should also make note of these to include in her lesson planning.
 	
• The consultant could have the mother watch the child during the week and see what are his <u>best times of the day</u> for attending, both auditorily and visually. These may be different from the times the child is engaged in his favorite activities or with his favorite toys. Some children become absorbed in their favorite activities making it difficult and frustrating for the mother and the child to interact. The teacher could make note of these "best times" to keep in mind when she is scheduling.
 	
• This discussion will need to be reviewed on a regular basis because, as the child matures, his interests will change.
	• <u>If Mother determines that her child is very responsive when he is just waking up from his nap,</u> she could engage in interactive behavior:
	  - reading a book,
	  - singing songs,
	  - saying rhymes,
	  - talking about things of immediate interest to the child.
	
	• <u>If Mother determines that her child is "out of sorts" just before supper,</u> that would be a good time to get out that bag of blocks he loves to play with by himself.
	
	• <u>If Mother determines that her child loves to help her in the kitchen or to play ball,</u> these would be important for the parent to note as activities that may interest him when they come up again.

OBJECTIVE: Parent's Talk Will Match The Child's Thoughts.

How the Teacher Helps	What the Parent Does at Home

Once parents have become physically responsive to the child, they may be at a loss for words. It is similar to being on stage in the spotlight and when it is your turn, you forget your lines. The teacher needs to take the parent out of the spotlight and arm her with some resources to put her at ease when she talks to her child.
 	
• The teacher could help the parent look carefully at all the "clues" the child gives to his meaning and even point them out if necessary:
  - facial expressions
  - eye gazes
  - tears
  - sounds
  - actions
  - situations
 	
Some parents feel that their child is not communicating anything to them. Therefore, they find it difficult to match their language to the child's thoughts.
 	
• The teacher could do a "How do you know?" activity:
  - How do you know when your child is hungry?
  - How do you know when he has to go potty?
  - How do you know when he is tired?
 	
• Almost every parent is going to have an answer for all of these questions. For each answer, the teacher can point out to the parent that the child communicated this to her in some way, with gestures, body language, facial expressions, shouts, cries or whines.
 	
(continued)
	Look for clues to meaning:
	• When his facial expression changes, Mother could say:
	  "Oh, Johnny, you look so sleepy."
	  "I see your silly face!"
	
	• When he looks at Mother, she might say:
	  "Peek-a-boo! I see you!"
	  "Hi, Johnny! Mommy's right here."
	
	• When he cries, Mother can say:
	  "What happened? Did you fall down?"
	  "That hurts!"
	  "I know you want to stay outside. Look, it is getting dark. It's time to go in the house."
	
	• When he makes sounds or vocalizes, Mother's talk might include:
	  "Ah-choo! What a big sneeze."
	  "I hear you laughing. What's so funny?"
	  "Da-da-da-da. Did you say, 'Daddy'?"
	
	• When he does something, Mother could say:
	  "Whoops! Johnny fell down."
	  "Are you waving? Bye-bye. Wave bye-bye."
	
	• When he is in a familiar situation, Mother says:
	  "Johnny wants up."
	  "Johnny wants a cookie."
	
	(continued)

OBJECTIVE: Parent's Talk Will The Match Child's Thoughts. (cont'd)

How the Teacher Helps	What the Parent Does at Home
• The intervener can encourage this watchfulness. She might say something like: "By watching your child, you are really getting to know him, his moods, his thoughts. You are already halfway there. Since you do such a good job of watching him and knowing what he wants, now it will be easier for you to use the appropriate language to match his thoughts." • The teacher can give some examples of language specific to the situations the parent has described. • The teacher can take a negative situation reported by the parent ("My child doesn't communicate anything.") and turn it into something positive ("Look how well you're able to know what he wants!") thus opening the door for more parental growth and confidence.	Looking for more clues to meaning: • When he bangs on the cupboard wanting a snack, the language match might be: "Johnny wants a cookie. Open the door, please." • When he wiggles, crosses his legs, and runs down the hall to the bathroom, the language match could be: "Johnny has to go potty. Quick! Go to the bathroom." • "When he yawns, rubs his eyes, and begins to fuss, the language match can be: "Johnny is tired. What a big yawn!" (Mother imitates yawn.) "Mommy is tired too."

OBJECTIVE: Parent Will Respond To The Child's Gazes, Smiles, Sounds, Gestures.

How the Teacher Helps	What the Parent Does at Home
Often when parents become used to the routines of every day, they conduct them almost as if they are on "automatic pilot." Things like diapering, feeding, bathing, zipping up jackets, putting on hats and mittens or wiping runny noses are repeated so often that they can be done while thinking about or doing something else. Since the parent is not thinking about the task at hand, she may be unaware of her child's actions at that time. • In order to build parent awareness, the teacher can ask the parent to observe while she (the teacher) interacts with the child in a very common, daily activity, e.g., feeding time. The teacher's instruction to the parent could be to tally every time the child does something to invite interaction, e.g., gaze, smile, make a sound, gesture, etc. • Another time, the teacher could ask the parent to observe the teacher and child engaged in some familiar activity. The parent is to ring a small bell every time the teacher misses an opportunity to respond immediately to the child. (The teacher can deliberately miss some obvious opportunities for interaction to stimulate parent-teacher discussion.) (continued)	To heighten awareness at home and become less automated during daily routines, the parent can remind herself to watch for signs of interaction from her child. • One day, she might concentrate on paying close attention to the interaction possibilities during mealtimes. • Another day, she might concentrate on interaction possibilities during dressing time. • Other times for concentration might include: – bathtime, – brushing hair, – putting on coats and hats, – tying shoes, – diapering or helping in the bathroom. After doing this for a week or two, the parent will probably be excited to see how many times the child invites interaction. She may even see an increase in opportunities for interaction as the week progresses. Her response to these attempts will reinforce the child and may cause these attempts to increase.

OBJECTIVE: Parent Will Respond To The Child's Gazes, Smiles, Sounds, Gestures. (cont'd)

How the Teacher Helps	What the Parent Does at Home
• Following the latter activity, the teacher can give the parent positive feedback on her participation in his exercise, e.g.: "You really caught me asleep at the wheel! I didn't notice Johnny reaching for more applesauce and you were right, that was a great time to respond to him," etc.)	

OBJECTIVE: Parent Will Make Frequent Eye Contact With The Child.

How the Teacher Helps	What the Parent Does at Home

Eye contact is an important social skill to establish. It also allows the child to get visual information from the speaker to supplement his incomplete auditory signals. At first, eye contact from the child may be fleeting, but as it is reinforced, the eye contact should become more frequent and also longer in duration to allow the child to take in longer verbal messages.
 	
• The teacher can demonstrate for the parent techniques that encourage eye contact:
  – bringing object up near speaker's mouth when talking to the child;
  – jiggling object in child's line of vision to get his visual attention. When he visually fixes on object, bring it up near speaker's mouth and the speaker's mouth movements may momentarily take his attention away from the object;
  – pausing in parent's activity. The child will look up to the adult to see why she has stopped her activity, then the parent can make eye contact.
 	
• The teacher can have the parent tally the number of times she gets eye contact during a specified period, e.g., mealtime or playtime. Teacher can suggest:
 	
(continued)
	To encourage eye contact at home:
	
	• When feeding the child, Mother can hold the spoon near her mouth and say: "More cereal?"
	
	• When cutting his meat, Mother can stop cutting and when child looks up to see why she stopped, she can say: "Mommy will cut the meat."
	
	• When dressing the child, Mother can hold each article of clothing up near her mouth to talk about it before she puts it on the child and say something like: "Here's Johnny's shirt."
	
	• When blowing bubbles, Mother can hold the wand up near her mouth but wait to blow until child looks at her and then say something like: "Mommy will blow bubbles," or "Blow the bubbles."
	
	• When turning on the lights, Mother can hold her hand on the light switch but wait until the child looks to turn the light on or off. She would then say something like: "Turn off the light."
	
	• When opening the door, Mother can take hold of the doorknob but wait to open the door until the child looks at her and then say: "Open the door."
	
	(continued)

OBJECTIVE: Parent Will Make Frequent Eye Contact With The Child. (cont'd)

How the Teacher Helps	What the Parent Does at Home
"He gave eye contact three times today. Let's see if by next week during the same activity we can increase the number of times to six!" (or whatever number is realistically attainable for that family). • A parent may express frustration with the fact that she just hasn't established eye contact with her child. When the teacher observes the mother-child interactions she might see that the child is often at an angle that makes it difficult to look at his mother. • Learning to position the child correctly will make it easier for the parent to naturally make eye contact. The teacher can make suggestions. • The key point for the teacher to point out to the parent is that the child needs to be FACE TO FACE ON EYE AND EAR LEVEL WITH THE ADULT. • If the parent can accomplish this principle, it will impact on many facets of development. It will be much easier for her naturally to respond to the child's signals, anticipate his interests, smile at him, return his smiles, talk to him, demonstrate affection as well as the point of this objective: make frequent eye contact.	When handing him a toy, Mother can hold the toy near her mouth and say: "Here's your ball." Positioning to enhance eye contact: • When bathing the child, position the child in the tub at an angle to enhance face-to-face contact of the adult and child. • When playing games with the child, the adult can get down on the floor. Sometimes to get eye contact, it may be necessary to bring the toy up to the adult's face level. • When Mother is doing household chores, the child can be positioned safely in an infant seat, highchair, walker, stool or chair next to Mother at an angle to enhance face-to-face contact and to enable the child to observe Mother's activities. • When the child is eating, he can be placed in a highchair, infant seat, stool or chair directly in front of Mother. She then positions herself on an appropriate chair to bring herself to his eye and ear level. • When going for a walk or pushing the stroller, Mother will need to stoop or squat down to the child's eye and ear level to talk to him. If the family has a stroller with a reversible handle, the handle can be put in the reversed position so the child faces the parent.

OBJECTIVE: Parent Will Smile Frequently At The Child.

How the Teacher Helps	What the Parent Does at Home
Hearing-impaired children who are limited in their comprehension abilities use other resources to supplement what they are missing. Facial expressions that show warmth and approval can be very important to the child. Some parents who are worried about their child, concerned about bills, or searching for a babysitter while Mother is at work, show this worry unconsciously. A child who is sensitive to facial expressions may perceive this as disapproval of him. • Teacher can point out things the child does that are "cute," looking at his hands, kicking, etc. Or she can hold up a toy and note his "clever" procedures. Mother will smile almost reflexively. • For the parent of the very young hearing-impaired child, it may be necessary to point out to her that she needs to get right in front of the child to make sure that he sees her warm smiles and looks of approval.	• The parent can SMILE at the child when eye contact is made: – when diapering, – when feeding, – when playing, – when dressing, – when waking up in the morning, – when bathing, – when greeting him when she comes home. • The parent can SMILE at the child and SAY something to match the child's thoughts or just to make "connection": "Hi, Johnny." "I love you." "Hi, there." "There's Mommy's big boy."

OBJECTIVE: Parent Will Return The Child's Smile.

How the Teacher Helps	What the Parent Does at Home
Some parents are thankful for having a happy child. Others, who aren't as fortunate to have a smiling, happy baby, are relieved when he's content because they get a break. In both instances, the parents are failing to see the child's smile as a powerful communicative tool. He's communicating: "Look at me, Mom, I'm a neat kid!" or "My tummy feels okay for a few minutes and boy, am I glad!" • Inteveners need to talk with the parent about the use of the child's smile as a way of communicating. • The teacher could ask the parent if she has ever smiled at an acquaintance she sees walking down the street and failed to have that smile returned. If this has happened, consider the feelings the situation evoked: Is she angry with me? Do you suppose something is wrong? Maybe she's not feeling well. Maybe she just didn't see me. • If a child reaches out to his parent with a smile he deserves to have a smile in return. • Teacher could have the parent tally the number of times the child smiles during a parent-infant session, or a portion thereof. This might heighten the parent's awareness of the child's smiles.	• Parent can enlist the help of other family members in helping her watch for the child's smiles and making sure that he gets a SMILE IN RETURN and perhaps some talk such as: "Hello, happy boy!" "Hi, Johnny!" "Gonna get you!" "Watcha doing?" • Parent might tally the number of times she (or other family member) returns the child's smile during a given period at home.

OBJECTIVE: Parent Will Frequently Demonstrate Affection

How the Teacher Helps	What the Parent Does at Home
A teacher may become concerned with the lack of affection a parent shows for her child. This is a difficult behavior for which to plan intervention strategies. • If the teacher sees that the parent and child are at a low point or having a bad day with each other, she might suggest that a hug and a kiss can be an effective soother. • In another session the teacher may see that tension is mounting between parent and child perhaps because an activity isn't going well, or because the child's behavior is less than desirable. The teacher can suggest that from time to time when this happens at home, the parent can just "break the cycle" by doing something entirely different and unplanned, going outside to play in the sand together or going to the park. The idea is to just have fun and enjoy one another's company—hugging and cuddling will then come naturally. • An example could be pointed out to the parent about how much better she feels when she has had a bad day if a little extra attention from her husband or parent or friend is shown. • A young child needs the reassurance of frequently demonstrated affection.	• The parent can become aware of how often she is taking time out of her busy schedule to give her child a hug, throw him a kiss, pat him on the back, or whatever she does to demonstrate affection. • She can make an effort to increase the amount of affection given to her child during the course of the day. • If she finds that she is not showing affection to him regularly or that things aren't going well enough so that she feels like demonstrating affection, then perhaps she needs to evaluate what is going on in her life that is preventing this from happening. If she can pinpoint the problem and do something to take better care of herself, maybe this will help to make her feel more affectionate toward her child.

OBJECTIVE: Parent Will Use "Love Talk."

How the Teacher Helps	What the Parent Does at Home
"Love talk" has a flavor all its own. The pitch and rhythmic qualities are characteristic of this type of talk between mothers and their babies. Mother's speech is very warm and loving in its message. • Teachers need to encourage parents to engage in this type of "talk." Often parents get so involved with <u>what</u> they're supposed to say and <u>how</u> they're supposed to say it that they lose sight of the times when "love talk" would be the most natural thing to do. • If possible, teachers could provide movies or videos of mothers and babies so that Mother can see and hear for herself how other parents talk. • If the parent has had other (hearing) children prior to the hearing-impaired child, maybe she can recall the type of "love talk" she used with them.	• At home, the parent can "do what comes naturally." If it feels more natural to get down on the floor and tickle, giggle, cuddle and coo with her child than to talk about putting on his pajamas, she should do it—or she could actually end up doing both! • Parent could plan some opportunities just to hold him in her arms and "wrap him in love." • Every time she changes him, she should accompany the activity with "love talk."

OBJECTIVE: Parent Will Display Pleasure In Interaction Activities.

How the Teacher Helps	What the Parent Does at Home
Frequently a mother brings in an activity to do with the child. She seats the child properly in the highchair and begins to feed him. Suddenly, she jumps up to get a spoon. A minute later, she remembers a washcloth, and then in a couple more minutes, she realizes she forgot to get him something to drink. After all this, she has lost his attention and it may be difficult to regain it. Mother may become frustrated and this makes it difficult for the two to have a pleasurable interaction. The teacher needs to help the parent plan ahead of time so she is free to enjoy the interaction and to display pleasure to her child.	Making minimal preparations prior to activities at home:
	• Preparing for his bath... Have all necessary items, e.g., towel, soap, washcloth, shampoo, clean pajamas close at hand.
	• Preparing to make toast... Place the loaf of bread, butter, knife, plate, jelly, toaster within easy reach of the adult.
	• Preparing to change diapers... Gather together the clean diaper, wipes, powder, lotion, change of clothing and put them within easy reach.
	• Preparing to make pudding... The adult will need the box of pudding milk, measuring cup, mixing bowl, egg beater, serving bowl, serving spoon, eating spoon.
• Making some minimal preparations ahead of time before feeding the child, for example, may insure a more pleasant interaction. If the adult has all the necessary items she will need within her reach, e.g., food, silverware, bowl, cup, napkin, then attention can be given to the <u>child</u> and not to rounding up needed items.	If parents have hobbies or special interests, there may be ways to enjoy that hobby with the hearing-impaired child.
The parent who may be feeling guilty for not making "special" time for the child may minimize the value of the routine interactions she has during the week.	• If Mother enjoys working in the garden, the child could have his own set of child-size garden tools, wheelbarrow, watering can, etc., so he can help Mother garden.
(continued)	• If Mother enjoys cleaning the house, the child could be involved by having his own cleaning supplies and tools, i.e., dustcloth, broom, paper towels, etc. Or he could use Mother's, i.e., "I'll dust and then you will dust."
	(continued)

OBJECTIVE: Parent Will Display Pleasure In Interaction Activities. (cont'd)

How the Teacher Helps	What the Parent Does at Home

• The teacher can have the mother and all family members note the things they enjoyed doing with the hearing-impaired child during the week, such as:
  – What were their favorite times with him?
  – When did they get special, warm feelings just being with him?
  – What do they enjoy doing with him?
 	
• The teacher needs to reinforce these times and let the parent know that these are wonderful learning opportunities.
 	
• Sometimes the insecure parent needs to hear, "See, look what a wonderful job you are doing already. That's a great activity to do with your child. Would you mind if I suggest it to another parent? I think her child would enjoy that too." What a vote of confidence this could be to a parent!
 	
• Helping the parent gain confidence with her child can allow her the freedom to enjoy the interactions and share that joy with the child.
 	
This is perhaps one of the most significant objectives. Once a parent can relax and have a good time with her child, many of the other skills will develop more naturally. Teachers can point this out.
	• If Daddy enjoys washing the car, the child could easily be involved with that activity.
	
	• If Mother enjoys painting or some other activity, the toddler could be given his own set of paints, paintbrushes and paper.
	
	• If Mother enjoys music, she can sing with the child, dance and sway to music, play the piano with him.

OBJECTIVE: Parent Will Set Limits.

How the Teacher Helps	What the Parent Does at Home
The parent can invite a very real problem with sibling rivalry if she fails to set limits for the hearing-impaired child. She excuses this lack of limits with: "I make his brothers share their toys with him because he doesn't understand that he shouldn't get into them." "I don't make him clean up his mess like the other kids because he doesn't understand." "If he hits his sister, I don't let her hit him back because he doesn't know that he's not supposed to hit." • The parents need to learn that they are not doing their hearing-impaired child any favors by treating him as "special" or "different." Not only will it prevent him from achieving all that he is capable of achieving, but they will also seriously damage the interpersonal relationships between the hearing-impaired child and his siblings. • During the parent-infant session, the teacher could model situations for the parents. The intervener could demonstrate setting limits by "showing and telling" him what is expected of him. • The child's actions will demonstrate to the parent that he does understand what is expected of him. (continued)	• At home, the parents need to take a look at the expectations they have for their children. They need to make sure that they are not making too many special concessions or excuses for their hearing-impaired child. • The siblings should not be carrying too much of the "load" around the house, for the household chores or for the care of the hearing-impaired child. • The hearing-impaired child can have a few clearly demonstrated expectations that are consistent from day-to-day. • The parent needs to give the child a secure framework in which to operate. Parent needs to assume role of authority figure with the child no matter where she is: at Grandmother's, at the neighbor's, in the doctor's office. • Parent could think ahead of time what she will do if the child throws a tantrum at Grandma's. If her strategy at home is to give him a "time out" on a chair, then she needs to do this at Grandma's house also.

OBJECTIVE: Parent Will Set Limits. (cont'd)

How the Teacher Helps	What the Parent Does at Home
• If the instructions are short and clearly demonstrated, the same expectations should be established for the hearing-impaired child as for the other children in the family. A pitfall that teachers need to come to terms with is that of: Who is the authority figure during the parent-infant session? • If the relationship that the teacher is trying to nurture is the parent-child relationship, then she needs to abdicate the authority role and leave it where it belongs—with the parent! • The teacher can "coach" the parent through rough times or make suggestions for what the parent might try the next time this situation occurs. • If the teacher keeps intruding and "rescuing" the parent from uncomfortable situations, the parent will only feel less capable of establishing authority with her child. Too, such behavior on the part of the teacher will interfere with the desired parent-child relationship. • The teacher needs to let the parent know that she (the parent) is to be the authority figure with her child during the parent-infant sessions and share with her the reasons why. • Parent can feel left out or demoted from her job if the teacher takes over.	

OBJECTIVE: Parent Will Demonstrate Consistent Authority.

How the Teacher Helps	What the Parent Does at Home
The parent can lack consistency in her authority. She sometimes says: "I can't explain to him why he can't have the candy, and he gets so upset if I don't let him have it." "I can't reason with him when he gets like this, so I just give in." • The intervener can provide information and instruction about what is normal behavior for a child the same chronological or developmental age as the hearing-impaired child. • A teacher can point out to the parent that a temper tantrum in the store for the candy at the check-out lane has nothing to do with the hearing impairment. An astute two-year-old can find out by the process of trial and error that just as his mother tries to write out the check, a loud and boisterous display of temper will be rewarded with the candybar of his choice. • Because the child senses he has control, he will ALWAYS stage the same display each and every time he approaches this situation. (continued)	Showing the hearing-impaired child as well as telling him <u>ahead of time</u> may prevent problems. • If fussing for candy at the check-out stand is a recurring problem, the mother may approach the candy as soon as she enters the store and point to it, shaking her head "no" as she says, "No candy today." • She completes her shopping and reminds the child, "No candy today," as she approaches the check-out lane, before he has the chance to ask. • She needs to be prepared for the inevitable: that one day he will again demand the candy. At that time, despite glowering looks or sympathetic comments around her, the mother removes it from his hand, puts it back and firmly says, "No." • If this or other similar situations are an every-time occurrence, the mother may need to make it a rule, "No candy at the grocery store. • If it is wrong once, it should be wrong forever more.

OBJECTIVE: **Parent Will Demonstrate Consistent Authority. (cont'd)**

How the Teacher Helps	What the Parent Does at Home
• Being able to explain to him that he can't have candy because Mommy doesn't have any extra money that day or because it decays his teeth or whatever the reason might be, will have absolutely no effect on preventing the temper tantrum. Consistency in these situations is probably one of the most important things a parent has to do.	

OBJECTIVE: Parent Will Respond In A Positive Way To The Child's Positive Behavior.

How the Teacher Helps	What the Parent Does at Home
Often a child can be observed to be playing quietly seemingly ignored by his mother. Once the child becomes restless and fusses, the mother gives him attention, negative though it is.	When positive behavior occurs, the parent can reinforce:
	• With verbal compliments:
	– "Thank you for helping Mommy."
	– "What a good job!"
• The teacher needs to point out what kind of behavior—positive or negative—the parent is reinforcing.	– "I like the way you made your bed."
	– "Wow! You really worked hard."
• The teacher needs to provide information and discussion about the role of reinforcement in establishing behavior.	• With body language:
	– a hug,
	– a kiss,
• The teacher needs to provide information about <u>positive</u> reinforcement.	– a wink,
	– a smile,
Too frequently, it is negative behavior that is being reinforced.	– a pat on the back,
	– clapping hands.

OBJECTIVE: Parent Will Handle The Child With Confidence.

How the Teacher Helps	What the Parent Does at Home
When the parent's confidence in handling the child is at a low point, often the teacher will find that the parent and child live in a household where life is pretty free of routine. The child and parent don't have any expectations of one another at any given time, therefore, things don't run very smoothly. In order to gain confidence, the parent needs to gain control. • The teacher can discuss with the parent the need for establishing a secure framework or routine in which to operate. For a child who may experience difficulty in communicating, knowing what usually happens at certain times of the day or in certain situations will help him use clues to supplement his incomplete comprehension. • Establishing this secure framework also helps the parent become more efficient and thereby frees her for more relaxed interaction with her child. It helps consistency, too. The parent can be more confident in knowing her role. • Routine helps the child become secure and safe with family rules and expectations. Without routines, it is often difficult to tell who is handling whom! If the parent feels confident in her overall handling of the child, then she is more likely to feel confident in making decisions regarding her child's future.	• Bedtime routines might include such activities as: – take a bath, – put on pajamas, – eat a snack, – brush teeth, – read a book, – sing a favorite song, – tuck him in, – turn out the lights. • Morning routines might include a sequence such as: – get up, – put on hearing aid(s), – eat breakfast, – get dressed. • Naptime routines might include such activities as: – read a book, – take a nap, – eat a snack when he wakes up. These rituals or routines can help the mother feel confident because she is in control of what is going to happen. The child may want to take over and go his own way, but Mother can confidently say: "No, it is time to take a bath now. First you will take a bath, <u>then</u> you may eat a cookie."

Some possible objectives that might be considered at this stage are:

- For the parent to see that the child is wearing his hearing aid(s). **235**
- For the parent to face the child frequently. **236**
- For the parent to hold the child in front of her when she talks to him. **238**
- For the parent to make eye contact with the child. **239**
- For the parent to follow the child's eye gaze. **240**
- For the parent to smile, wink or give a look of pleasure when she gets the child's eye gaze. **241**
- For the parent to talk and use the child's name when she gets his eye gaze. **242**
- For the parent to play reciprocal eye-contact games with the child. **243**
- For the parent to play reciprocal, imitative games with the child's vocalizations. **244**
- For the parent to match language to the child's feelings and moods. **245**
- For the parent to match language to the child's ideas and interests. **246**
- For the parent to use the child's name whenever talking to him. **247**
- For the parent to use the child's name to get his attention. **248**
- For the parent to stop activity to respond to the child. **249**
- For the parent to respond promptly to child's crying, cooing or babbling. **251**
- For the parent to use reinforcement effectively. **253**

OBJECTIVE: **Parent Will See That The Child Is Wearing His Hearing Aid(s).**

How the Teacher Helps	What the Parent Does at Home
The important message for the parent is that the child has to develop a "sound" memory just as a hearing child does. The hearing aid delivers a signal that would sound imperfect to us, but for the hearing-impaired child, it is quite valid. Therefore, all the messages spoken to him must be delivered with the signal which he is learning. Thus, he must use his hearing aid(s) consistently. • The teacher-counselor could plot the child's audiogram showing the child's unaided responses. Then she should superimpose the responses with the aided ears. This visual representation helps the parent see what differences the hearing aid(s) makes. If a child needs glasses to perceive images, would anyone think of not letting that child use his glasses? Of course not! Therefore, the child who needs amplification to perceive sound must not be deprived of it. He cannot learn to understand language if he has the aid on one day and not the next. He is truly being deprived when he does not get the needed amplification.	The parent needs to be reminded to put the child's hearing aid(s) on when: • he gets up in the morning; • he gets up from his nap; • he finishes his bath so he can take full advantage of the rest of the bedtime ritual; • he is in the car, even if the aid has to be turned down or covered with a cap so he doesn't fiddle with it; • he goes on errands or outings so he can take full advantage of the experience; • he plays outside, even if this means keeping a more watchful eye. He needs to hear the talk of his family and friends as he plays; • he goes to school; • he watches television.

OBJECTIVE: Parent Will Face The Child Frequently.

How the Teacher Helps	What the Parent Does at Home

The parent may find it awkward at first to remember to face her child.
 	
• The teacher can give the parent suggestions for positioning the child and herself in the environment to allow for maximum face-to-face contact.
 	
• It is important for the teacher to have the family investigate their own home and find safe ways of positioning the child so he can be included in many activities throughout the day. The family needs to find out what works for them.
 	
• The teacher needs to remind the parent that confining the child for long periods of time in any way can be unhealthy. If the child spends a few minutes watching his mother peel potatoes, for example, and then wants down to go do something else, that is reasonable.
 	
• The goal is to help the adult find ways of effectively engineering a few minutes of good face-to-face situations many times throughout the course of the day's activities. In that way, Mother can go on with her necessary chores but still have many meaningful interactions with her child without having to interrupt her work. She will, however, have to make a few modifications and undoubtedly things will take a little longer.
	Suggestions for face-to-face positioning:
	
	• <u>When putting on socks and shoes</u>, the child can sit on a chair or bed and the adult can kneel on the floor in front and face the child quite easily.
	
	• <u>When watching his mother put on make-up or dry her hair</u>, an infant could be strapped securely in an infant seat and placed safely on the bathroom counter. An older child, perhaps, could be seated on the counter facing the mother.
	
	• <u>When looking at books</u>, an infant could sit in an infant seat, stroller, walker, highchair or infant swing and the adult could seat herself on the floor or low stool in front of the child. The adult could hold the book open with the pages facing toward the child or place the open book on the highchair or walker tray. That way the child has a full view of the book <u>and</u> the adult's face.
	   An older child could nestle in the corner of the couch or in a beanbag chair and the adult could again seat herself on the floor in front.
	   For a taller adult with adequate lap space, the child can be seated on the adult's knees, facing the adult. The adult can lean the open book against her chest facing the child.
	
	(continued)

OBJECTIVE: **Parent Will Face The Child Frequently.**
(cont'd)

How the Teacher Helps	What the Parent Does at Home
	• <u>When cleaning the house</u>, an infant can be securely positioned in a walker, infant seat, highchair or swing so he can be near the mother and face her for maximum interaction.
	A stroller may wear a path in the carpet, but for the mother who is rushing about from room to room doing laundry, washing dishes, vacuuming or dusting, the stroller can allow her the option of bringing the child along.
	A playpen strategically positioned can also be useful. The mother can, for example, dump a load of clean towels to be folded into the playpen. Consistent face-to-face contact can be established as she pulls each towel out of the playpen, plays peek-a-boo, tickles the child's cheek with them, talks about their warmth and folds them.
	• <u>When dressing or undressing the child</u>, he should be positioned on a bed or floor facing the parent. The parent will again need to bring herself down to his eye and ear level.

OBJECTIVE: Parent Will Hold The Child In Front Of Her When She Talks To Him.

How the Teacher Helps	What the Parent Does at Home
This objective refers mainly to the positioning by the mother of her infant. Many mothers can be seen picking up the infant from behind with the mother's arm about the infant's waist. After picking up the infant, many mothers then poise the child on their hip with the infant facing outward. Also, many infants are carried in carriers on their parent's back. These are all to be discouraged. • The teacher needs to talk to the parent about the value of picking up the hearing-impaired infant and young child so that he is in front of her: — he can see his mother's face, — if held closely against the chest, he can receive tactile stimulation as she talks to him. — he participates in an interaction that can be perceived as more accepting, rather than the facing-out body positioning which prohibits rather than promotes interaction. — his gazes and eye contact are much easier to reinforce in this face-to-face position.	The applications of this objective at home include: • Attempting to modify routines or habits where necessary to pick the child up so that he is in front of the mother whenever possible. • Holding the child in front when talking to him. • Holding the child close when singing to him. • A child can learn to lip-read as well as hear when parents talk while holding him in a face-to-face position.

OBJECTIVE: Parent Will Make Eye Contact With The Child.

How the Teacher Helps	What the Parent Does at Home
If the adults have made many attempts to modify their environment and routines to enhance face-to-face contact as suggested previously, they are well on the way to establishing good eye-to-eye contact. • The teacher can "coach" the parent when she sees the child gaze at his mother's face. • The teacher might say, "He gave you great eye contact just then. It looked like you were surprised and that you didn't know what to say. You don't have to say something special each time your child looks at you. You could simply smile at him and say: "Hi, Johnny. I love you." • The teacher could remind the parent of the techniques suggested on pages 219 and 220. • Since this objective deals with the parent making eye contact with the child, the teacher could tally the number of attempts the parent makes to obtain eye contact over a given period of time. If it is five times over a fifteen-minute period, for example, the teacher could challenge the parent to increase those attempts to eight to ten the next time they do this activity. • The teacher could also note the techniques the parent uses to obtain eye contact. They could then discuss these techniques and determine which were the most effective. The teacher could then suggest some others to try, if appropriate.	Techniques to establish eye contact: • observe effective face-to-face positioning • get down on the child's eye level • bring the child up to the adult's eye level • call the child's name • hold object of interest near speaker's mouth • pause in activity and wait for child to look up Parents need to respond to child's gaze immediately.

OBJECTIVE: Parent Will Follow The Child's Eye Gaze

How the Teacher Helps	What the Parent Does at Home
Because the child's eyes focus on the thing he is thinking about, this is the quickest way for Mother to understand the child's thought. • The intervener may hang a mobile in the room within the child's view and then wait to see if the child looks at it. If the child looks toward the mobile, Mother could then go and point to it, talk about it and allow the child to touch it. • The teacher may present other objects within the child's view and follow the same procedure. • To make the mother aware, the teacher could ask the parent as the child looks at the object, "What do you suppose he is thinking?" • The teacher could make a mental note of whether the parent's language is appropriate in length and concepts. The adult wants to know what the child is seeing in order to know what the child is thinking about.	Every time the child looks at something, the mother would say: — "That's a doggie." — "Here's a pillow." — "Look at the kitty." — "There's Daddy. Hi, Daddy." — "There's Johnny's book. Open the book."

OBJECTIVE: Parent Will Smile, Wink Or Give A Look Of Pleasure When She Gets His Eye Gaze.

How the Teacher Helps	What the Parent Does at Home
Since you want the eye gaze to be a rewarding experience for the child, he needs to receive positive reinforcement when he gives eye gaze. That positive reinforcement might be a smile, a wink or a look of pleasure. • The teacher will discuss positive reinforcement with the parent. • The teacher will tell the mother why she should reinforce eye gaze. • During a planned activity, the teacher will note the type of reinforcement the mother uses to reinforce the eye gaze. Is there variety in her reinforcement? Are there other reinforcement techniques she could use? • The teacher reinforces the mother for these attempts. This interaction transpires all day long, not just during an activity at school. The parent has many opportunities throughout the day to reinforce eye gaze.	• Child looks when Mother walks in the room, Mother smiles and says: "Hi, Johnny. Mommy's home!" • Child looks up as Mother approaches the child to pick him up. Mother smiles and says: "Let's go, Johnny." • Child looks up as Mother starts to dress the child. Mother smiles and says: "Time to get dressed." • Child looks at Mother as she pulls shirt over his head. Mother winks and says: "Peek-a-boo! I see Johnny."

OBJECTIVE: Parent Will Talk And Use Child's Name When She Gets His Eye Gaze.

How the Teacher Helps	What the Parent Does at Home
When a child plays, he often will pause in his activities to look up to the adult. The child may have a quizzical look, a look of frustration or a look of satisfaction on his face. Whatever the purpose for the gaze, the child is inviting interaction and he needs to be immediately reinforced. • The teacher can again "coach" the parent in these situations. When the gaze occurs, she can say: "He just gave you a nice long gaze. I don't think you saw him, but it looked as if he wanted you to see how well he did the puzzle. Watch and when he looks up again, try and smile and tell him what a good job he did." • When the parent talks to the child as he looks up at her, she is reinforcing his eye contact. If the reinforcement comes often enough, eye gazes will become more frequent and meaningful.	Reinforcing eye gazes by talking to the child: • If the child looks puzzled, the adult might say: – "What's that?" – "Where does it go?" • If the child looks frustrated, the adult might say: – "Johnny, do you need help?" – "That's hard to do, isn't it?" • If the child looks satisfied or pleased, the adult might say: – "Johnny, I like that." – "Oh, Johnny, what a good job." – "I see your puzzle. You worked hard.

OBJECTIVE: **Parent Will Play Reciprocal Eye-Contact Games With Child.**

How the Teacher Helps	What the Parent Does at Home
Reciprocal eye contact is an essential step in conversation. I talk, you look at me and listen. You talk, I look at you and listen, and so on back and forth in a ping-pong-like fashion. The listener shows interest in the speaker. The hearing-impaired child needs to learn that the parent is interested in him and what he is doing. • The teacher will ask the parent what kinds of eye contact "games" she plays with her child at home. • The teacher will suggest eye games for the parent to do at home: – "Peek" – "Gonna Get You" – "I See You" Parent and child exchange playful glances as child teasingly does something he knows he shouldn't, i.e., touching the dials on the TV. Reciprocal eye contact, in addition to being a basis for conversation, is also an indication of social/emotional development.	Mother will make an attempt to sustain back and forth, ping-pong type of eye gaze and "conversation" during such activities as: bathtime mealtime playing ball dressing

OBJECTIVE: Parent Will Play Reciprocal, Imitative Games With The Child's Vocalizations.

How the Teacher Helps	What the Parent Does at Home
While reciprocal eye contact is an essential step in conversation, reciprocal vocalization is certainly the basis of it. • Learning reciprocal vocalization through games as a young child will set the stage for appropriate conversational skills later. • Imitating the child's sounds and babbling back to him is one technique that is effective in setting up this back-and-forth characteristic of "conversation." • Parents may feel silly imitating the child's sounds and babbling. However, if the parent understands the values of these imitative games, some of the self-consciousness may subside. The teacher needs to talk to the parent about imitation. • By imitating what the child does, the adult shows him that she values his attempts at communication: 　　You talk, I listen and 　　then I'll comment on 　　what you just said. • Imitation is a skill that also becomes valuable to the child later on when he is able to imitate the adult model and match the rhythm, time and intonation. • Imitation is is the tool teachers will use to shape the child's speech sounds when he is in school. Parents will use it to correct spoken language at home.	Imitative games to play: 　"Copy Cat" • If the child is babbling or vocalizing, the parent can be instructed to wait until the child stops and then take her turn and babble back to the child, setting up the ping-pong like pattern of conversation. • If the child says "mah-mah-mah," the adult can say "mah-mah-mah" back to him. • The next time, she might imitate the child's sounds, "mah-mah-mah," but say them on a higher or lower pitch or in a loud, soft or whispered voice. • Another time, the mother might imitate his sounds, "mah-mah-mah," and then give him another sound to listen to, e.g., "gah-gah-gah." 　"You Scared Me" • The parent can have fun with the child's vocalizations. 　– A response to a child's playful vocalization can be a jump or a startled reaction and a <u>very</u> animated comment, e.g., "Oh, you scared me!" 　– This often sets up a playful game between the parent and child because the child wants to see his parent repeat the "scared" action again and again.

OBJECTIVE: Parent Will Match Language To The Child's Feelings And Moods.

How the Teacher Helps	What the Parent Does at Home

Hearing-impaired children can be very "physical" in their expression of feelings and moods until they acquire the language to express them. However, recognition of and empathy for those feelings can do a lot to defuse some powerful emotions. Parents need to learn to identify feelings and talk about them with their child.
 	
● Earlier, it was suggested that the teacher could assemble a set of magazine pictures or photographs of children communicating through body language, facial expressions, or gestures in familiar, everyday situations. The teacher could expand this to include some that very obviously depict strong feelings and moods.
 	
● The teacher and the parent or a small group of parents could look at these pictures as a stimulus for discussion. The teacher could ask questions like:
  – "What do you think the child is feeling?"
  – "What would you say to this child as an appropriate language model?"
 	
● The teacher could indicate whether or not the model the parent gives is too complex or too simple for her child at his particular level of language development.
 	
● Teachers need to help the parents be aware of and model language for happy times as well as negative.
	Matching language to feelings and moods at home:
	
	– "We are going to Grandma's house.
	I love Grandma.
	Are you happy to see Grandma?"
	
	– "Tell Suzy to stop that!"
	
	– "You don't like spinach."
	
	– "You don't want to get up, do you?
	Johnny is so tired!
	Sorry. Time to get up!"
	
	– "Do you like the cookie?
	Ummm. That looks good!"
	
	– "I see what you did.
	You have been working hard.
	What a good job!"
	
	– "You don't want anymore meat.
	Is your tummy full?"
	
	– "You are angry with Mommy!"
	
	– "I love you, Johnny."

OBJECTIVE: Parent Will Match Language To The Child's Ideas And Interests.

How the Teacher Helps	What the Parent Does at Home
Learning to match language to the child's ideas requires a lot of practice and guidance. The teacher cannot merely offer a generic statement such as, "Now you need to talk to Johnny all the time and give him the language for what he is trying to say." The mother <u>needs to be shown</u> how to do this in many different situations, on many different occasions. • "Coaching" the parent through a familiar activity or situation is effective. For example, when the child is tugging at his mother's skirt and fussing, the teacher could ask, "What do you think he's trying to tell you right now?" The mother may say, "Probably that he wants to be picked up." The teacher could reply, "I think you're right. Now would be a good time to say something like, 'Do you want up? Mommy will pick you up. Up-up-up.' " • The teacher can share her pleasure in seeing that the child is trying to communicate. • She can demonstrate to the parent that now she can follow <u>his</u> lead and it will be easier to model his language or communication attempts.	Examples of matching language to ideas: • The child smacks his lips as he and his mother drink a milkshake. Mother might say: (Mother imitates smacking noises.) "Mmmmm good! This milkshake tastes good. Do you want more?" • The child is in his highchair. After he has finished eating a cookie, he makes a grasping gesture toward his mother and vocalizes, "uh-uh-uh-uh." Mother might say: "I hear you. Oh, Johnny's cookie is all gone! Do you want more? Yes. Johnny wants more cookies." • The child laughs in response to his mother playing Peek-a-Boo. Mother could say: "I see you. Oh you are such a silly boy! Cover your eyes. Johnny! Where's Johnny? Peek-a-boo!"

OBJECTIVE: Parent Will Use The Child's Name Whenever Talking To Him.

How the Teacher Helps	What the Parent Does at Home

Young children are ego-centered and it is very reinforcing for them to hear their own name used often.
 	
• The teacher can remind the parent to use the child's name often when talking to him.
 	
• It can be very confusing for the child if everyone in the family has a different "pet" name for the child. Until he truly knows his name, it would be easier for him if everyone called him by the same name or nickname.
 	
• Using his name prior to giving directions or asking questions is an effective way to get the child's auditory and visual attention.
	Examples of situations where the child's name can be emphasized:
	
	• When modeling language for what the child is trying to say:
	  – "Johnny wants up."
	  – "Johnny wants a cookie."
	  – "Johnny wants a turn."
	
	• When modeling language for what he is doing:
	  – "Johnny is pushing the truck."
	  – "Johnny is swinging. Up and down, up and down."
	  – "Johnny is eating his lunch."
	
	• When giving directions:
	  – "Johnny, get your book."
	  – "Johnny, finish your sandwich."
	  – "Johnny, drink your milk."
	
	• When asking questions:
	  – "Johnny, do you want more?"
	  – "Johnny, are you all finished?"
	  – "Johnny, are you ready for bed?"

OBJECTIVE: Parent Will Use The Child's Name To Get His Attention.

How the Teacher Helps	What the Parent Does at Home
It is is not unusual to see many strategies used for getting the hearing-impaired child's attention. • Some of these strategies for gaining the child's attention are disturbing to the child. The teacher could point these out to the parent: grabbing his face and turning it toward the speaker or tapping him on the arm or shoulder. • Other strategies are visual and infringe on the concentration of other people in the room, such as flicking lights on and off or stomping on the floor. • In an emergency situation, any of these might be necessary. • On a daily basis, it would be more appropriate to train the child to auditorily respond to his name.	Situations where the child's name can be used to get his attention: • When calling him: "Joh——neee!" • When needing his attention: "Johnny. Look at Mommy." • When calming him down: "Johnny. It's okay, Johnny. Tell me what happened." • When pointing out a significant sight or sound to him: "Johnny. Listen!"

OBJECTIVE: Parent Will Stop Activity To Respond To The Child.

How the Teacher Helps	What the Parent Does at Home

Response is a valuable skill to master. It requires the adult to shift her attention away from the important task at hand.
 	
• The teacher can make it clear that the parent doesn't have to completely drop what she is doing. She only needs to pause, respond to the child and then resume her activity.
 	
Many hearing-impaired children have the tendency to interrupt conversations.
 	
• Sometimes they are not aware that the people are talking.
 	
• Other times, they are so used to having their needs gratified immediately that they interrupt without thinking.
 	
• A parent can respond to the child in such a way that she is demonstrating her appreciation of his verbal communication, but also helping him learn appropriate manners.
	Appropriate responses when engaged in an activity:
	
	• If the mother is talking to a friend or another child, she might say to the hearing-impaired child:
	    "I hear you Johnny. Just a minute. Mommy is talking........Okay, Johnny What did you want to say?"
	
	• If the mother is on the phone, she could say to the hearing-impaired child:
	    "Just a minute. Mommy is on the telephone. You have to wait....... Okay, Johnny. What do you want?"
	
	• If another child is talking to the mother and the hearing-impaired child interrupts, the mother could say:
	    "Johnny, Kathy was talking first. You have to wait........Okay, Johnny What did you say?"
	
	• If Mother is engaged in an activity and the hearing-impaired child is requesting attention, the mother could say:
	    "I hear you Johnny. Mommy is busy. You will have to wait.......Okay, Johnny. Now I can help you."

A pitfall that teachers often fall into is that of doing a lot of talking to the parent "over the child's head," as it were. For example, the child may be sitting on the floor between his mother and teacher. He could (continued)	At home the parent can evaluate her situation and determine if a lot of "talking over the child's head" is going on there also. (continued)

OBJECTIVE: Parent Will Stop Activity To Respond To The Child. (cont'd)

How the Teacher Helps	What the Parent Does at Home
be playing with blocks while the mother and teacher are actively engaged in a discussion about hearing aids. In this situation and many like it, the teacher unfortunately is demonstrating how to "tune out" the child rather than "tune in" to him and his needs. • It might be suggested that if the teacher needs to do a great deal of talking to the parent or if the parent brings up a topic that requires a lengthy discussion, that a session be scheduled without the child. • If this is not possible, perhaps the child could be placed off a little distance from the teacher and mother and given something something to do so that he knows that he is not to be included in the discussion. • The teacher should evaluate from time to time and if a lot of parent-teacher talking is going on, maybe the sessions are turning into a social chat rather than a learning situation for all involved. If this is so, adjustments need to be made—always in favor of the parent-child relationship.	• Unless it is something that cannot wait, perhaps the parents could postpone lengthy discussions until after the hearing-impaired child is in bed. • If company comes, the parents will obviously want to visit with their friends. They could find something for the child to do and place him off a little distance from the group so he knows that he is not to be included in the discussion.

OBJECTIVE: Parent Will Respond Promptly To The Child's Crying, Cooing, Or Babbling.

How the Teacher Helps	What the Parent Does at Home
Often when a parent is not responding to the child's vocalizations, it is due to a lack of awareness. The teacher can do much to heighten the parent's awareness. • The intervener can comment on the child's vocalizations, i.e.: "Oh, that's a new sound, isn't it? That's great! I haven't heard that one before. Does he always use that sound when he's trying to get your attention?" • The teacher can talk to the parent about responding to the vocalization. She could say: "You know, whenever you can, you need to respond to that vocalization immediately in the same manner as you would if he said, 'Mommy come here!'" • The teacher needs to explain why prompt response is necessary: "We want to reinforce that vocalization immediately so he will do it again and again until he realizes that it was <u>his voice</u> that brought you running." (continued)	• The parent can keep an on-going list of sounds the child makes. She can also note when these sounds occur. • Once a month the parent can tally the number of vocalizations she heard during a specified amount of time. She can check and see if the amount of vocalization is increasing over time. • The parent can ask for help from other members in the family to make sure that someone is responding promptly to the child's crying, cooing or babbling.

OBJECTIVE: Parent Will Respond Promptly To The Child's Crying, Cooing, Or Babbling. (cont'd)

How the Teacher Helps	What The Parent Does at Home
• The teacher can ask the parent to tally every time the child vocalizes for a fifteen-minute play period. At the end of the period, they can count the number of vocalizations. The teacher and parent can discuss the results: "Is this amount of vocalization typical for your child? Did we respond to these vocalizations every time they happened? Let's really make a big response every time he makes even a little sound and see if the amount increases."	

OBJECTIVE: Parent Will Use Reinforcement Effectively.

How the Teacher Helps	What the Parent Does at Home
Many of the techniques described previously are effective types of positive reinforcement. If these are being used consistently, then the parent is meeting this objective. • The intervener may need to explain reinforcement. • The teacher can discuss the effect of positive reinforcement in establishing desired behavior. • The teacher can review with the parent effective ways to give positive reinforcement.	Natural mothering techniques used by many are effective reinforcement strategies: • Responding promptly to distress calls • Responding to gazes, smiles, sounds, gestures • Smiling at the child • Returning the child's smile • Demonstrating affection • Using "love talk" • Parent displaying pleasure in interaction • Responding in a positive way to child's positive behaviors • Ignoring child's negative behaviors • Smiling at the child when getting eye gaze • Stopping activity to respond to the child • Responding promptly to child's crying, cooing, babble

Some possible objectives that might be considered at this stage are:

- For the parent to see that the child is wearing his hearing aid(s). **257**
- For the parent to use appropriate intonation prominently in her talk. **258**
- For the parent to utilize statements, questions and exclamations in her self-talk. **259**
- For the parent to read the child's signals regarding turn-passing. **260**
- For the parent to wait after vocalizing; using stress and intonation to signal to the child that it's his turn to talk or vocalize. **261**
- For the parent to express feelings of love, surprise, sadness, joy, etc. with appropriate tone. **262**
- For the parent to play games such as Pat-a-Cake and Peek-a-Boo providing intonation and prosodic features. **263**
- For the parent to use a <u>variety</u> of the prosodic features in length, pitch and loudness in her talking. **265**
- For the parent to imitate the child's intonations in her vocalizations. **266**
- For the parent to imitate the child's utterances. **267**
- For the parent to use relatively short sentences. **268**
- For the parent to speak more slowly than she does with an adult. **269**
- For the parent to say something when the child's eyes are on her face. **271**
- For the parent to repeat the self-talk frequently. **272**
- For the parent to repeat activities and language about the activities often. **273**
- For the parent to apply similar language to a variety of situations. **274**

OBJECTIVE: **Parent Will See That The Child Is Wearing His Hearing Aid(s).**

How the Teacher Helps	What the Parent Does at Home
If the parent has been consistent with hearing-aid use up to this point, the child will become dependent on the hearing aid(s) and may begin to ask for them as soon as he awakens. Some children even want them on at bedtime and the parents remove them as soon as the child falls asleep. Others leave them on all night. Consistent hearing-aid use cannot be stressed enough.	Reminders:
• As the verbal input from the parent becomes more and more sophisticated, the need for hearing a clear language signal becomes crucial.	• The child's hearing aid(s) should be the FIRST article of "clothing" placed on the child every morning.
• The meaning carried by the auditory features of intonation, length, pitch and loudness will be enhanced by the hearing aid.	• The hearing aid(s) should be the LAST thing taken off before the child falls asleep.
• For many hearing-impaired children, these features would be completely absent if they were not wearing their hearing aid(s).	• If the parent and child will have an opportunity for interaction following the child's bedtime or bath, the hearing aid(s) should be put back on the child so he can have full advantage of the language opportunities of the bedtime routines.
• For others, the effects of these features would be diminished if not wearing their aid(s).	
Consistent hearing-aid use is mandatory if the hearing-impaired child is to reach his full potential.	
• The intervener can ask questions about the aid to check if the child is using it at home, i.e., "How many batteries does it use per month? When does he take it off? Does he wear it for breakfast?" Etc.	

OBJECTIVE: Parent Will Use Appropriate Intonation Prominently In Her Talk.

How the Teacher Helps	What the Parent Does at Home

Some parents are not very animated or dramatic in their talking. For them this may be a difficult skill to accomplish. However, if they have a basic understanding of how their child can gain meaning through changes in intonation, it may be more motivating for them to work to attain this objective.
 	
• A teacher can demonstrate to the parent how the meaning of identical words within a phrase or sentence can be changed if the intonation is varied.
 	
• She can ask the parent to say, "Oh, my!" to convey surprise. Next she can ask the parent to say the same two words, "Oh, my," to convey disappointment, concern, sadness or love. It should be evident to the parent that, in this situation where the words remained the same, the intonation contours have carried the meaning.
 	
• The teacher can stage another demonstration with nonsense syllables. She can tell the parent that she is going to say four different sentences in nonsense syllables conveying different meanings which she is to identify, such as excitement, anger, disappointment and sadness. Again, the parent should be reminded that she is identifying these on the basis of intonation alone.
 	
• Since intonation is an auditory component of language, this further reinforces consistent hearing aid use, no matter how profound a child's hearing loss might be.
	Meaning can be communicated through appropriate intonation in natural situations throughout the day:
	
	• Love
	  "I love you."
	  "Give Mommy a big hug."
	  "You're my sweet baby boy."
	
	• Concern
	  "Uh-oh! The egg is broken."
	  "Oh, Johnny. What happened to your finger?"
	  "Did you fall down?"
	
	• Excitement
	  "Johnny! Look at the hot-air balloon!"
	  "Hurry! The balloon is landing!"
	  "Johnny is walking! What a big boy!"
	
	• Disappointment
	  "I'm sorry you can't go."
	  "I know you want to play, but we have to go home now."
	  "I know you want candy, but Mommy said, 'No'."

OBJECTIVE: Parent Will Utilize Statements, Questions And Exclamations In Her Self-Talk.

How the Teacher Helps	What the Parent Does at Home
• The message that the intervener needs to give the parent is that children need to have appropriate experiences with different sentence types. There is much valuable information carried in the different intonation contours. • The teacher can demonstrate this to the parent. She can tell the parent that she is going to say three different nonsense sentences, one a statement, one a question and one an exclamation. The parent is to identify the type of sentence based on the intonational pattern used. The teacher can then "babble" a question with a rising contour, a statement with a falling contour, and a command with a choppy, steady contour. It should be easy for the parent to identify these sentence types and therefore see the value of emphasizing this auditory information for her child.	Utilizing statements, questions and exclamations in daily activities: When Bathing • How parents utilize statements: "Mommy turned on the water." "We will wash your arms." "Johnny poured the water." • How parents utilize questions: "Do you want bubble soap?" "Can Mommy help?" "Did you wash your face?" • How parents utilize exclamations: "Oh, no! Mommy is all wet!" "Be careful! The water is hot!" "Ooops! Johnny spilled the water." When Eating • How parents utilize statements: "Mommy poured the milk." "Mommy will cut your meat." "Mommy likes mashed potatoes." • How parents utilize questions: "Do you want more?" "Are you all finished?" "Is the soup too hot?" • How parents utilize exclamations: "Be careful! The knife is sharp!"

OBJECTIVE: Parent Will Read The Child's Signals Regarding Turn Passing.

How the Teacher Helps	What the Parent Does at Home
The parent-child interactions progress in a rather orderly fashion. At first, the parent responds in a general way to anything the child does. Then those responses become more specific as she responds to the child's vocal efforts with a verbal attempt to match the child's thoughts. Next turn-taking is established. The child should begin to initiate these interactions. • The teacher should help the parent recognize these signals. • The teacher can "coach" the parent through routine activities by pointing out the child's signal that it's the parent's turn to talk.	Parent will observe child at home to determine the child's signals regarding turn-passing. These signals might include: • pausing or looking at the parent's face as if seeking an explanation or comment • bringing something to the parent and then waiting for a comment • taking the parent by the hand and leading her to something that he wants to show her • early questioning either through intonation or early question words, "dah?" or "whazat?" This initiative on the child's part is the development the parent wants. Of course these signals, indicating that the child wants the parent to take a turn, require an immediate response.

OBJECTIVE: **Parent Will Wait After Vocalizing, Using Stress And Intonation To Signal The Child That It Is His Turn To Talk Or Vocalize.**

How the Teacher Helps	What the Parent Does at Home
A bad habit that a parent (and teacher) can fall into is that of doing too much talking and not having any expectations for the child. If one goal is to establish the back and forth ping-pong-like pattern of conversation, then the parent needs to learn to wait to give the child an opportunity to take his turn. <ul><li>The teacher can "coach" the parent through natural experiences and indicate to her when she needs to pause and wait for the child to respond.</li><li>The teacher can engage the parent or another teacher in a "nonsense" conversation to demonstrate how intonational contours signal to the listener the turn-taking aspect of our language. First speaker: "Duh-duh-duh-duh-duh?" Next speaker: "Duh. Duh-duh-duh-duh." First speaker: "Duh-duh-duh-duh-duh!" Next speaker: "Duh. Duh-duh-duh-duh!"</li></ul> If the parent (or teacher) says of a child that he just isn't attempting to talk or vocalize, the adults need to evaluate if anyone is giving him the chance. If everyone is always talking for him and not waiting for him to respond, he will not have any need to talk.	At home does the parent pause and wait for a response: <ul><li>when she asks him a question?</li><li>when she comments on something he is doing?</li><li>when she comments on something she is doing?</li><li>when she shares her feelings with him?</li><li>when she talks about what he is seeing?</li></ul> The child's "responses" at this point may not be complete. They may only be a vocalization or attempt at a word. The important point for the child to learn is that his mother values what he has to "say" no matter what it is.

OBJECTIVE: Parent Will Express Feelings Of Love, Surprise, Joy, Etc., With Appropriate Tone.

How the Teacher Helps	What the Parent Does at Home
A parent can give a child "mixed messages" if the intonational contour she uses to talk to the child doesn't match her feelings. For example, Mother has just come into the Center with her hearing-impaired toddler by the hand and a new baby in her arms. As they sit down to wait, the toddler's love pats to the baby's face become pinches and the baby begins to cry. Mother's response to the toddler is, "Be nice," spoken in a sweet, soft tone. Mother is undoubtedly boiling inside, but the intonational message to the toddler was a pleasant one, so he toddles off down the hall unscathed. The parent should be encouraged to let the child know her feelings with <u>appropriate</u> intonational clues.	The parent should share her feelings with the child. – "That makes me angry." – "Wow! What a good job!" – "Don't pull my hair!" – "Stop that!" – "I don't like that!" – "I like that!" – "I'm sorry." – "Mommy is tired." – "Oh, how sad. Your teddy's leg fell off." – "I love you so-o-o-o much!" – "That was fun!" – "The .... was so good!"
• The teacher could encourage the parent to verbally share her feelings with the child.	
• The teacher could discuss with the parent that the child needs to hear language put to the feelings that he sees conveyed so that he will then learn how to convey his feelings in the appropriate way.	
• Intonational contours carry much meaning and when used by the hearing-impaired child they will enhance the intelligibility of his speech. He needs to hear these contours prominently used by his parents in appropriate, meaningful expressions.	

OBJECTIVE: **Parent Will Play Games Such As Pat-A-Cake And Peek-A-Boo Providing Intonation And Prosodic Features.**

How the Teacher Helps	What the Parent Does at Home
Often a mother of a hearing-impaired child will be observed singing and playing games with the new (hearing) baby that were never observed with the hearing-impaired child at that stage. A parent may comment that she stopped playing these games when she learned he was hearing impaired because she felt he couldn't hear them or understand. • Parents should be encouraged to play such games because of the valuable intonational information. • The teacher should encourage the parent to play the games because they also offer good opportunities for face-to-face contact. • Games are enjoyable for the child and enhance parent-child bonding. • It isn't necessary to understand the words of the rhymes. They are fun to hear and say. What's a "hickory-dickory" anyway?	The following are some suggestions for games and rhymes. There are many wonderful books available in bookstores or at the library. • Peek-A-Boo. Mother can start by covering her face, "Where's Mommy?" She uncovers her face and says, "Peek-A-Boo!" Then if the child approves, cover his face, "Where's Johnny?" Uncover his face and say, "Peek-A-Boo!" After he catches on to the game, he will wait to hear his name and then will uncover his own face. • S-o-o-o Big!. Say, "How big is Johnny?" and then help him answer by saying, "So-o-o-o big!" as Mother raises his hands above his head. He should learn that when Mother says, "How big is Johnny?" he is to answer by raising his hands above his head. • Ahh————Boo!. Mother says, "Ahh————" as she slowly brings her child up to her face and then gently says, "Boo!" He will learn to anticipate the "Boo!" and eventually say it himself. • This Little Pig. Mother points to the child's toes one by one and says: "This little pig went to market, This little pig stayed at home, This little pig had roast beef, This little pig had none. (continued)

OBJECTIVE: **Parent Will Play Games Such As Pat-A-Cake And Peek-A-Boo Providing Intonation And Prosodic Features. (cont'd)**

How the Teacher Helps	What the Parent Does at Home
	This little pig cried, 'Wee, wee, wee, wee!' all the way home."
	These rhymes are fun for Mother to say while bouncing the child on her knees. The underlined words indicate the rhythmic pattern of the bouncing.
	● Ride a Cock Horse Ride a cock-horse to Banbury Cross To see a fine lady upon a white horse. Rings on her fingers and bells on her toes, She shall have music wherever she goes!
	● Baby Rides (Slowly) This is the way the baby rides Walking, walking, walking, walking... (Quickly) This is the way that Mommy rides, Trot, trot, trot, trot, trot.... (Fast and very bouncy) This is the way that Daddy rides, Galloping, galloping, galloping, galloping.
	● Trot to Boston To develop an anticipatory response, when Mother gets to the last line, she can spread her knees apart so the child "falls in" (holding his hand so he doesn't get hurt). Trot, trot, trot to Boston, Trot, trot, trot to Lynne. Watch out, little boy (girl)! So you don't fall in!

OBJECTIVE: Parent Will Use A <u>Variety</u> Of The Prosodic Features In Length, Pitch And Loudness In Her Talking.

How the Teacher Helps	What the Parent Does at Home

Many teachers of the hearing impaired create a variety of artificial games and activities to work on length, pitch and loudness. They have been observed tossing a baby up in the air on a blanket so they can have the parent use ascending and descending pitch as he goes up and down. They have been observed to have the mother say, "b-b-b-b-b-b-" for a toy sail boat as they push it across the water. Where is the <u>meaning</u> behind these activities? When there are so <u>many natural times</u> throughout the day that pitch, loudness and duration can be <u>meaningfully and appropriately used</u>, there seems to be no reason for dreaming up artificial activities.
 	
● The teacher can point out natural uses of these prosodic features when talking about:
   – eating
   – playing
   – going up and down stairs
   – calling the child's name
   – being quiet when someone is sleeping
 	
● The parents should incorporate pitch, loudness and duration in ways that feel natural to them.
	Daily activities that encourage the natural use of prosodic features:
	
	● <u>When the child is eating</u>, Mother can say:
	   "Mmmmmmm good!"
	   "Ooooooooh! It's hot!"
	   "It's toooooooo hot!"
	   "Moooore."
	   "Aaaaall gone."
	   "All gone!"
	
	● <u>When playing</u>, Mother might blow bubbles with the child and say:
	   "Blow."
	   "Pop-pop-pop-pop-pop."
	
	● <u>When going up and down the stairs</u>, Mother might say:
	   "Up-up-up" with an ascending pitch.
	   "Down-down-down-down" with a descending pitch.
	
	● <u>When calling the child's name throughout the day</u>, parents can be encouraged to call their child's name varying the volume appropriately with the situation and distance.
	
	● <u>When someone is sleeping</u>, parents can whisper with the child and tiptoe around quietly. Later, the parents can request the child's help in waking up the sleepyhead by using loud voices.

OBJECTIVE: Parent Will Imitate The Child's Intonation In Her Vocalizations.

How the Teacher Helps	What the Parent Does at Home
It is often said that "imitation is the sincerest form of flattery." By imitating the child's intonations, the parent is saying in effect, "I like to hear that, will you do it some more?" This is reinforcing a behavior that the parent wants to encourage. • The parent can be instructed to lay the foundation for later imitation abilities by imitating the child's actions in a playful manner. • The teacher can encourage the parent to recognize the intonational patterns in the child's vocalizations and then to imitate them. • Sometimes the child is just playing with his voice and these intonational patterns can be playfully imitated in a back and forth exchange. • Other times, the child is communicating something with the intonation paired with a word approximation. For example, the child may point and say, "Dah?" with a rising intonation indicating that he is asking a question. The parent can take the child's appropriate intonation contour and put it to the proper language as in, "What's that?"	• If the child is in his bed babbling, the adult can stick her head in the door and imitate the babble, i.e., "Muhmuhmuhmuhmuh. Mommy hears you!" • If the child is "scolding" his Teddy Bear for getting all muddy, Mother can give him the language for what he is trying to say and preserve his appropriate intonation: "No-no, Teddy. Stay out of the mud!" • If the child is very insistent on getting a toy that is out of reach and says, "Duh-duh-duh-duh-duh!" Mother can get him the toy and say: "Johnny wants the car right now!"

OBJECTIVE: Parent Will Imitate The Child's Utterances.

How the Teacher Helps	What the Parent Does at Home
Imitating a child's utterances is one way of verifying that the adult has understood the child's meaning. It says to the child, "I am interested in you and what you say. Now is this what you wanted to tell me?" Once the <u>meaning</u> is verified, the adult can shape the child's utterance and use it in a meaningful context. • The teacher can point out that sometimes if an adult imitates the child's utterance and looks carefully at the situation, it can clear up the adult's confusion. For example, the child points down the stairs and says, "up." Mother says, "Oh, do you want to go <u>down</u> the stairs?" Child shakes head no and again says, "up" as he points down the stairs. Mother looks down the stairs and suddenly understands the child's meaning and says, "Oh, you want the <u>cup</u>. Did the <u>cup</u> fall down the stairs? Let's go get the <u>cup</u>."	Other examples: • Child is standing by the back door saying "Ow." Mother investigates and asks, "Do you have an owie?" Child shakes head and says, "No!" He now stomps his foot and points outside and again says, "Ow." Mother suddenly understands and says: 　<u>"Outside</u>? Do you want to go <u>outside</u>? Okay. Mommy will open the door. Let's go <u>outside</u>." • Child points to a picture on the wall and says, "doggie." Mother looks where the child is pointing and says: 　"<u>Doggie</u>? Yes, I see the <u>doggie</u>. Look at the <u>doggie's</u> nose. The <u>doggie</u> has a big nose. Where's Johnny's nose? Yes. Johnny's nose and <u>doggie's</u> nose." • Child says, "Uh-oh." Mother looks to see what happened and says: 　"Uh-oh! Johnny dropped the ice cream. What a mess! Let's wipe it up."

OBJECTIVE: Parent Will Use Relatively Short Sentences.

How the Teacher Helps	What the Parent Does at Home

Talking in relatively short sentences doesn't always come easily for parents, especially parents who are used to conversing with adults all day long about very complex subjects. The teacher needs to share with the parent some of the reasons that she should use short sentences with her child.
 	
• The language spoken to the child should be about one step above what he is capable of using. We want to be challenging him at all times.
 	
• Young hearing-impaired children at this point in their parent-infant program may be using a few labels and familiar expressions. Therefore, if this parent only speaks in single words and echoes these expressions, she is "rubber stamping" the child's language and isn't "stretching" his ability.
 	
• On the other hand, if the adult talks in long, complex sentences, she will lose his attention and he will be unable to pick out the words he knows from the long string.
 	
• If the parent talks in relatively short sentences, about the here and now:
    – the child can visually attend to the speaker for the length of the sentence;
    – the child may be able to pick out from the short sentence a few key words that he understands.
	The following are some examples of utterances spoken by a child and demonstrations of appropriate and inappropriate sentences spoken in response.
	
	The child is looking at a truck in the street and he says, "truck."
	
	• An appropriate adult response would be:
	    "Johnny sees a truck. Look! The man will drive the truck."
	
	• An adult response that would be too long might be:
	    "I see the man driving the big blue truck. That truck looks like Uncle Jimmy's truck, doesn't it?"
	
	• An adult response that "rubber stamps" the child's language would be:
	    "Truck. That's a truck."
	
	The child is looking at a broken chair and says, "broke?"
	
	• An appropriate adult response would be:
	    "Yes. The chair is broken. Daddy will fix the chair."
	
	• An adult response that would be too long might be:
	    "Daddy will fix the broken chair tonight after he comes home from work."
	
	• An adult response that "rubber stamps" the child's language would be:
	    "Chair broken. Daddy fix."

OBJECTIVE : Parent Will Speak More Slowly Than She Does With An Adult

How the Teacher Helps	What the Parent Does at Home
There has been a lot of talk in this text about using natural rhythm and intonation and speaking in complete sentences as you would with a hearing child. We are referring to talking distinctly and of slowing down the pace. Phrasing and emphasis should be used effectively the way any "super mother" does. • The teacher can encourage the parent to emphasize key words of the sentence. • The teacher can demonstrate to the parent that if she wants to share more information on a topic than can be contained in one simple sentence, she can use several short sentences. These sentences can be separated by pauses that allow the child the opportunity to receive one thought before he is presented with another one. • Observe nine- or ten-year-old children talking to a toddler. They naturally fall into the "motherese" without being coached. Their sentences get shorter than those they use with their peers, the pitch of their voice often gets higher and they speak significantly slower. • Observe the slower pace used when adults are talking to children on "kids shows" on educational television. This is the kind of pace that we are suggesting. It doesn't distort the rhythm, it only emphasizes the key thoughts and gives the child a little more time to think about it. (continued)	• The parent can note the time (on the second hand) when she talks to an adult and when she talks to a young child. • The parent can visit a day-care center or a preschool and note the teacher's rate of talking. • The parent can look in a mirror and observe what she does when she imagines her husband is the listener and contrast this with what she does when she imagines her child is the listener.

OBJECTIVE: Parent Will Speak More Slowly Than She Does With An Adult. (cont'd)

How the Teacher Helps	What the Parent Does at Home
• Evaluate the rate that Mother uses with the child and determine if it is appropriate. Do the same with all family members. Ask for their help in talking a little slower if necessary.	

OBJECTIVE: **Parent Will Say Something When The Child's Eyes Are On Her Face.**

How the Teacher Helps	What the Parent Does at Home
If the parent says something when the child's eyes are on her face, she is reinforcing his eye contact. If this reinforcement comes often enough, eye contact will become more consistent, spontaneous and of longer duration. • The teacher can point out that if the child is now looking spontaneously to the adult for information, his effort needs to be rewarded immediately and every time it happens. • If the child has progressed to the point that he is looking to the adult spontaneously, it can mean that the child realizes that the information he gets from watching the speaker is helpful. • If the child is looking spontaneously, the adult will have many more opportunities to give information to the child. Spontaneous eye contact must be rewarded by saying something meaningful every time it occurs.	When the child spontaneously looks at the adult's face, she can: • talk about what the child is doing • talk about what she is doing • use "love talk" • ask the child to help her • share her feelings At the point in the child's development when the adult was reinforcing any eye gaze with a wink, a smile or a word or two, it wasn't as important then <u>what</u> was said, only that <u>something</u> was said or done. Now, however, since the child is looking spontaneously for information, it is important that whatever the adult says be <u>tied to some meaning</u>.

OBJECTIVE: Parent Will Repeat The Self-talk Frequently.

How the Teacher Helps	What the Parent Does at Home
Most parents of young children talk to themselves naturally as they go about the house. It needs to be made part of their consciousness. They need to realize that their child can "tune in" to them. Some parents find it helpful to focus on one time of the day until the talking becomes more second nature to them. • The teacher and parent may decide that Mother will concentrate on meaningful talk centered around mealtimes throughout the coming week. • As a preparation for the week of talking about mealtime, the teacher could plan an eating activity to demonstrate appropriate self-talk to use during mealtime. • The next session, the teacher could ask the parent how things are going and even ask her to bring in an eating activity to demonstrate what she has been doing. • If the parent felt that she had given the previous area of emphasis her best effort, she could move on to another time of the day, e.g., dressing activities, as her area of concentration for the upcoming week.	Times of the day that may be good times for talking with the child: • getting dressed • eating breakfast • playing with Mommy • cleaning the house • doing the laundry • eating lunch • reading a book • going for a walk • fixing supper • eating supper • watering the flowers • playing with Daddy • taking a bath • going to bed Anything that is worth doing is worth talking about with the child.

OBJECTIVE: Parent Will Repeat Activities And Language About The Activities Often.

How the Teacher Helps	What the Parent Does at Home
A parent's life is by nature very repetitious. She does the same things at the same times, day in and day out. Parents need to use similar language at these repetitious times. <ul><li>The teacher can point out to the family a few examples to illustrate the natural availability of repetition in the home: The child eats at least three times a day, 7 days a week. In one week's time, similar language can be repeated about mealtime <u>21 times</u>. The child is involved in dressing activities at least twice a day, 7 days a week. In one week's time, similar language can be repeated about dressing <u>14 times</u>. The child bathes at least once a day, 7 days a week. In one week's time similar language can be repeated about bathtime <u>7 times</u>.</li><li>The family can be encouraged to repeat familiar phrases and expressions often.</li><li>The parent can be encouraged to read to the child because reading can provide many, many opportunities for natural repetitions of language.</li></ul>	Twenty-one times a week at mealtime: <ul><li>Think of all the foods to talk about..... They get cut, stirred, chewed, swallowed, cooked, peeled and buttered. Some are eaten with a fork or spoon, others are drunk out of a cup. They taste good, sour, bitter, spicy, salty, delicious.</li><li>Parents need to say: "It's time to eat. Mommy will cut the meat. Do you want more? Would you like some milk? Wipe your mouth. Look at Johnny eat all of his food!"</li></ul> Fourteen times a week at dressing time: <ul><li>Think of all the clothing— shirts, pants socks, pajamas ... They get put on, zipped up, buttoned, tucked in, pulled down. One arm goes in, another arm goes in. One leg goes in, the other leg goes in too. The belt buckles, shoes tie. He looks nice, handsome, clean, like a big boy.</li><li>Parents need to say: "It's time to get dressed. Put on your shirt. Where is your hand? There it is! Here are your pants. Put your leg in. Now put your other leg in, too. Tuck in your shirt. Where are your socks? Did you find your shoes?"</li></ul>

OBJECTIVE: Parent Will Apply Similar Language To A Variety Of Situations.

How the Teacher Helps	What the Parent Does at Home

The parent can be shown how repetitions of the same word or phrase in many different situations can be of benefit.
 	
 • The teacher and parent can brainstorm to think of how many times "Open the__" could be repeated in natural activities throughout the day:
  – Open the box.
  – Open the milk.
  – Open the cupboard.
  – Open the refrigerator.
  – Open your eyes.
  – Open your mouth.
  – Open the car door.
  – Open the garage door.
  – Open the mailbox.
  – Open the closet.
 	
 • The teacher could suggest that the parent set aside a special kitchen drawer or cupboard for the child. One week, the parent might put in a collection of items that "roll." As the child plays with the items, Mother can talk about:
 "The ball is rolling. Roll the can. Does the block roll? No. The block does not roll. The marbles can roll."
 	
 • Another time she might put in a variety of containers to "open" or toys to "push." She can give the child experience with similar language while she's busy in the kitchen.
 	
 • Using similar language in a variety of situations will reduce the occurence of a child saying, "Open the door," whenever he wants help opening anything, from doors to boxes to cereal.
	Similar language can be used again and again in different situations:
	  – Let's put on your jacket.
	  – Let's put on your pajamas.
	  – Let's put on your sunglasses.
	  – Let's put on your hearing aid.
	  – Let's put the milk on the table.
	  – Let's put the food in the dog's dish.
	  – Let's put the dog outside.
	
	  – Where is Tommy?
	  – Where is your ball?
	  – Where is Daddy?
	  – Where is the dog?
	
	  – Peek-a-boo (when he looks up from the floor)
	  – Peek-a-boo (when you peek around the corner)
	  – Peek-a-boo (when you pull his shirt over his head)
	  – Peek-a-boo (when he hides under his bed covers)

AREA D:
TALK *FOR* THE CHILD

Some possible objectives that might be considered at this time are:

- For the parent to see that the child is wearing his hearing aid(s). **277**
- For the parent to label in complete sentences the child's: food, clothing, playthings, body, actions, feelings and perceptions (smells, tastes, sounds, etc.). **278**
- For the parent to point out perceptual characteristics of an object. **280**
- For the parent to provide activities at the child's interest level. **281**
- For the parent to provide linguistic models for the child through parallel talk. **282**
- For the parent to make a special effort to include structure words in her language models. **283**
- For the parent's utterances to deal with the child's interest in the here and now. **285**
- For the parent to participate in verbal activity with the child such as reading, singing songs or playing games. **286**
- For the parent to give the child the linguistic form that she believes to express his thought, and wait for him to imitate it. **288**
- For the parent to use prosodic features prominently to help the child imitate. **290**
- For the parent to reinforce the child's efforts in a positive manner. **291**
- For the parent to express the same idea in many different ways. **292**
- For the parent to see that experiences are repeated. **293**
- For the parent to ask questions. **294**

OBJECTIVE: Parent Will See That The Child Is Wearing His Hearing Aid.

How the Teacher Helps	What the Parent Does at Home
At this point, hearing-aid use should be mandatory during all waking hours. • The teacher should monitor the hearing aid. • The teacher can check to see how often the mother checks the characteristics of the hearing aid(s). • The teacher can check the mother's ability to troubleshoot the hearing aid(s). • Does the mother check the fit of the earmolds? What does she do if they are too loose and causing feedback? turn the aids down? or make an appointment to have new molds made? • Does the mother understand the necessity of maintaining the recommended volume setting? • Does the mother monitor the hearing aid? i.e., try it on herself to check for volume, static and other manifestations of malfunctions. If consistent hearing-aid use and care has been the way of life for the child, he should reach for his aid(s) as soon as he gets out of bed in the morning in order to be tuned in to his family's talking.	The teacher can help the parent develop a home program where the child becomes more responsible for wearing his own hearing aid(s). • He can learn to put on hearing aid(s). • He can learn to adjust the volume (either to the correct number, color or mark made on the volume control). • He can clean his earmolds. • He can learn to check the batteries with a tester that clearly shows the condition of the batteries. • He can report to his teacher or parent when his hearing aid(s) is not functioning.

OBJECTIVE: **Parent Will Label In Complete Sentences The Child's: Food, Clothing, Playthings, Body, Actions, Feelings, Perceptions (Smells, Tastes, Sounds, Etc.)**

How the Teacher Helps	What the Parent Does at Home
Everything in the child's environment has a name and the child needs to have experience with these "things" in meaningful situations accompanied by complete sentences. • The teacher can model many typical activities and demonstrate the labeling process using complete sentences. • The parent can plan activities to conduct with the child to demonstrate her understanding of the language to be used. • During the parent's activity, the teacher can coach her and make other suggestions for language input. • The teacher may make suggestions to the parent for activities to do at home.	• <u>Foods</u> can be identified and discussed as they are used in cooking: "I need an <u>egg</u>. Will you get an <u>egg</u>? The <u>egg</u> is in the refrigerator. Can you crack the <u>egg</u>?" • <u>Clothing</u> can be <u>identified</u> as Mother sorts the laundry. Then Mother can follow up with things like: "Put Daddy's <u>shirt</u> on the <u>shirt</u> pile. Put the <u>towel</u> in the basket." • <u>Playthings</u> can be discussed as Mother and child clean up the playroom. Mother can say: "Where does the <u>truck</u> go? Put the <u>truck</u> on the shelf. Put the <u>blocks</u> in the can. The <u>cars</u> go in this basket." • <u>Body parts</u> can be identified as the child takes a bath. "Wash your <u>foot</u>. Did you wash the dolly's <u>foot</u>? You have soap on your <u>nose</u>. Shall I scrub your <u>back</u>?" • <u>Actions</u> can be discussed as Mother and child play. "<u>Catch</u> the ball. You <u>kicked</u> the ball over the fence. Can you <u>bounce</u> the ball?" (continued)

OBJECTIVE: **Parent Will Label In Complete Sentences The Child's: Food, Clothing, Playthings, Body, Actions, Feelings, Perceptions (Smells, Tastes, Sounds, Etc.) (cont'd)**

How the Teacher Helps	What the Parent Does at Home
	• <u>Places</u> where the parent and child frequently go can be photographed. The photos can be kept in a small snapshot album in Mother's purse or in the car. Mother can show the child and talk about where they are going: "We will go to the <u>grocery store</u>." "It's time to go to <u>school</u>." "First we will go to <u>ShopKo</u>, then we will go to <u>McDonald's</u>."
	• <u>Concepts</u> can be reinforced by making a scrapbook of photographs and magazine pictures organized into categories: – Clothes I Wear – Foods I Like to Eat – Toys I Play With – People I Know – Things I Do
	Mother and child can talk about these pictures and point out perceptions, such as: "Those shoes are called <u>sandals</u>. You have a pair of <u>sandals</u> to wear in the summer." "The boy is <u>jumping</u>. Do you like to <u>jump</u>?"

OBJECTIVE: Parent Will Point Out Perceptual Characteristics Of An Object.

How the Teacher Helps	What the Parent Does at Home

A hearing-impaired child once entered a program and could identify numerous pictures but could not identify real objects which the pictures represented. She obviously had not experienced the <u>real</u> objects and their perceptual characteristics of sight, smell, touch, taste, sound and use.
 	
• Words cannot be taught from pictures because perceptual characteristics must be experienced.
 	
• The teacher can set up a situation so the parent understands that her knowledge of a word depends on her previous perceptual experiences.
 	
• The teacher can show the parent a picture of a baby. The parent's knowledge of the word and her perception of its "babyness" is based on:
  – holding it
  – smelling its lotion, powder, formula
  – feeding it
  – changing it
  – hearing it cry, goo, gurgle
 	
• The teacher and parent should discuss the perceptions of smell, touch, taste, sight, sound, use.
 	
• The teacher and parent will discuss the perceptual characteristics to be pointed out prior to parent activities.
 	
• The teacher must monitor that the parent stays within the child's interest and developmental age.
 	
Children learn when the perceptual characteristics are pointed out. The more things they can notice about an object, the sooner the word becomes the child's.
	Parent points out perceptual characteristics of objects:
	
	• <u>Milk</u>
	Here's the milk. The milk is cold.
	The milk is in a big carton.
	The milk carton is heavy.
	Do you want chocolate milk? or white milk?
	The milk smells sour.
	The milk carton is empty.
	Pour some milk for _____(the kitty).
	Help _____ buy a quart of milk.
	Do you want milk on your cereal?
	Mix _____ with some milk.
	
	• <u>Teddy Bear</u>
	The teddy bear is soft.
	The teddy bear can sit.
	Make Teddy walk.
	The teddy bear's arms can move.
	His eyes are made of glass.
	The teddy bear's ears are on top of his head.
	The teddy bear has a music box inside.
	Look. His tongue is sticking out.
	
	• <u>Pants</u>
	Here are the pants. They have long legs.
	The pants have three pockets.
	One pocket has a penny in it. This pocket is turned inside out.
	The back pocket has a hole in it.
	The pants have belt loops.
	You put a belt through the loops.
	We have to wash your dirty pants.
	Hang up your pants.
	Fold your pants and put them away.
	You can wear your blue pants today.

OBJECTIVE: Parent Will Provide Activities At The Child's Interest Level.

How the Teacher Helps	What the Parent Does at Home
The child's interests grow out of his chronological (or developmental) age. His language grows out of his linguistic age. These two "ages" may not be synonymous. • The intervener can review with the parent child development and appropriate activities and toys for the developmental age of her child. • The teacher can help the parent to know what language to use at the child's linguistic level while stimulating his interests. • If the child demonstrates an interest in a concept, the teacher can point out this interest to the parent and then "brainstorm" with her to determine other situations throughout the day where this interest could be experienced again. • For example, if the child has just learned to cut with scissors and is interested in cutting things, he could be provided with a variety of experiences such as cutting paper, carrots, potatoes, toast, pancakes, fingernails, toenails, coupons, playdough, slice and bake cookies and so on. It is important to keep the child's mind stimulated by being at his interest level even though he may be at a lower language level.	Parents have special advantages because they can see first hand the changing interests of each child. Parents can take advantage of these interests at the moment when they are at their peak. For example: • A trip to the library to check out books about dogs because he loves dogs • A walk with the child because he wants to collect rocks • A night at the ball game because he is learning to play • A visit to a construction site because he loves big machines and tools • A trip to the Fun Center to ride on bumper boats because everyone at school is talking about them • A visit to the airport to watch the planes take off and land because he is fascinated with airplanes • A stop at the park to kick a soccer ball around a real soccer field because he thinks he might like to join the team.

OBJECTIVE: Parent Will Provide Linguistic Models For The Child Through Parallel Talk.

How the Teacher Helps	What the Parent Does at Home
Parallel talk involves talking at the child's interest level about what he is experiencing or what the mother wants him to experience. • The teacher can stress to the parent that this needs no extra props. It can be done with something as mundane as eating lunch or with something planned, such as carving a Jack-O-Lantern. • The parent simply describes what the child is doing or experiencing at the moment it is happening. • The teacher can monitor the parent's language to make certain it is neither too simple nor complex for the child at his level of linguistic development. • The teacher can model parallel talk for the parent during planned activities. • If the child is in a classroom, the parent can observe the child in class and pay close attention to the kind of parallel talk the teacher uses with her child during classroom experiences.	<u>Getting Dressed</u> Johnny, it's time to get dressed. Where are your shorts? You found them. They were in the top drawer. You put on your shorts all by yourself. Which shirt do you want to wear? That one? Okay. Johnny is wearing a blue shirt. Where are your socks? You were sitting on your socks! Can you get them on by yourself? Here are your shoes. Oops. You put that shoe on the wrong foot. There. You are all dressed. Look in the mirror. You look very nice. <u>Carving a Jack-O-Lantern</u> Here's your pumpkin. Do you know what you call a pumpkin with a face? Yes. It's a Jack-O-Lantern. Would you like to make a Jack-O-Lantern? Let's cut the eyes. The Jack-O-Lantern has two round eyes. Johnny wants a triangle for his nose. What kind of mouth should we make? Let's make a happy mouth. Johnny drew five teeth in his mouth. There! We made a smiling Jack-O-Lantern. Johnny put a candle in the Jack-O-Lantern. Mommy will light the candle.

OBJECTIVE: Parent Will Make A Special Effort To Include Structure Words In Her Language Models.

How the Teacher Helps	What the Parent Does at Home
Because of the importance of functors or structure words to the meaning of language, the hearing-impaired child needs to have many, many opportunities to hear these used in context. Structure words are words in the sentence that convey syntactic (see pp. 51, 90-91, 144-148 in Part I) meaning. At this point, these structure words are not expected to appear in the child's own speech. However, just as the parent of a hearing child would be talking to him at a level a year above his speaking age, so should the parent of a hearing-impaired child. • At this point when the parent is making a special effort to include structure words in her language models, hearing-aid use is mandatory because of the limited acoustic power and low visibility of these words. • The child may not hear them but he can note the length or time envelope of the modeled sentence and try to imitate it. • The teacher can remind the parent that the child needs to hear his <u>own</u> production of complete phrases or sentences. Does his production match what he hears? • The teacher can read to the parent and then ask her to list the function words used. (continued)	These structure words can be naturally included in a wide variety of household experiences. • Tie your shoelaces <u>so</u> you won't trip <u>on</u> them. • <u>If</u> you eat your meat, you <u>may</u> have <u>a</u> cookie. • Put <u>the</u> butter <u>in the</u> refrigerator. • I'm <u>in a</u> hurry. • You <u>may</u> get <u>the</u> milk <u>and</u> pour it <u>in the</u> pan. • The pudding <u>will</u> be ready <u>in a</u> minute. • You <u>could</u> empty <u>the</u> dishwasher while you are waiting. • You <u>can</u> go outside, <u>but</u> don't get your shoes wet. • Put <u>some</u> gravel <u>in the</u> fishbowl. • Be careful <u>so</u> it <u>doesn't</u> overflow. • <u>Did</u> you feed <u>the</u> fish <u>or</u> do you want me to? • There's <u>only a</u> little food left <u>in the</u> box. • You <u>may</u> take <u>some</u> cookies <u>to your</u> friend, <u>but</u> leave <u>one for</u> me.

OBJECTIVE: Parent Will Make A Special Effort To Include Structure Words In Her Language Models. (cont'd)

How the Teacher Helps	What the Parent Does at Home
• The teacher can read to the parent using "nonsense" words and then ask the parent to fill in the appropriate words, i.e. "The kams gambled on the glo but the keen gaged the oop." She should be able to do this task with fairly high accuracy because of her knowledge of the linguistic code which enhances the predictability of our language. The hearing-impaired child needs to hear natural sentences appropriate to the situation so he can accumulate knowledge of the linguistic code. • These structure words cannot be taught in isolation, they must be experienced in meaningful context. (See structure words pp. 51, 90-91, 144-148)	

OBJECTIVE: Parent's Utterances Will Deal With The Child's Interest In The Here And Now.

How the Teacher Helps	What the Parent Does at Home
Many are the eager parents who bring their children to school and want them to "show off" for the teacher. Mother says, "Tell Mrs. Jones where you went last summer." The child stares blankly at his distraught mother who took him on this educational trip. The trip was wonderful and a very valuable experience for the child, but the time to talk about it was while they were there or while they are looking at pictures that clearly represent things they did and talked about together.	Look around and tune in to the world and what is happening <u>right now</u>. There are interesting things to talk about all the time.
• A more successful approach to the above scenario would be for the parent and child to come to school with a meaningful treasure the child got while on his trip. The "treasure" is "here and now" and the child can talk about it successfully.	• the bug crawling up the wall • the leaves blowing off the trees • the bird feeding its babies • the worm crawling across the driveway • the sprinkler that goes slowly one direction and then twirls quickly back the other way • the neighbor mowing the grass
• Trips and experiences are extremely valuable for the child to build his cognitive base. They also provide many opportunities to use familiar language in a variety of situations. Just because he won't talk about them to teachers and relatives, it does not mean that he didn't receive any benefit from them.	• the dog playing catch with his master • the kite high up in the air • the man across the street sawing firewood • the neighbor up the street fixing his mailbox • the bulbs that Daddy is planting in the yard • the flat tire on big sister's bicycle
• Daily here-and-now activities are more important to the child at this level than are past events. He's more interested in the bug crawling up the wall than the ride he went on at Disneyland last summer. Parents need to capitalize on these rich cognitive experiences <u>at the time they are happening</u>.	• the twigs that blew down out of the tree in last night's rain storm OBSERVE—POINT IT OUT TO THE CHILD—TALK ABOUT IT!

OBJECTIVE: Parent Will Participate In Verbal Activity With The Child Such As Reading, Singing Songs Or Playing Games.

How the Teacher Helps	What the Parent Does at Home

Reading, singing songs or playing games are valuable activities for the parent and child. The teacher and parent can discuss their value:
 	
• There is much repetitive language in books and songs.
 	
• There are fun rhythms to hear and say in rhymes and songs.
 	
• Reading is an easy way to provide experiences with new people, places and ideas.
 	
• Games can provide a fun way to practice using certain language or concepts.
 	
• Books, games and songs allow for one-to-one time for the parent and child.
 	
• The parent can recite nursery rhyme, story or song and show pictures as a representation.
 	
• Later the parent can have children identify which rhyme, story or song she said or sang by selecting the correct picture.
	• Reading nursery rhymes. There are many beautifully illustrated nursery rhyme books at local bookstores or libraries.
	
	• Acting out fingerplays or rhymes with actions. Young children love to learn these. A familiar fingerplay would be the Eency Weency Spider. There are many others dealing with certain topics or seasonal subjects. Again, Fingerplay books are available at bookstores or libraries.
	
	• Playing games such as Follow the Leader or Ring Around the Rosie. Consult your local library for those that are of interest to children the age of your child. Also, Mother can check with her friends to see what games their children are playing.
	
	• Sports provide an opportunity to use a variety of language and concepts. The parent can provide inexpensive equipment and have fun. The language will be as varied as the games, the equipment and the rules.
	
	• Reading a book. The technique for reading to hearing-impaired children proceeds through a series of stages:
	  1. Labeling the pictures. "See the doggie. Show me the kitty. Nice kitty."
	  2. Picture descriptions. "The doggie is chasing the cat. The cat ran up a tree."
	
	(continued)

OBJECTIVE: **Parent Will Participate In Verbal Activity With The Child Such As Reading, Singing Songs Or Playing Games. (cont'd)**

How the Teacher Helps	What the Parent Does at Home
	3. <u>Paraphrase the story</u>. "This is a story about three bears: Daddy Bear, Mommy Bear and Baby Bear. One-two-three bears. Mommy and Daddy and Baby Bear lived in this house. There's Mommy Bear's chair. There's Daddy Bear's chair. And there's Baby Bear's chair. Where's your chair?" and so on... **4.** <u>Read the story as it is printed</u>. At this point, the child is probably at the "Picture Description" stage or at the stage where Mother "paraphrases the story." Don't read the actual story at this stage.

OBJECTIVE: **Parent Will Give The Child The Linguistic Form That She Believes To Express His Thought And Wait For Him To Imitate It.**

How the Teacher Helps	What the Parent Does at Home
Adults must continue to take their cues for language input from the child's attempts at communication. The adult listens to what the child says, examines the situation to get clues for his meaning, and then expands the child's incomplete utterance into a complete phrase or sentence.	Many opportunities come up throughout the day when the parent could expand the child's language. <u>Child Language with Adult Expansion</u>

Adults must continue to take their cues for language input from the child's attempts at communication. The adult listens to what the child says, examines the situation to get clues for his meaning, and then expands the child's incomplete utterance into a complete phrase or sentence.

- This takes practice and guidance because the expansions required from the parent are constantly changing as the child's language develops. The parent needs to keep changing because she wants to be challenging him and exposing him to language one step above his present level of development.

- The teacher can ask the parent to bring in a language sample of spontaneous language used by the child during a given period of time.

- The teacher and parent can discuss the language sample. What did Mother do about the incomplete utterances? Did she expand them? What would have been some of her expansions?

- The teacher and parent can discuss how to put linguistic form to these utterances.

(continued)

Many opportunities come up throughout the day when the parent could expand the child's language.
<u>Child Language with Adult Expansion</u>
CL: "me does"
AE: "This is what I do."
CL: "my touch that?"
AE: "Can I touch that?"
CL: "big ball?"
AE: "Where is the big ball?"
CL: "big ladder...out"
AE: "I want to get the big ladder out."
CL: "outside...swing"
AE: "I want to go outside and swing."

Parents can observe the child at home and determine if the child is lacking common expressions to communicate some of his needs. For example, if the child's brother takes his car away, the child's immediate reaction may be to respond physically with hitting or grabbing it away. A more socially acceptable solution would be to say, "That's mine! Give it back!"

- The hearing-impaired child needs to have these types of expressions modeled for him <u>when the situation occurs:</u>
    "Move over."
    "I was there first."
    "That makes me angry."
    "Don't do that!"
    "It's my turn."
    "May I have another one?"

OBJECTIVE: **Parent Will Give Child The Linguistic Form For That She Believes To Express His Thought And Wait For Him To Imitate It. (cont'd)**

How the Teacher Helps	What the Parent Does at Home
• The teacher could set up some "worksheets" for the parents to help them gain practice in expanding their child's language attempts. The teacher can write the child's language attempts on the left side of the page (based on a language sample taken during the session at the center) and leave some spaces on the right side of the paper for the parent to write in how she would model that language.	

OBJECTIVE: Parent Will Use Prosodic Features Prominently To Help The Child Imitate.

How the Teacher Helps	What the Parent Does at Home
When the parent is modeling a sentence for the child to imitate, she phrases it into thought concepts and puts the emphasis where appropriate to stress the meaning. After the child has imitated the sentence, the parent puts it back together and says it once again so the child can hear the whole. • The teacher demonstrates breaking the sentences into thought concepts. This is different from just chopping the sentence into words. Each phrase must have meaning that "stands alone." • For example, take the sentence: "I don't want to go to bed." If it were chopped into words, the child would be imitating something like this: (I don't) (want to) (go to) (bed.) The meaning of the sentence gets lost. However, if the sentence is phrased into thought units, it retains and even emphasizes its meaning: (I don't want) (to go to bed).	Sample sentences that may occur at home: • I want to go outside and swing. (I want) (to go outside) (and swing). • Where is the big ball? (Where is) (the big ball)? • Johnny put the candle in the Jack-O-Lantern. (Johnny put) (the candle) (in the Jack-O-Lantern). • Johnny wants a triangle for his nose. (Johnny wants) (a triangle) (for his nose). • I don't want to go to the doctor. (I don't want) (to go) (to the doctor). Remember: after the child has imitated the phrases, put the sentence back together and say it once again so the child can hear the whole.

OBJECTIVE: **Parent Will Reinforce The Child's Efforts In A Positive Manner.**

How the Teacher Helps	What the Parent Does at Home
Learning to talk is hard work for the child as well as for the parent. The child constantly needs to be reinforced for his efforts. • Teacher can suggest to the parent that she does not give negative reinforcement, such as: "No, not like that." "I can't understand a thing you say." "Your speech is horrible." • Instead, a parent can reinforce the child's effort in a positive manner by: – listening to him – expanding his sentence for him to hear – giving him a hug, a kiss, a pat on the back, a wink – giving him eye-to-eye contact – giving him undivided attention – repeating his utterances • If the parent wants the child to talk, then she needs to make it worth his time and effort. This effort needs to be rewarded. We are reminded of a child who wouldn't wear his hearing aid. When asked why he didn't wear it, his reply was that it was because all he ever heard when he wore it was "no."	Parent can reinforce the child in verbal and nonverbal ways: – a hug – a pat on the back – with clapping – a wink – by giving him your undivided attention – by putting down what you are doing or turning off the TV to listen to him – by commenting on what he has to say – by helping him find books or pictures to supplement his information – by writing down what he says and drawing an illustration to make a little story Parent can reinforce the child by giving encouragement: – Good job! – I like the way you did that! – That's exciting. Let's go tell Daddy. – You said that just right! – Good for you! – I like the way you said that. – Good sentence!

OBJECTIVE : Parent Will Express The Same Idea In Many Different Ways.

How the Teacher Helps	What the Parent Does at Home
Parents often find a particular way to say something and because the child understands it easily, they continue to use the same expression. This is much as if they had a "rubber stamp" that was used over and over. i.e., "Received in Shipping." Natural language used by hearing children is never stereotyped. • The teacher can help the parents avoid "rubber stamping" their child's language by exposing him to more colorful language and giving him different ways of saying the same things. • The teacher can point out situations where the parent can give the child an alternative way of saying something.	The parent should help the child's expressions "grow up." What was acceptable six months ago should be "updated" now. "<u>I have an owie.</u>" becomes... 　"I have a bruise." 　"I have a hangnail." 　"I scraped my knee." 　"I skinned my elbow." "<u>It's time to go bye-bye.</u>" becomes... 　"It's time to go home." 　"It's time to go to school." 　"It's time to leave." "<u>Fall down...</u>"becomes... 　"The blocks fell over." 　"The blocks fell off the table." 　"You knocked the blocks down." "<u>All gone...</u>" becomes... 　"The cup is empty." 　"There is no more juice." 　"I can't find it." 　"Mommy put it away." The parent should become more specific or colorful in her description of things. If the child uses "good," she should begin to talk about "delicious cookies," "wonderful pie," "scrumptious cake." If he uses "big" and "little," the parent could begin to talk about a "large dog," "a small cat," "an enormous elephant," "a tiny little mouse."

OBJECTIVE: Parent Will See That Experiences Are Repeated.

How the Teacher Helps	What the Parent Does at Home

Children learn through repetition.
• Teachers need to point out to parents that they don't need to create this, it comes about naturally just through the repetitive quality of our daily lives.
• The most meaningful experiences are nothing different from daily living. The experiences don't have to be contrived.
• The intervener needs to be constantly aware of the environment of each family. If she wants the experiences to be repeated at home, then the experiences she demonstrates or models for the parent have to be ones out of that particular family's daily life.
• For example, she should not be making peanut butter in the food processor with an inner city family that is struggling to make ends meet with welfare payments and food stamps. This is not <u>their</u> reality!
	There is much repetition in "round the clock" activities.
	<u>Rise'n Shine</u>
	  get dressed
	  eat breakfast
	  clean up the kitchen
	
	<u>Helping Mommy</u>
	  do the laundry
	  put the clothes away
	  vacuum and dust
	  wash the floor
	
	<u>Playtime</u>
	  play with toys
	  read a book
	  play games
	
	<u>Lunchtime</u>
	  fix lunch
	  eat lunch
	  clean up the kitchen
	
	<u>Outings</u>
	  grocery shopping
	  go to the bank
	  put gas in the car
	  go to the car wash
	
	<u>Dinnertime</u>
	  fix dinner
	  eat dinner
	  clean up the kitchen
	
	<u>Time with Daddy</u>
	  mow the grass
	  go for a walk
	  play ball
	  read a book
	
	<u>Bedtime</u>
	  take a bath
	  put on pajamas
	  have a snack
	  brush teeth
	  read a book
	  turn out the lights
	
	ALL IN A DAY'S WORK!

OBJECTIVE: Parent Will Ask Questions.

How the Teacher Helps	What the Parent Does at Home
One of the most important elements in a child's advanced language is his ability to ask and answer questions. Providing him experience with questions now will help lay the foundation for more advanced forms of questions later on.	These are routine questions used to get information that is readily available to the child. The information sought is either within the child's visual field or well-known to him.

More detailed correspondence:

How the Teacher Helps

One of the most important elements in a child's advanced language is his ability to ask and answer questions. Providing him experience with questions now will help lay the foundation for more advanced forms of questions later on.

- The teacher can be aware of:
  What kind of questions does Mother ask?
  What kind of response does the child give?
  Does Mother wait for a response?
- The teacher can make suggestions for the types of questions the parent should be asking.
- At this point, the parent may need to give the child alternative answers to choose from. For example, Mother asks "Where is your jacket?" The child looks puzzled. She gives him alternative answers to choose from or to give him the idea of the type of answer she is looking for: "Is it in the closet? on your bed?" The child then gets the idea he is to give a response that indicates a location and he is then able to respond, "In the garage."
- If the child doesn't give a verbal answer to the above question, but indicates his understanding by responding appropriately and going to get his jacket out of the garage, Mother will need to model his answer: "In the garage" or "My jacket was in the garage."

What the Parent Does at Home

These are routine questions used to get information that is readily available to the child. The information sought is either within the child's visual field or well-known to him.

- What's that noise?
- What's that? (an object for identification)
- What does a doggy say?
- What do you want?

- Where's Daddy?
- Where's your ball?
- Where's your nose?
- Where are you going?

- Who's that?

- Which one do you want? (choices presented)

- Yes/No Questions
- Do you want more?
- Are you finished?

- Why do you want ___?

- How will you get the cookie?

- When did Grandma come?
- When will we go to see Santa Claus?

Some possible objectives that might be considered at this time are:

- For the parent to take the child's utterances and expand them into complete and/or correct language. **297**
- For the parent to expand the child's sentence to include appropriate structure words. **298**
- For the parent to model new ideas related to the child's utterances. **299**
- For the parent to keep a scrapbook. **300**
- For the parent to use drawings to serve as a reference. **301**
- For the parent to point out perceptual characteristics (e.g. of smell, touch, taste, sight and sound) while talking about items. **302**
- For the parent to expand the child's experiences by trips into the community. **304**
- For the parent to provide experiences that naturally promote active learning and talk about the concept of <u>classification</u>. **307**
- For the parent to provide experiences that naturally promote active learning and talk about the concept of <u>causality</u>. **309**
- For the parent to provide experiences that naturally promote active learning and talk about the concept of <u>contingencies</u>. **310**
- For the parent to provide experiences that naturally promote active learning and talk about the concept of <u>spatial relations</u>. **311**
- For the parent to provide experiences that naturally promote active learning and talk about the concept of <u>time</u>. **312**
- For the parent to ask questions (information—seeking, open-ended and choice questions). **313**
- For the parent to provide experiences to further the child's social development. **314**

OBJECTIVE: **Parent Will Take Child's Utterances And Expand Them Into Complete And/Or Correct Language.**

How the Teacher Helps	What the Parent Does at Home
As the child's language develops, the parent's expansions increase in difficulty. The parent wants to remember to challenge the child and present language to him one step above his current level of development. • The teacher can monitor the parent's expansions to make sure that she isn't "rubber stamping" the child's language. • The teacher can ask the parent to bring in a language sample of the child's spontaneous language. The teacher and parent can discuss possible expansions of his incomplete or incorrect language. • The teacher can present a language sample taken in the session or class of the child's spontaneous language. The teacher and parent can discuss possible expansions of his incomplete or incorrect language. • The teacher can request that the parent observe the child in class on a regular basis and observe the type of expansions the teacher is using with the child.	Many opportunities for expansion of the child's language will occur throughout the day. The parent will need to take her child's language attempt as her guide to the difficulty of the expansion. • Child is searching through Mom's purse while Mom is putting on her coat to go. Child says, "Keys?" Expansion: "Where are your keys?" • Child is giving a doll a bath and the doll falls down in the tub. Child says, "Baby fall down." Expansion: "The baby fell in the water." • Child could not open closet door. Mother opens it to get a toy out. Child says, "Door....big." Expansion: "The big door is hard to open." • Child is going to pound on a pan lid with a wooden spoon. He says, "Mommy cover that ear—that ear." Expansion: "Mommy will cover both ears."
The expansion must preserve the original thought of the child. Match the language to the thought!	Sometimes if a child consistently uses an incorrect expression, the parent can use a different strategy. • Child consistently says, "Me do" to indicate he wants to do it himself. Mother can say, "When you want to do it, you can say, 'I want to do it!' Can you say that?"

OBJECTIVE: Parent Will Expand Child's Sentence To Include Appropriate Structure Words.

How the Teacher Helps	What the Parent Does at Home

Structure words are important to the meaning of our language. The hearing-impaired child needs to have many opportunities to perceive these words used in context. One way of doing that is for the parent to expand the child's sentence to include those appropriate structure words that he has left out.
 	
• Since these structure words cannot be taught in isolation, there is no better time to experience them than at the time the child has the need to use them.
 	
• The teacher can remind the parent that the child needs to hear his own production of complete phrases or sentences including these structure words in the appropriate place. Does his production match what the adult has said? In length? In stress? In number of units?
 	
• The teacher needs to remind the parent to listen carefully for the structure words that have been left out. Our own ears have the unique ability to "fill in" many of the little words that have been left out because we're so used to hearing them and we know where they go. We want the hearing-impaired child to have the same advantage: that of being able to predict which word was used— to use Information Theory.
	Parent can listen carefully for the child's omission of these structure words and then give him the expansion of his sentence to include them.
	
	Child Language with Adult Expansion
	CL: "My touch that?"
	AE: "Can I touch that?"
	CL: "My down Jesse's house."
	AE: "I'm going down to Jesse's house."
	CL: "My watch movie Tommy house."
	AE: "I watched a movie at Tommy's house."
	CL: "Put baby bed."
	AE: "Put the baby in the bed."
	CL: "Me ride skateboard."
	AE: "I ride on a skateboard."
	
	At this point many of these child utterances are perfectly understandable. Adults have the tendency to respond appropriately to the meaning of the child's sentence and don't notice the structure words that have been left out.
	
	For example, if the child said, "My watch movie Tommy house." The parent might respond, "You did? What movie did you watch?" This is an appropriate response. However, we are suggesting that she also "slip in" an expansion of the child's utterance. It might go something like this:
	    "You watched a movie at Tommy's house?
	    What movie did you watch?"

OBJECTIVE: Parent Will Model New Ideas Related To The Child's Utterances.

How the Teacher Helps	What the Parent Does at Home
At this stage, language is becoming conversation—the talk <u>with</u> the child. The nature of a conversation between two people is that it flows back and forth with each person adding comments. The critical factor is that they stay on the same topic. If a person can only give one sentence on a topic, he cannot be a part of that conversation for very long, and communication breaks down. Children often talk in fragmented thoughts and have difficulty staying on topic. A "super mom" would help her child learn this important conversational skill by offering new ideas related to what the child has just said. The "almost mother" would usually keep to the single utterance per topic. • The teacher can observe and make certain that these new ideas are at the child's interest and age level. • The parent will use appropriately sophisticated language in her conversations with her child.	This is where the title, "Talk WITH the Child" comes into action. That is what this objective is all about: sharing a time with the child and sharing information that you have that he might be interested in. This modeling of new ideas can be used alone or in combination with expanding the child's incomplete utterance. Here are some examples. The new idea that has been modeled will be underlined. Child says: "Man drive truck." Adult says: "The man is driving the truck. <u>Look at the dirt in that truck. That's a dump truck.</u>" Child says: "Dog barking." Adult says: "The dog is barking. <u>I think he sees the mailman walking up the street.</u>" Child says: "Blow nose." Adult says: "You need to blow your nose. <u>Do you have a bad cold?</u>" Child says: "Telephone ringing." Adult says: "I hear the telephone ringing. <u>Maybe Daddy is calling.</u>" Child says: "All done puzzle." Adult says: "Are you all done with the puzzle? <u>Look at all the animals in that puzzle. Which one do you like?</u>"

OBJECTIVE: Parent Will Keep A Scrapbook.

How the Teacher Helps	What the Parent Does at Home

Scrapbooks can be used very successfully to reinforce general life experiences as well as important events. They give the child a "here and now" way of recalling and retelling past events.
 	
• Sometimes the teacher can help parents get started making a scrapbook.
 	
• If the teacher takes the child on a fieldtrip, she can demonstrate how she would make a scrapbook page to reinforce that trip.
 	
• The teacher can show the parents samples of scrapbooks that parents have made in the past. If they see that scrapbooks don't have to be elaborate, maybe they will feel more ready to tackle the project.
 	
• The teacher can encourage the parents to be "scavengers" and look for anything that may serve as a memento of a trip or event:
  – placemats, napkins
  – postcards
  – ticket stubs
  – brochures
  – photographs
  – T-shirts
 	
• The teacher can encourage the parent to be tuned in to the child's interests. The parent may be intent on teaching the child about the mountains, but if the child is more interested in the semi-trailer trucks seen along the highway, these need to be talked about too.
	Parents can make scrapbooks to reinforce everyday experiences. The scrapbook can be organized into categories:
	  – Things I Wear
	  – Things I Like to Eat
	  – Things I Don't Like to Eat
	  – Things I Like to Play With
	  – Sports I Like
	  – People I Know
	  – My Family
	  – Things I Like to Do
	
	• A large scrapbook can be used as an ongoing experience book. The pictures, postcards and souvenirs that have been collected can be organized into places or events, i.e., Dairy Farm, The Zoo, Picnics, Birthday Parties, Holidays, etc.
	
	• A Summer Vacation Scrapbook can be made effectively with some pre-planning. Parents can write to the Chamber of Commerce in the city where they will be visiting and ask for brochures and information about the area. If they have motel reservations, the motel could be asked to send a postcard ahead of time. Parents can cut out the most descriptive pictures of the area and begin a trip book. They can cut out pieces of cardboard to put together for a book or do something as simple as pasting the pictures in a spiral notebook. This book can be taken on the trip along with some glue, tape, pencils and pens so it can be added to as they go along. As always, parents need to be tuned in to the child's interests, and reinforce these in the book.

OBJECTIVE: Parent Will Use Drawings To Serve As A Reference.

How the Teacher Helps	What the Parent Does at Home
A parent can write some simple experience stories with her child about something that happened (or is going to happen) of particular significance to him. Those trips to the zoo, airplane rides to Grandma's house, experience with the new baby, a trip to the hospital, a bus ride or even a visit to the neighborhood playground could be reinforced with the child after they are finished. • Photographs, postcards, train tickets, hand-drawn pictures or any souvenir to help the child recreate the experience can be used in making experience stories. • In writing these stories, the parent can choose five or six of the most significant things that happened and write one sentence and illustration on a page. • The parent can use cardboard so the child can easily turn the pages. The pages can be hooked together with rings or yarn. If desired, she could cover these pages with clear self-adhesive vinyl for durability. • Parents who are not "great artists" do not need to worry. Children will accept almost any representation if they have had the experience and can help with drawing. Parents can ask, "What do we draw here?"	A simple story about a trip to the playground might look something like this: Mommy and Amy went to the playground. / Amy slid down the slide five times! Mommy pushed the swing so high! / Amy fell in the mud and got all dirty. Amy got dizzy on the merry-go-round. / The water in the fountain was cold.

OBJECTIVE: Parent Will Point Out Perceptual Characteristics (Of Smell, Touch, Taste, Sight And Sounds) While Talking About Items.

How the Teacher Helps	What the Parent Does at Home

Perceptual characteristics of an object must be experienced to help the child learn the language and make it "his." The optimal time for the parent to point these out to the child is while they are talking about and using a particular item.
 	
 • The intervener can remind the parent to become aware of the perceptions of smell, touch, taste, sight, and sound and use them in relation to the things the child is interested in and relating to.
 	
 • There are fascinating things to point out to a child about even the most mundane items. He needs to have the language to talk about these things and the curiosity to find out more information.
 	
 • Pointing out perceptual characteristics helps a child to become more observant and interested in his environment. An interested, curious child is more motivated to learn.
 	
 • The teacher can suggest to the parent that she can play guessing games such as, "I'm thinking of something with four legs. What is it?"
 	
 • The teacher can suggest to the parent that she could play "I Spy" as another variation of a guessing game. Mother says, "I Spy with my eyes something that is green." The child can look around the room and guess everything that he perceives as green or else ask for more clues.
 	
 (continued)
	The parent has the raw materials and resources for wonderful perceptual experiences right in her own back yard and even the living room!
	
	 • Take a look at that caterpillar crawling across the driveway:
	
	   – He is crawling slowly.
	   – He is fuzzy.
	   – He tickles your hand when he crawls across it.
	   – He is dark orange and brown—some people think this means we will have a hard winter.
	   – He doesn't make any noise.
	
	 • When you water the plant in the living room, have you noticed that:
	
	   – Some of the leaves are wilted.
	   – Some of the leaves have fallen off.
	   – The dirt is very cracked and dry.
	   – The leaves feel fuzzy.
	   – The water sits on top of the dirt before it soaks down into the dirt
	   – Some of the water runs through and comes out the bottom.
	   – A little while after you water it, the leaves perk up.
	   – The plant is leaning toward the window.
	   – If you turn the plant around, it will lean toward the window the other way in a couple of days.

OBJECTIVE: **Parent Will Point Out Perceptual Characteristics (of Smell, Touch, Taste, Sight And Sounds) While Talking About Items. (cont'd)**

How the Teacher Helps	What the Parent Does at Home
• The parent and child could take a "Walk" through the house and find things that roll, things that grow, things that are blue, etc.	

OBJECTIVE: Parent Will Expand The Child's Experiences By Trips Into The Community.

How the Teacher Helps	What the Parent Does at Home
It has been said that when a person goes about the task of learning to read, for example, he brings to that task the bag and baggage of his experiences. These past experiences help him to know more about his world so when he reads a story, he can apply this prior knowledge and read with some comprehension, grasp the implications of what he has read as well as surmise from the context what isn't written down.	THINGS TO DO AND PLACES TO GO
	• <u>Going to a shopping center</u> just to explore, not necessarily to buy. As the child looks at things, handles some, the parent is stimulating him and learning about his interests.
• Hearing-impaired children need as broad a base of experiences as possible.	• <u>Sitting on a river bank</u> watching the boats, the trains, or cars over the bridges. It's a fun place for learning.
• Going on experiences into the community will give the child the opportunity to apply his language to a variety of situations	• <u>Picking peaches, apples or strawberries</u> at any number of farms in many areas. Watch the newspaper for notices of when these fruits are available for picking.
• The teacher can help the parent pursue the resources of the community.	• <u>Going to the pumpkin patch</u> to select just the right pumpkin for that special Jack-O-Lantern. Watch the paper for notices of when the patches are open. Some also have other special related activities like hayrides or hot-dog roasts that would also provide lots of language and wonderful memories.
• One of the authors spent a summer visiting all the local parks and recreation areas in the community in an effort to have first-hand knowledge of their benefits to the child. She then compiled a list of these and included a brief description of each. This list was organized according to categories: Places to go to learn about vehicles, animals, foods, outdoor sports and so on. This could be done in any community.	• <u>Finding a real farm</u> not far away. Seeing farm animals and things growing can be information that will be worthwhile and help build a firm foundation for his subsequent social studies. Call your County Extension Office or Chamber of Commerce for possible suggestions.
(continued)	((continued)

OBJECTIVE: **Parent Will Expand Child's Experiences By Trips Into The Community. (cont'd)**

How the Teacher Helps	What the Parent Does at Home
• As sophisticated language begins to emerge, the parent's role expands beyond the home. Up to now, we have stressed that parents have all the resources they need within the scope of their daily experiences. Now they need to add to their resources by taking full advantage of the learning potential of their community.	• Visiting the airport is lots of fun. Try parking where the child can watch the planes land and take off. Some airlines will allow a parent and child to board a plane to look around if you call and make arrangements for times when they are not busy. • Watching a construction site is fascinating. It seems that shopping centers are popping up everywhere and it's interesting to watch the large equipment and men guiding huge steel beams into place with ease and accuracy. • Visiting a zoo is always fun for children. Many zoos have train rides, petting areas and lots of animals who look different, sound different, move differently and live in different environments. • Visiting an art museum is an experience in beauty and tranquillity and exposes children to art forms they might not otherwise have the opportunity to see. • Visiting a state fair is a great way to see all types of farm animals in abundance. Also, you can watch livestock judging, riding competition, tractor pulls, etc. Contact the State Fair Office for schedules of events that may be of special interest to the child. (continued)

OBJECTIVE: Parent Will Expand Child's Experiences By Trips Into The Community. (cont'd)

How the Teacher Helps	What the Parent Does at Home
	• <u>Visiting a park</u> offers varied experiences. Hungry ducks and geese are waiting to be fed in some parks. Ice skating can be watched or enjoyed at some locations. Fishing is allowed in some area parks. Picnics are always a must for a visit to the park. Pack the picnic basket together for more fun. Playground equipment usually comes with the territory at a park. Check out different parks in the area for more variety of play opportunities.

OBJECTIVE: **Parent Will Provide Experiences That Naturally Promote Active Learning And Talk About The Concept of <u>Classification.</u>**

How the Teacher Helps	What the Parent Does at Home
Classification is a cognitive skill that assists learning and is one of the fundamental skills of learning. When new language can be filed under appropriate classifications, it can be retrieved more easily. • Stories of experiences are one way of classifying things that go together. • Nouns need to be classified with the right verbs and adjectives so as to prevent language errors of "burry tree," "noisy moon," etc. • The teacher can remind the parent of the way adults use classification: We classify blue, gray, aqua as cool colors. We classify red, orange, yellow as warm colors. We classify run, skip, jump as action verbs. We classify I, you and me as personal pronouns. We classify 75 to 90 dB as severely deaf. We classify 90dB+ as profoundly deaf. We classify Mercedes and Rolls Royce as cars belonging to rich people. • The teacher can remind the parent of the way classification can be used with children: A child classifies pens, pencils crayons as things that write. He classifies boots, shoes, slippers, socks, sandals as things to wear on his feet. (continued)	• To introduce classification at home, Mother can talk about things as she uses them: "Mommy will put in an apple, a banana and some grapes. These are all fruits. Put the bowl of fruit on the table." "Let's put away your toys. Here's your truck, your blocks and your puzzles. You have lots of toys. Put your toys on the shelf." "What kind of cereal do you want? Here's Frosty O's, Freaky Flakes, Crunchy Munch. Is Freaky Flakes your favorite cereal? Can you put away the rest of the cereal?" • In using classification at home, Mother can say: — Get me something to write with. — Go find something to play with. — I need something to cut with. — You need to put something on your feet. — Can you find something I can use to wrap this? — You may eat a piece of fruit. — What vegetable shall we have for dinner? — What toy do you want to get for your friend? — What clothes do you want to wear? — What friends do you want to come to your party? — Put the fruit in the refrigerator and the cereal in the pantry.

OBJECTIVE: **Parent Will Provide Experiences That Naturally Promote Active Learning And Talk About The Concept of <u>Classification</u> (cont'd)**

How the Teacher Helps	What the ParentDoes at Home
He learns to classify apples, bananas, pears, grapes as fruit. He classifies dolls, trucks, blocks as toys. He classifies shirts, pants, sweaters, dresses as clothes. He classifies Johnny, Jimmy, David and Bradley as friends. • The child needs to learn the fundamental cognitive skill of classification to help him learn more effectively, to share his ideas ("I like fruit"), to manipulate his environment ("Please get some fruit at the store") and to store the information mentally.	

OBJECTIVE: Parent Will Provide Experiences That Naturally Promote Active Learning And Talk About The Concept Of <u>Causality</u>.

How the Teacher Helps	What the Parent Does at Home
Causality is the relation of effect to cause. If I do this, it will cause something to happen. • Learning to deal with causality requires the child to "think" with his language and to draw on his past experiences. • This will allow him to sharpen his skill at predicting outcomes of experiments, of stories, of his actions. • This cognitive skill will allow him to answer the question: What will happen if.........?	Causality can be expressed and discussed many times throughout the day. • <u>At breakfast</u>: If you spill the juice, the floor will be sticky. • <u>At playtime</u>: If you don't stop fighting, you will go to your room. • <u>Helping Mommy</u>: If you don't water the plant, it will die. • <u>At bedtime</u>: If you unplug the clock, the alarm won't ring in the morning.

OBJECTIVE: Parent Will Provide Experiences That Naturally Promote Active Learning And Talk About The Concept of <u>Contingencies.</u>

How the Teacher Helps	What the Parent Does at Home
• Contingency is the interrelation of two actions, not caused by one or the other but happening together. • Contingency is a cognitive experience that children can learn so easily in their experiential world and is so difficult when deductive examples must be used.	Contingencies can be expressed and discussed many times through the day. • We will eat dinner when Daddy gets home. • Grandma rode in an airplane when she came to visit. • The dusting was done before we ran the vacuum. • After we stirred the pudding, we ate it. • While we watched television, Daddy went to sleep. • Johnny played with his trucks while Mommy fixed supper. • When Tom comes over, we can watch television.

OBJECTIVE: **Parent Will Provide Experiences That Naturally Promote Active Learning And Talk About The Concept Of <u>Spatial Relations.</u>**

How the Teacher Helps	What the Parent Does at Home
This involves helping the child to understand the relationship of things and people. • Describing the positions of things in relation to each other (in, on, under, over, on top of). • Describing the movement of things and people (toward, from, to, into, out of). • Describing relative distances between things (close, next to, near, far). • Learning to find things around the house, at school, in the neighborhood. • Describing the relative size dimensions of people, animals and objects. All of these concepts require cognitive ability. Putting language to these concepts is necessary for the child to learn, share his ideas and manipulate his environment.	The concept of spatial relations can be discussed and experienced throughout the day. • At breakfast: Put the bowl <u>on</u> the table. Put the milk <u>in</u> the refrigerator. Put the spoon <u>next to</u> the bowl. This spoon is <u>bigger than</u> that one. • At playtime: Put the doll <u>between</u> the teddy bear and the giraffe. Put the books <u>on</u> the shelf. The car rolled <u>under</u> the chair. Back the car <u>out of</u> the garage. This <u>little</u> car fits <u>inside</u> the <u>big</u> moving van. • When helping Mommy: Take the dirty clothes <u>out of</u> the hamper. Spray the polish <u>on</u> the table. Put the vase back <u>on top of</u> the mantle. Plug the vacuum in here, that plug is too <u>far</u>. • Outside in the neighborhood: Johnny lives <u>next to</u> David. We can't walk to Tommy's house, he lives too <u>far</u>. The <u>enormous</u> airplane flew <u>over</u> the house. That new house is the <u>largest</u> one in the neighborhood. • At bedtime: Crawl <u>under</u> the covers.

OBJECTIVE: Parent Will Provide Experiences That Naturally Promote Active Learning And Talk About The Concept Of <u>Time.</u>

How the Teacher Helps	What the Parent Does at Home
The child who is probably in preschool now, needs to understand and describe the relationship of people and events in time in order to understand and manipulate his environment which is becoming more and more abstract. • The teacher can encourage the child to make plans and discuss with him his plans and experiences. • The teacher can encourage the parent to anticipate and describe future events for her child and help him prepare for them. • The parent can talk about the order of things. • The parent can help the child understand and talk about conventional time units (yesterday, today, tomorrow, hour). • The parent can help the child understand and talk about seasonal changes as they occur.	The concept of time can be experienced and verbalized as the child goes through his day. • <u>At breakfast:</u> "Eat your egg first before it gets cold." "After you finish eating breakfast, we will go to the park." "We should eat the donuts we bought yesterday before they get stale." • <u>At playtime:</u> "Today I am going to build a house. First I will make a floor, then I will make some walls, and last I will put on the roof." "Can Tommy come over to my house tomorrow?" "After you are finished with the playdough, please clean it up." • <u>At bedtime:</u> "It's time to go to sleep." "You will have to turn out your lights in a few minutes." "When you're finished with that book, turn off your lights."

OBJECTIVE: **Parent Will Ask Questions (Information Seeking, Open-ended And Choice Questions.)**

How the Teacher Helps	What the Parent Does at Home

The ability to ask and answer questions is an important element in a child's advanced language system. Questioning is an integral component of the back-and-forth quality of conversations. In order to be able to sustain the conversation, a child must be able to answer questions appropriate for his linguistic age. He needs experience with questions used for different purposes that include:
    – questions used to seek missing information
    – questions to pose problems and seek acceptable solutions
    – questions to make choices
    – questions to determine the child's knowledge of a subject
    – open-ended questions where there are no "right" or "wrong" answers
 	
• Many questions are asked when a child gets to school.
 	
• Before a child encounters these questions in the abstract realm of the formal classroom, it is important that they are used in reality situations now.
 	
• For the development of his understanding of question forms, a child must experience a large number of meaningful conversations that include questions and answers. Without this experience, he cannot know when it is appropriate to ask certain questions or what constitutes an appropriate answer.
	The following are some examples of questions that can be asked. The answers may need to be modeled for the child at this point.
	    What is he eating?
	    Why is he eating?
	
	    Which one do you want?
	    Why did you choose that one?
	    What would you do if all the chocolate cookies were gone?
	    What do you think might happen if we all wanted chocolate cookies and there weren't enough?
	
	(looking out the window)
	    What kind of day is it today?
	    How can you tell that it's rainy? windy?
	    What should you wear on a rainy day?
	    Why do we wear coats and boots made of plastic or rubber in the rain?
	    Do you know where the sun is on a cloudy day?

OBJECTIVE: Parent Will Provide Experiences To Further The Child's Social Development.

How the Teacher Helps	What the Parent Does at Home
No matter how well a hearing-impaired child has developed oral language, if he does not have the social skills to apply that language ability, he will not be able to reach his full potential. • Providing social experiences where the child can have success at an early age will help prevent walls from forming around the child • Carefully guiding the child, talking about problems he encounters and possible solutions will be necessary. • Investigating mainstream social opportunities ahead of time can save frustration and disappointment later on. • The adults in charge of the social activity must be accepting and willing to take the extra time and effort required to interact with a hearing-impaired child. If the adult is not receptive to the child, another social situation should be sought. • Mainstreaming of hearing-impaired children does not "just happen." It takes careful guidance on the part of loving, caring adults to make it successful. Adults who know when to intervene as well as when to let go. • The parent needs to realize that she can't fight all of her child's battles for him. There will be times when things don't go so well. But maybe that's true of all children and not just hearing-impaired children.	The following are some suggestions for parents to explore: – inviting a friend over – having a play group where the responsibly for hosting the group rotates among a small group of mothers – religious school (Sunday School, Bible School) – Scouting organizations – dance classes – gymnastics – library story time – classes at the local Children's Museum – classes at local community colleges are sometimes held for young children – enrolling in a preschool for normally hearing children At all times the parent should remember that nothing is "etched in stone." If one situation is not working out, maybe there is another situation with fewer language expectations that might be better for the present time. It needs to be fun for the child if he is to receive any benefit from the experience.

Some possible objectives that might be considered at this stage are:

- For the parent to understand the <u>importance</u> of wearing hearing aids. **317**
- For the parent to establish consistent, hearing-aid use during all waking hours. **320**
- For the parent to maintain the hearing aid in good working order. **322**
- For the parent to respond promptly to questions about hearing-aid function. **323**
- For the parent to respond appropriately to questions about the workings of the hearing aid. **324**
- For the parent to describe the problem when the hearing aid is malfunctioning. **325**

OBJECTIVE: **Parent Will Understand The <u>Importance</u> Of Wearing Hearing Aid(s).**

How the Teacher Helps	What the Parent Does at Home
In order for a parent to understand the importance of wearing hearing aid(s), she needs to have a thorough knowledge of her child's hearing loss and how a hearing aid can affect that loss. • The teacher can provide materials and discussion about the normal ear and how it functions. Diagrams are available from some hearing aid dealers and some elementary science texts give very clear and satisfactory explanations. • After the parent has a knowledge of how the ear works, the teacher can discuss where the hearing system is impaired in the case of her child, i.e., the inner ear, the middle ear, or mixed problems. • An audiogram can be explained to demonstrate how hearing function is measured. The parent needs to have a basic familiarity and understanding of: – pitch (frequency) Which is high? low? – loudness (measured in decibels) – audiometer – tympanometry (tympanogram) – sound field – head phones – pure tones, warble tones – bone conduction/air conduction – speech range – SAT (speech awareness threshold) (continued)	There are many terms, machines, tests and professionals that the parent of a newly-identified hearing-impaired child must learn about. • Parents need to realize that they can ask questions when they don't understand: – what someone has said to them, – what someone's role is with their child, – what someone's qualifications are, – what a test is for, – what the results mean, – what is expected of their child, – what is expected of them, – how something works. • Parents shouldn't feel silly about asking questions because they are not expected to know about these things when they are encountering them for the first time. Also, if they are to become their child's best advocate, they need to have a thorough knowledge on which to base future decisions. • Whenever possible, both parents should attend the audiological appointments during the early days of diagnosis and hearing-aid recommendation. If the parent is alone, perhaps another supportive person could go along. There is a great deal of information to absorb and digest and it is difficult for the mother to handle it all and then try to relate what she has been told to the father or other family members. (continued)

**OBJECTIVE: Parent Will Understand The *Importance*
Of Wearing Hearing Aid(s). (cont'd.)**

How the Teacher Helps	What the Parent Does at Home
She needs to discuss this in general—at first not in relation to her own child's audiogram.	• Mother should discuss findings with her spouse if he was unable to attend.
• The teacher cannot assume that the audiologist has explained all this or that the parent "heard" it.	• The parent should discuss findings with in-laws and parents.
• After the teacher and parent have discussed audiograms and hearing testing, then the teacher can discuss the child's actual audiogram.	• The family collects their questions and asks the teacher.
Sometimes it is helpful for the parent to see the child's thresholds plotted on a graph that shows the speech range and the pitch and loudness of common environmental sounds. The importance of wearing aids takes on practical applications.	• The parent needs to begin to keep a file at home of copies of the child's audiograms and any other diagnostic reports.
	• Copies of the signed IFSP or IEP might be added.
• After the teacher and parent have discussed the child's un-aided responses, the teacher can then superimpose the child's aided responses on the audiogram form. Then it will be clear to the parent how the hearing aid helps the child.	• The parent should take note of the recommended volume setting of each aid. <u>It is important that the child wear the hearing aid at the recommended volume setting at all times</u> if he is to receive maximum benefit from the hearing aid. In some cases the child may be receiving <u>no</u> benefit from the aid if he is wearing it at a lower volume.
• The teacher needs to guard against the common misunderstanding that putting on a hearing aid is like putting on glasses. You put on glasses and you may have 20/20 vision. The teacher needs to explain that in the case of a sensorineural hearing loss, putting on a hearing aid can bring some sounds and pitches into the child's range of hearing, but that he will not have "20/20 hearing."	
(continued)	

OBJECTIVE: **Parent Will Understand The _Importance_ Of Wearing Hearing Aid(s). (cont'd)**

How the Teacher Helps	What the Parent Does at Home
• The teacher must have a cooperative relationship with the audiologist. If the parent has specific questions about the tests or the way they were conducted, the teacher needs to refer the parent back to the audiologist. • Teacher and audiologist need to develop communication channels. • At this stage, the audiologist will have written a report. The teacher needs to go over the report with the parent. Just giving a hearing-impaired child a hearing aid without training to listen is futile. The training to listen must pervade his entire day. Listening is not something done at a given time with a set procedure.	

OBJECTIVE: Parent Will Establish Consistent Hearing-Aid Use During All Waking Hours.

How the Teacher Helps	What the Parent Does at Home

When consistent hearing-aid use is <u>not</u> established right away, it may be due to a lack of familiarity with the hearing aid.
 	
• The teacher needs to practice <u>with</u> the parent putting in the hearing aid until the parent feels more at ease.
 	
• The teacher needs to practice putting in the hearing aid with the father, older siblings, grandparents, friends, babysitters and anyone else available until it becomes second nature.
 	
• The teacher can assist the parent in marking the earmolds and the aids with identifiable markings so it is readily apparent which aid and mold goes in which ear.
 	
• The teacher can give the parent some strategies to use to get started:
  – start with a few, short periods of wear each day during which time the child is actively engaged in interesting activities.
  – lengthen and increase these times as quickly as possible.
  – while the parent is watchful at the bonding stage, she should watch the aid also and what the child does about it.
  – anticipate when the child is getting anxious about the aid being in place.
 	
(continued)
	Parent needs to make a special place to keep extra batteries, battery tester and any other related materials. If Mother is away, someone else would know where the materials are kept.
	
	• Hearing aids should always be put in the same spot when removed from the child.
	
	• The parent should post a card clearly indicating:
	  – volume setting (for each aid),
	  – setting to indicate that the aid is on, whether "M" or "O" or whatever,
	  – how to tell which aid goes in the right or left ear,
	  – any other pertinent information.
	
	• Those in charge when Mother is away <u>must</u> assume responsibility for the child's hearing-aid wear. They should receive help from Mother on its use and care.
	
	• When the parent is establishing gradually increasing periods of wear each day:
	  – she might put some toys in a box that are only to be played with during these times.
	  – she might plan to do something special on another occasion, e.g., play with playdough or blow bubbles.
	
	(continued)

OBJECTIVE: **Parent Will Establish Consistent, Correct Hearing Aid Use During All Waking Hours. (cont'd)**

How the Teacher Helps	What the Parent Does at Home
• The parent must remember her role as an authority figure. She should adopt the attitude that <u>she</u> is in charge of the hearing aid(s) and when they are worn.	– when the child becomes anxious about wearing the aid, the adult needs to intervene and praise him for wearing it and remove it <u>before</u> he pulls it out. – if he removes the aid, the parent should replace it, praise him for wearing it and then a little later take it out herself.

OBJECTIVE: Parent Will Maintain The Hearing Aid In Good Working Order.

How the Teacher Helps	What the Parent Does at Home
In order for the parent to maintain the hearing aid(s) in good condition, she needs to know how it works and how to maintain it. • The teacher can use the child's hearing aid or a similar hearing aid and demonstrate to the parent each of the parts of the hearing aid. • The teacher can provide a diagram of a hearing aid and draw in and clearly label all the parts specific to the child's own personal hearing aid: – the microphone – the battery compartment – the volume control switch – the sound hook – the earmold – any tone switches – function settings, i.e., telephone coil – tubing, cords or wires – any special adaptations of aid, i.e., venting of molds, etc. • The teacher can help the parent establish a program of daily hearing-aid check which would include: – a sound check (listening to the quality of the aid through a stethoscope or the parent's own earmold) – a battery check (with tester) – earmold check—are they clean, cracked, fitting properly? – tubing or cord check • Intervener will give reading material to the parent.	• Parent will assemble necessary equipment for daily hearing-aid check and keep on hand: – stethoscope or own personal earmold – battery tester – supply of extra batteries – extra cords (if used) – solution for cleaning earmolds (if desired) – dry-aid kit to use if aid becomes damp – typewriter eraser to brush dust or food crumbs out of controls • Parent will ask audiologist for instructions on the use and care of the child's hearing-aid. • Parent will establish a system of daily hearing-aid check and will realize the importance of doing this <u>every day</u>. • If the child is at a babysitter's home, day-care center or school, the parent will provide them with extra batteries. • The parent will instruct the babysitter, day-care workers or teachers in simple hearing-aid maintenance, i.e., how to put it back in if it falls out, how to push the mold in if it begins squealing, how to change the batteries if they go dead. • The parent will check into insurance on the aid(s). • Parent will take the aid in for repairs as needed.

OBJECTIVE: Parent Will Respond Promptly To Questions About Hearing-Aid Function.

How the Teacher Helps	What the Parent Does at Home

Many times parents are faced with questions from family members, friends and passers-by in the grocery store about the hearing aid.
• The teacher can prepare the parent by giving her clear information about the child's hearing loss and hearing aids in many different ways and over time.
• The intervener needs to discuss the advantages of two hearing aids versus one; body aids versus behind the ear models, etc.
• The teacher can help the parent "rehearse" answers to these questions:
  – "What is that thing in your child's ear?"
  – "What good is a hearing aid anyway if he is deaf?"
  – "How come he doesn't talk if he can hear with that hearing aid?"
 	
These can be difficult and very emotional questions for the parent to answer. If she is prepared with factual answers, not only will she feel more comfortable in answering them, but she will also be doing a public service by informing the public.
• The parent needs to become her child's best advocate. In order to do that, she needs to be able to answer questions that other people dealing with her child might ask. These people may play a significant role in her child's life, i.e., babysitters, grandparents, relatives, neighbors, teachers, etc. If she can give clear answers to these "significant others" they will be able to help her child learn.
	Many parents resent the questions they are asked by relatives and "well-wishers." They need to have factual answers they can give and recognize that the questions are prompted by lack of understanding. People usually are not asking the questions to be critical.
	
	Mother could discuss with the teacher questions and/or criticisms that she receives. Many times the teacher can help know how to deal with these situations. Also, the teacher could put the parent in touch with another parent or parents who have hearing-impaired children and have "been there."

OBJECTIVE: Parent Will Respond Appropriately To Questions About The Workings Of The Hearing Aid.

How the Teacher Helps	What the Parent Does at Home
As the child's advocate, the parent may be asked questions by teachers, neighbors, babysitters, and relatives pertaining to the working of the hearing aid(s).	All significant caregivers in the child's life need to have information about the hearing aids and and how they work.

How the Teacher Helps

- The intervener needs to be conversant with current developments in the areas of audiological testing and advancements in hearing aids.
- The teacher can help prepare the parent to answer these questions by playing a "What would you do if" quiz game. She can pretend to be the babysitter calling the mother at work and asking a question pertaining to the workings of the aid. She can help the parent work through answers to questions such as:
    - The hearing aid won't work, what should I do?
    - The battery is dead. How do I put in a new one?
    - The earmolds came off the aids. How do I tell which one goes on which aid?
    - How do I turn it on?
    - What volume setting do I turn it on?
    - He wants to talk on the telephone. Do I do something special with his aid?
    - What does the "M" on the switch mean?
- The parent needs to be able to answer questions effectively and appropriately if she expects others to help her child maintain consistent, all-day hearing-aid use.

What the Parent Does at Home

- The parent can spend time with each one, going over the hearing aid, its parts and answering questions.
- The parent can have each person practice putting in the earmold(s) until he becomes comfortable with the task.
- The parent can inform everyone where the aids are to be kept so they can be found and put on the child in the mother's absence.
- Caregivers need to regularly check and see if the hearing aid is working (especially the batteries).

OBJECTIVE: **Parent Will Describe The Problem When The Hearing Aid Is Malfunctioning.**

How the Teacher Helps	What the Parent Does at Home
In order for a child to establish and maintain consistent, all-day hearing-aid use, the parent will need to know what to do when the hearing aid is malfunctioning.	At home, if the parent has assembled extra cords, batteries, dry-aid kits, etc., as described earlier, then she can try some things if the hearing aid isn't working. By eliminating the things she tries, i.e., replacing batteries or cords, she can narrow down the problem.

How the Teacher Helps

- The intervener will help the parent establish some hearing aid "trouble-shooting" techniques.

- In addition to learning how to check the hearing aid on a daily basis, the parent needs to be able to go one step further: to develop the ability to describe the problem and then try to fix it.

- During the parent-infant sessions, if hearing-aid problems arise, the teacher and parent could examine the hearing aid together, diagnose the problem and try some things to fix it.

- The teacher can give the parent a "trouble shooting" sheet that describes hearing-aid malfunctioning problems and recommends remedies to try. If the teacher does not have access to these materials, she could check with audiologists or hearing-aid dealers in her area.

- Teachers might have some aids that are malfunctioning. The parent can figure out the problem and correct it, if possible.

What the Parent Does at Home

- The parent can ask the teacher to call the hearing-aid dealer or audiologist, describe the problem and what she has tried and see if he has any other suggestions.

- Once the parent has determined that the problem is something she cannot fix, she will take the hearing aid to be repaired immediately.

- If the hearing-aid repairs are going to take more than a couple of hours, the parent could see if the hearing-aid dealer or audiologist has another hearing aid with the same specifications for the child to borrow. Sometimes the child's school has a stock of hearing aids the child can borrow for a short period of time.

Some possible objectives that might be considered at this stage are:

- For the parent to provide the child with the best listening environment. **329**
- For the parent to close the doors, turn off the TV or radio, shut off the mixer, etc., to cut down on ambient noise. **330**
- For the parent to be close to the child when talking to him. **332**
- For the parent to get the child's attention before speaking. **333**
- For the parent to speak at the child's ear level. **334**
- For the parent to call the child by his name and wait for him to look. **335**
- For the parent to continually increase the distance from the child when calling him by name. **336**
- For the parent to provide verbal auditory input with affectionate intonation. **337**
- For the parent to hum, sing and play games with sounds with the child. **338**

OBJECTIVE: Parent Will Provide The Child With The Best Listening Environment.

How the Teacher Helps	What the Parent Does at Home
This objective refers to the physical environment of the child's home. • The teacher will talk about things important for good listening: — carpeted floors to cut down on noises — draperies to cut down on reverberation — overstuffed furniture rather than chrome and glass to reduce reverberation • Intervener might borrow a sound-level meter from an audiologist. Since they are inexpensive, she might order one for her center. Using it near the child, she can show how the volume of ambient noise is affected by the environment. • With a noise-level meter, the intervener can show how kitchens are noisier than living rooms, or why basements can be poor listening environments, and so on.	Of course, a parent can't be expected to remodel her entire home when she learns that her child is hearing impaired. However, perhaps some simple modifications can be made, particularly in the rooms where she spends the most time with her child. • Could curtains or drapes be added as a window treatment over the miniblinds? • Could an area rug be placed under the kitchen table where most of the talking goes on? • Could pillows be added to the chairs and couch in the living room to absorb some sound and reduce reverberation?

OBJECTIVE: Parent Will Close The Doors, Turn Off The TV Or Radio, Shut Off The Mixer, Etc., To Cut Down On Ambient Noise.

How the Teacher Helps	What the Parent Does at Home
A hearing aid is not selective—everything is amplified, not just the important sounds of voices. For this reason, parents need to pay close attention to preparing the auditory environment. Parents need to be alert to the noise level of their home. • The teacher can have the parent listen to the noises of the center or school through the child's hearing aid (at a comfortable volume level for the parent). They will become aware of all the noises that are going on around them. She could also use a noise-level meter to demonstrate these noise levels. The teacher can ask them to listen at home for noises: televisions, radios, doors slamming, sounds coming through open windows, air conditioners or fans running, dishwashers or washing machines going through their cycles. These sounds can mask out the <u>important sounds of voices</u>.	One thing common to every home everywhere is that whenever there are people in that home there will be noise. It is impractical to think that a parent can provide a perfectly quiet environment in which to talk to the hearing-impaired child. However, there are some things the parent can do to <u>improve the listening environment when she is talking to the child</u>: – turn off the TV when no one is watching it, – turn down the volume momentarily if she needs to say something important to the child, – turn off the radio running in the background, – turn off the mixer, vacuum, dishwasher, etc., while talking to the child, – turn off the TV or radio during mealtimes, – turn off the dishwasher at a time she wants to do something with the child in the kitchen, – turn off the washing machine or dryer at a time when she wants to talk to or with her child if those appliances are near, – move away from another conversation, – move away from stationary appliances such as air conditioners, fans, humidifiers, etc., when they are running, – find good, quiet talking places for those special talks. (continued)

OBJECTIVE: **Parent Will Close The Doors, Turn Off The TV Or Radio, Shut Off The Mixer, Etc., To Cut Down On Ambient Noise. (cont'd)**

How the Teacher Helps	What the Parent Does at Home
	– When household and other noises cannot be controlled, the parent can get closer to the child's hearing aid to make her voice the most important signal.

OBJECTIVE: Parent Will Be Close To The Child When Talking To Him.

How the Teacher Helps	What the Parent Does at Home
Learning to position the child so he is close to his mother may require a few modifications in the home environment. • The teacher can demonstrate ways of positioning the child for closeness during experiences at the center. • The teacher can coach the parent when she is doing an activity with her child. She could say something like, "You might want to move him over in that chair so he would be closer to you," or "You might want to get down on the floor so you would be closer to him." • Prior to an activity, the teacher can ask the parent, "Where will you have Johnny sit?" "Where will you position yourself so you can be as close to him as possible?" • Intervener can have a tape recorder and demonstrate speaking a few inches from the mike and several feet from the mike. Play it back and let the parent see how weak the latter recording is.	At home, Mother may need to look at her environment and arrangement of furniture to see if it allows for preferable seating and positioning of the hearing-impaired child. • Where does he sit at the table? • Does he sit close to her so she can talk to him? • Does she have a stool or something he can sit on to be near her when she is working in the kitchen? • Is there a space big enough on the floor in the living room or family room so the two of them can get down on the floor together when playing? • Could she fold clothes on her bed so there would be room for the clothes and him so they could be close for this activity? • If he is an infant or toddler, could the playpen be moved from room to room or kept in the room where Mother is likely to be? • Could he have a toy basket or area in the corner of the kitchen or other work area so he could be near Mother when she is working rather than off in his room alone playing?

OBJECTIVE: Parents Will Get The Child's Attention Before Speaking.

How the Teacher Helps	What the Parent Does at Home

If the hearing-impaired child is going to receive maximum benefit from the talking directed to him, the parent will need to get his auditory (and visual) attention before speaking to him.
 	
• The teacher can demonstrate techniques to get the child's attention.
 	
• Initially, the attention-getting techniques may need to be visual, i.e., getting into the child's line of vision, pausing in activity to wait for the child to look up, etc.
 	
• Parents and intervener both have been observed employing all of the techniques listed here and the child still does not look. Many times the parent and teacher may have their own agenda and have forgotten to tune in to his interests and his agenda. They may be trying too hard to establish something that comes naturally when both child and parent are on the same "wave length."
 	
• Mother may be trying to get the child to look at her so she can show him some other feature of a toy and talk to him. However, the child may be intent on his present activity. Mother would have a much better chance of getting his attention if she were to take his lead and join HIS activity.
	At home, this will require some modifications in activity and talking style. Many of the objectives developed in this and in the language section will aid the parent in getting the child's attention before speaking, such as:
	  – face-to-face contact,
	  – bringing the child to the room where she is working,
	  – getting close to the child when speaking,
	  – providing the child with a good listening environment.
	
	The following are some additional techniques the parent might use to get the child's attention:
	  – follow the child's lead and join his activity,
	  – call the child's name,
	  – pause in Mother's activity to wait for the child to look up,
	  – jiggle an interesting object in child's line of vision and then bring it slowly up by the speaker's mouth,
	  – practice good face-to-face positioning techniques.
	
	Getting the young child's auditory and visual attention takes a lot of effort on the part of the parent but will be rewarded later as conversation develops.

OBJECTIVE: Parents Will Speak At The Child's Ear Level.

How the Teacher Helps	What the Parent Does at Home
Speaking at the child's ear level will help for the same reason being close to him does. Speech must be delivered to the hearing aid. • The teacher can demonstrate techniques for speaking at the child's ear level. • The teacher can coach the parent during parent activities to suggest how she could change her position or the position of the child to enhance speaking at the child's ear level. • The teacher can tally the number of times during a play period that the parent gets to the child's ear level to speak to him. • If the child is wearing only one aid, Mother can position herself on the child's side nearest the aid.	At home, Mother can make a few modifications to make it easier to speak at the child's ear level: • When the child is playing on the floor, Mother can get down on the floor with him. • When the child is sitting in a highchair, Mother can lower herself by sitting on a chair or stool. • When they are reading a book, Mother can seat the child on the couch and she can sit on the floor in front of him. • When it is not possible to get down to the child's ear level, Mother can bring the child up to her by picking him up or placing him safely on a stool or countertop.

OBJECTIVE: Parents Will Call The Child By Name And Wait For Him To Look.

How the Teacher Helps	What the Parent Does at Home

Training the child to respond to his name yields benefits when the child achieves this task. With the advancement in hearing-aid technology, most hearing-impaired children will be able to achieve this goal.
 	
• The teacher can demonstrate to the parent how to call the child and then wait for him to have the opportunity to respond by looking up.
 	
• The teacher can suggest that the parent start with the simplest task and then increase in difficulty:
  – call the child when directly in front of him (if he is looking away)
  – call the child when directly behind him
  – call the child from one to two feet away
  – call the child across a quiet room (six to eight feet)
  – gradually increase the distance
 	
• The teacher needs to remind the parent to call the child's name and then wait for a look. If the parent keeps calling the child's name over and over in succession, the child may tune this out as insignificant noise.
 	
• At first, if the child is having difficulty responding to his name when called at an unexpected time, the teacher can alert him to "listen" and then Mother can call him.
	The parent can take many opportunities throughout the day to call the child's name and wait for him to look. Of course, when the child looks, the mother should reinforce him by talking, blowing him a kiss, giving him a wink or showing surprise.
	
	• The parent can call the child when he is at play if she wants to talk to him.
	
	• The parent can call the child to tell him that she's going to a different room.
	
	• The parent can call the child to tell him it's time to eat.
	
	• The parent can call the child to wake him from his nap.
	
	• The parent can call the child in games:
	  – Peek-a-Boo (cover his eyes and he is to uncover them when he hears his name)
	  – hiding games.
	
	The parent can keep a tally at home of the number of times she calls his name and he looks. She could mark down each time she calls his name and circle those when he looks up. She could repeat this in a month to see if the number of responses has increased.

OBJECTIVE: **Parents Will Continually Increase The Distance From The Child When Calling Him By Name.**

How the Teacher Helps	What the Parent Does at Home

Once the child is responding to his name called unexpectedly at close range, the mother can gradually increase the distance between the speaker and the child.
 	
• The teacher can indicate when she feels the child is ready to progress to this step.
 	
• If the child is having difficulty responding to his name when called from increasing distances, the teacher can alert him and then Mother can call him.
	The parent can <u>gradually</u> increase the distance from the child when calling him around the house:
	  – from one to two feet behind him
	  – from four to six feet behind him
	  – from across the room (in quiet)
	  – from just outside the doorway of a quiet room
	
	Depending upon his hearing level, Mother can increase the distance from the microphone, i.e., from adjacent rooms, from down the hall or from outside.

OBJECTIVE: Parents Will Provide Verbal Auditory Input With Affectionate Intonation.

How the Teacher Helps	What the Parent Does at Home
The most significant sound for the child to tune in to is the sound of the human voice. Since he should be consistently responding to the voice, his experiences with vocal sounds should be pleasurable and reinforcing. • The teacher can discuss with the parent that some of the earliest meanings the child perceives are those conveyed by intonation. • The early talk any mother uses with her (hearing) baby is "love talk." The early sounds a hearing-impaired child hears through his hearing aid(s) should be of the same quality—"love talk." • The teacher should monitor the parent-child relationship so that she uses "love talk." • This affectionate verbal intonation should be reinforcing to the child and encourage him to "tune in" for more. • This exchange of loving vocal sounds should enhance mother-child bonding which is so very important to language development.	Mother can evaluate the interactions with the child at home. • Does she find herself taking time out to just snuggle, cuddle and "coo" with the child? • Does Dad "rough and tumble" with Johnny in the same manner as he does with the other children? • Does she allow herself the "luxury" of relaxing and having fun with her child?

OBJECTIVE: Parents Will Hum, Sing, And Play Games With Sounds With The Child.

How the Teacher Helps	What the Parent Does at Home

A lot of time is spent with a young (hearing) child humming, singing, and playing with sounds. This kind of interaction enhances language growth. The hearing-impaired child needs to receive the same kind of interaction.
 	
• The teacher can share with the parent appropriate songs, fingerplays and rhymes. The teacher could make up some song sheets with the words (and instructions for motions) for different ages of children.
	If the parent doesn't know many songs, fingerplays or rhymes, she could find books of them at local libraries.
	
	Some possible times for singing:
	— before naps: quiet songs
	— before bed: lullabies
	— when dressing: "This Is The Way We........"
	    put on our pants
	    put on our shirt
	    put on our socks
	    tie our shoes
	    comb our hair
	    brush our teeth
	    and so on
	— at playtime: movement songs
	    "Ring Around the Rosie"
	    "Row, Row, Row Your Boat" (Mother and child sit on floor facing one another, clasp hands and rock back and forth to make a boat.)
	
	The parent should make sure the child has his hearing aid(s) on during these times. In fact he should wear it during all his waking hours.
	
	If the child does not have his aid(s) on, the parent can hold the child close to her chest so he can feel the vibration, and she can sing directly into his ear.

Some possible objectives that might be considered at this time are:

- For the parent to recognize the need for the child to have pleasurable experiences with sounds. **341**
- For the parent to notice what sound the child is seeking and show him. She may label the sound, i.e., "The dog is barking." **342**
- For the parent to associate meaning with the noise. "The telephone is ringing. I'll answer it." **344**
- For the parent to call attention to noise such as the popping of popcorn in the popper. **345**
- For the parent to start and stop mixer, blender, vacuum, etc., to get the child's attention, not as a learning situation. **346**

OBJECTIVE: Parent Will Recognize The Need For The Child To Have Pleasurable Experiences With Sounds.

How the Teacher Helps	What the Parent Does at Home
If any child has a pleasurable experience with something, he will want that experience repeated. If he has pleasurable experiences with sounds, he will want to repeat those experiences and hear those sounds again. • Pleasurable experiences with sound assist in establishing consistent hearing-aid use. • The child who hears negative messages will not be motivated to wear the aid. • The authors are reminded of an older hearing-impaired child who would not wear his hearing aids. When asked why, he said that all he heard was fussing or scolding and he didn't like it.	At home, pleasurable experiences with sounds can be accomplished in a variety of ways: • most importantly, using pleasurable loving tones when talking to the child as much as possible • playing with toys appropriate for his age and demonstrating for him the sound potential of the toy when meaningful in the context of the play • singing and humming songs • reading books to him • talking to him about the things he is interested in • swaying and dancing to different types of music on the radio or record player • letting him hear "love talk" from the people who are important to him

OBJECTIVE: **Parent Will Notice What Sound The Child Is Seeking And Show Him. She May Label The Sound, i.e., "The Dog Is Barking."**

How the Teacher Helps	What the Parent Does at Home
In the section on language, there was an objective where the parent was instructed to follow the child's eye gaze to see what he was interested in and then go to the object and comment on it. This is the auditory correlate of that objective. Here the parent will notice by the child's facial expression or gestures that he has heard something. The parent will then identify what it is that he has heard, take the child to the source of the sound and label it for him. • Sometimes, the parents need to be helped to watch for indications that their child is hearing something. Initially, these indications will be very subtle, i.e., in the infant, it may be a pause in sucking, a wide-eyed gaze. In an older child, it may be a pause in activity, a puzzled look, or eyes searching to see what is going on. Teachers need to help parents recognize these signs and learn to respond to them. • Interveners can demonstrate to parents how to respond to a sound when their child has shown signs of hearing something. If the young child stops his activity to look up, the parent can say: "Did you hear that? Let's go see." (continued)	When the parent notices evidence that the child has heard something, she can: • take the child to the source of the sound • talk about the sound with the child • show the child how the sound is made (if it is a machine that can be turned on and off) • show the child what the machine does (i.e., the vacuum cleans the floor, the lawn mower cuts the grass, etc.) Environmental sounds are only important in that they have meaning for the child as related to his daily life. Speech sounds are far more important.

OBJECTIVE: **Parent Will Notice What Sound The Child Is Seeking And Show Him. She May Label The Sound, i.e., "The Dog Is Barking." (cont'd)**

How The Teacher Helps	What the Parent Does at Home
The parent takes the child to the source of the sound if possible and then labels it for him. "Oh, look at the dog. The dog is barking. Woof! Woof! I hear the dog." • Sometimes the teacher needs to heighten the parent's awareness of sounds occurring around the home. She could do this by emphasizing a different room of the house and ask the parent to watch the child and to see what he responds to in that particular room.	

OBJECTIVE: Parent Will Associate Meaning With The Noise: "The Telephone Is Ringing. I'll Answer It."

How the Teacher Helps	What the Parent Does at Home
A child hears a sound. He then needs to know what that sound means in relation to what it tells him about his environment, or in relation to what it tells him to do next. Sounds must have <u>meaning</u>. • For example, the child hears the phone ring. He needs to have <u>meaning</u> attached to that sound: "The telephone is ringing. I'll answer it," or "The telephone is ringing. Maybe Daddy is calling." • The teacher can demonstrate these situations when they occur during parent-infant sessions.	<u>In the kitchen:</u> • "The buzzer is sounding. Let's see if the cake is done." • "The telephone is ringing. I'll answer it." • "The mixer is running. Mommy is making a cake." • "The blender is running. Daddy is making a milkshake." <u>In the living room:</u> • "The doorbell is ringing. Go see who is at the door." • "The television is on. Please go turn it off." <u>In the bedroom:</u> • "The alarm is ringing. It's time to get up." • "The baby is crying. Let's go see what she wants." <u>Outside:</u> • "I hear a fire truck. There must be a fire." • "I hear an ambulance. They must be taking a sick person to the hospital."

OBJECTIVE: Parent Will Call Attention To Noise Such As Popping Of Popcorn In Popper.

How the Teacher Helps	What the Parent Does at Home
The most meaningful time to call attention to a sound is during the course of a "hands-on" experience in which the child is engaged. <ul><li>The teacher can point out that the sound of a popcorn popper only has relevance to the child's life when he and his mother are popping popcorn for him to eat. That is the time to point out the sound the popper makes.</li><li>The intervener should caution against planning activities to make sounds—just for the sake of making sounds. She must always be sure that they are meaningful to the child.</li><li>The teacher should also avoid planning activities to "test" the child's responses to sounds. For example, teachers have been observed setting an alarm clock to ring sometime during a session. When the alarm rings, the teacher and parent wait anxiously to see if the child hears the sound and then searches for it. However, what is this teaching the child? The appropriate meaning attached to a ringing alarm clock is that, "It's time to get up." So why, in the middle of a parent-infant session at school and in the middle of the day when they're not asleep, is an alarm ringing? Then, he is supposed to search for it and find it so his mother and teacher will clap their hands! Where is the meaning in this activity?</li><li>The teacher can plan many activities that include sounds within a meaningful context.</li></ul>	<ul><li>When Mother and child are making toast for breakfast, Mother can alert the child to listen for the sound of the toast popping up. This indicates the toast is done.</li><li>When Mother and child are running bath water in the tub, Mother can alert the child to the sound of the running water. This is one indication that the water is on and filling up the tub.</li><li>When Mother and child are folding clothes, Mother can alert the child to the sound of the dryer buzzer. It is an indication that some more clothes are dry and need to be folded.</li><li>When Mother and child are cleaning the house, Mother can alert the child to the sound of the vacuum. This sound means that the rugs are being cleaned.</li><li>Mother and child lie down to take a nap and set an alarm to wake them up. Mother alerts the child to the sound of the alarm ringing because it is telling them to wake up. It is also telling them to turn it off.</li></ul>

OBJECTIVE: Parents Will Start And Stop Mixer, Blender, Vacuum, Etc., To Get The Child's Attention, Not As A Learning Situation.

How the Teacher Helps	What the Parent Does at Home
If the mother is in the kitchen mixing a cake with a mixer when the child comes into the room, she may need to turn off the mixer to get the child's attention, tell him that she is mixing a cake, and then turn on the mixer for him to hear. • Again, the teacher must always place the emphasis on the <u>meaning</u> associated with the sound. • Teachers have been observed displaying a collection of appliances on a table in front of a young child. The child turns his back, the teacher turns on one of the appliances, and then the child is to turn back around and identify which appliance he heard. Where is the <u>meaning</u> in this activity? For the young child, environmental sounds must be meaningful to his life and his interests not an unnatural drill. • The intervener can demonstrate to the parent how she can stop what she is doing (i.e., vacuuming, mixing, mowing, etc.) to get the child's attention so she can talk to him, and then turn the noise-making appliance back on for him to listen to.	• When Daddy is shaving with <u>his electric razor</u>, he can turn off the razor to get the child's attention, talk to him about what he is doing, and then turn the razor back on for him to see and hear it working. Daddy might say: "Daddy is shaving. The shaver makes a noise. Listen. Daddy will turn it on. Now Daddy can shave." • When Mommy is drying her <u>hair with a blow dryer</u>, she can turn off the dryer to get the child's attention, talk to him about what she is doing, and then turn the dryer back on for him to see and hear it working. Mommy might say: "Mommy is drying her hair. See, Mommy's hair is wet. Mommy will turn on the dryer. The dryer blows Mommy's hair." • When the clothes dryer is <u>running</u>, Mommy can turn it off and open the door, talk to him about the dryer drying the clothes, and then turn the dryer back on for him to see and hear (and feel) it working. Mommy might say: "The dryer stopped. Mommy will open the door. Feel the clothes. The clothes are hot. The dryer dries the wet clothes. Mommy will turn it back on. The dryer is drying the clothes."

Some possible objectives that might be considered at this stage are:

- For the parent to use voice rather than non-voice auditory or sensory stimuli. **349**
- For the parent to rely on voice as an attention getter. **350**
- For the parent to use the child's name in positive, vocal tones. **351**
- For the parent to call attention to the speaker. **352**
- For the parent to engage in vocal play with the child. **353**
- For the parent to *consistently* use the child's name as a means of getting attention. **354**
- For the parent to *expect* the child to respond to his name. **355**

OBJECTIVE: **Parent Will Use Voice Rather Than Non-voice Auditory Or Sensory Stimuli.**

How the Teacher Helps	What the Parent Does at Home

The human voice is the most important auditory signal. Therefore, the parent should do everything possible to help the child respond to speech.
 	
• If the teacher plans meaningful games with sounds, the auditory stimuli should be voices <u>not</u> noisemakers, drums or bells.
 	
• The stimuli used to help a child alert to sounds should be the stimuli that the parent wants the child to alert to at home. Those stimuli would be:
  – voices, when he is called,
  – voices, when someone is talking to him,
  – voices, when he is asked to do something.
	In order to make her voice the most important auditory signal, Mother will:
	
	• position the child effectively on eye and ear level,
	
	• get close to the child when talking to him,
	
	• wait for the child to look before speaking to him,
	
	• eliminate background noise when talking to her child.
	
	In order to use her voice as an auditory stimulus, Mother can:
	
	• call her child often and wait for a response,
	
	• sing to her child,
	
	• talk to her child about what he is interested in at the moment,
	
	• read to her child,
	
	• play verbal, interactive games with her child, i.e., Peek-a-Boo.

OBJECTIVE: Parent Will Rely On Voice As An Attention Getter.

How the Teacher Helps	What the Parent Does at Home

As has been mentioned before, the human voice is the most important auditory signal to which the child can attend.
 	
• The intervener and parent together should work toward the child responding to his name when called.
 	
• Attention-getting devices to be avoided:
   – tapping the child
   – pulling his face toward the speaker
   – flashing lights
   – stomping on the floor
   – hitting the table
 	
• Parent needs to assist child in awareness that someone is talking and who that someone is.
 	
• Parent needs to make child aware of other voices pointing out when Daddy, brother, intervener, etc., are speaking.
	The parent's voice must take on significance and be used to get the child's attention in a meaningful situation.
	
	If the child responds to his mother's voice, he needs to be rewarded with a smile, a hug, some talk about something he is interested in.
	
	• Often the parent is observed calling the child's name over and over to get his attention. Each time the intensity is louder and the tone is more frustrated. The human ear is able to "tune out" sounds that are irritating or nonsignificant to the listener. Often a sound that is heard over and over becomes just that—irritating and nonsignificant.
	
	• When the parent calls the child's name, she should wait and allow him the opportunity to respond. Then if she calls him again and he does not respond, she should employ an additional strategy, such as moving closer or moving into his line of vision.

OBJECTIVE: Parent Will Use Child's Name In Positive Vocal Tones.

How the Teacher Helps	What the Parent Does at Home

One form of positive reinforcement would be positive vocal tones. The child hears his name spoken with pleasant intonation and he will want to "tune in" again.
 	
• Positive vocal tones are reinforcing to the child.
 	
• Negative or harsh vocal tones may have the opposite effect of what is wanted. The child may decide to "tune out" the undesired tones.
 	
• Teacher can model positive vocal tones.
 	
• Teacher can suggest ways in which parents can use positive vocal tones.
 	
• The intervener could talk to the parent about the comforting power of the human voice. She can show the parent how the exclamation, "Yes, Johnny. Mommy will be right there!" can be a valuable source of comfort to the hearing-impaired child.
 	
• Mother may need to say, "Mommy's coming!" until she gets in the same room and near him.
	At home, parent can use positive vocal tones when:
	  – calling the child's name
	  – talking to him about his interests
	  – reading to him
	  – singing to him
	  – using "love talk"
	
	• Parent can use pleasant tones when calling the child.
	
	• Parent should use child's name pleasantly in other connections such as:
	  – "Thank you, Johnny."
	  – "Here's your coat, Johnny."
	  – "Johnny, let's go outside."
	  – "Let's take Daddy a cookie, Johnny."

OBJECTIVE: Parent Will Call Attention To The Speaker.

How the Teacher Helps	What the Parent Does at Home
Sometimes, in order for a hearing-impaired child to follow a conversation or to receive the message someone is saying to him, it may be necessary for the parent to call attention to the speaker. • The teacher can model this behavior by saying to the child, when appropriate: "Look at Mommy." "Mommy wants to tell you something." • Other times, the teacher can alert the child to listen for the speaker: "Listen. Do you hear Mommy?"	At home, the parents can make sure that the child is aware of people talking to him: – "Johnny, look at Grandma." – "Daddy is talking to you, Johnny." – "Johnny, listen. I hear Daddy." – "Johnny, Daddy wants you. He is in the garage."

OBJECTIVE: Parent Will Engage In Vocal Play With The Child.

How the Teacher Helps	What the Parent Does at Home
Parent needs to connect voice with tones of pleasurable interaction. • Vocal play is of the "coochy-coochy-coo" variety that every parent the world over plays with her child. It is important for bonding. • Vocal play is having fun with sounds with the child. • The teacher can encourage the parent to engage in vocal play with the child. Sometimes the parent becomes so serious with her role as language provider for her child that she may think simply playing with sounds would be a waste of time. • The teacher can demonstrate to the parent how to imitate the child's vocalizations to set up a playful exchange with the child.	Parent can playfully repeat the child's babbling or other spontaneous vocal sounds. • When the child playfully babbles, the parent can imitate this and then wait for the child to do it again. • If the child sneezes or coughs, the parent can imitate the sneeze or cough and say, "Ah-choo! Johnny sneezed." • When the child blows bubbles or "raspberries," the parent can imitate this behavior and then wait for the child to do it again.

OBJECTIVE: Parent Will *Consistently* Use The Child's Name As A Means Of Getting Attention.

How the Teacher Helps	What the Parent Does at Home
In order for a hearing-impaired child to learn to respond to his name when called, the parent will need to consistently use the child's name as a means of getting attention. • The teacher can chart the number of times the parents use the child's name to get his attention during a session or a specified period of time during a session. • The teacher can challenge the parent to increase the number of times the parent uses the child's name as a means of getting attention. • The parent can listen to a tape of her own talking to the child and count the number of times she used the child's name. • Video taping can also be used to alert the parent to the frequency with which she uses her child's name.	At home, the parent can evaluate her technique for getting the child's attention. • How often does she call his name to get his attention? • Does she find herself using any physical means for getting his attention, i.e., tapping him or turning his face? • Does she find herself stomping on the floor or flipping the lights to get his attention? The parent may need to modify her techniques to eliminate any undesirable methods of getting the child's attention and replace them with acceptable ways.

OBJECTIVE: Parent Will *Expect* The Child To Respond To His Name.

How the Teacher Helps	What the Parent Does at Home

Parental expectations influence parental behavior. If the parent believes that the child will some day be capable of reciprocal communication, then she must believe that the child will respond to his name when called.
 	
• If the parent has doubts that the child will ever respond to his name, she will be less likely to be motivated to call his name consistently.
 	
• The teacher can demonstrate to the parent that the child should be able to learn to respond to his name. She can do this by reviewing the child's audiogram. The teacher and parent can plot the aided responses on the audiogram to see how these responses fall within the speech range.
 	
• The teacher and parent together can develop some realistic strategies for ensuring that Mother's calls fall within the auditory capabilities of the child.
 	
    Initially, Mother may need to be right behind the child to be within his auditory capabilities.
 	
    Or, it may be the case that the child can probably hear her if she waits until she gets in the same room before she calls his name.
	Mother will expect the child to respond to his name when she:
	
	• calls him from six to twelve inches behind him,
	
	• calls him from three to four feet behind him,
	
	• calls him from across the room,
	
	• talks to him at the dinner table,
	
	• talks to him when playing with him,
	
	• talks to him when dressing him,
	
	• first puts his hearing aid on and begins talking to him.

Some possible objectives that might be considered at this stage are:

- For the parent to give the child intonation patterns. **359**
- For the parent to wait for some response, such as cooing or a smile. **360**
- For the parent to ask the child for one or two items that the child has among his playthings, clothing, food, etc. **361**
- For the parent to use certain phrases such as: "Turn the light on/off," "Get your coat," and expect the child to recognize them. **362**
- For the parent to *expect* the child to respond to words, phrases or sentences within a restricted set. **363**
- For the parent to expect the child to comprehend freely from unlimited numbers of rhymes, objects and sentences about experiences. **364**

OBJECTIVE: Parent Will Give The Child Intonation Patterns.

How the Teacher Helps	What the Parent Does at Home

Intonation is the first vocal output to which children universally respond. Since auditory recognition proceeds from the general to the specific, initially this skill will involve recognizing the <u>difference</u> in intonation patterns. Does Mother sound happy, loving, angry or tired?
 	
 • As an exercise in the power of intonation to transmit <u>meaning</u>, the teacher can ask the parent to participate in demonstrating this. She can take a sentence, similar to anything that might be spoken to a young child, and ask the parent to say it with varying intonational patterns. For example, take the sentence:
 	
   "What's the matter with the baby?"
 	
 Ask the parent to say this sentence with happy, loving, angry and tired intonational patterns. How did the <u>meaning change</u>? The teacher can point out that this meaning was transmitted purely through intonational patterns because the words remained the same.
 	
 • The teacher can encourage the parent to use these intonation signals to meaning prominently in her talking with the child.
 	
 • The teacher can remind the parent that this meaning through intonational patterns was transmitted <u>auditorily</u> and therefore consistent <u>hearing-aid use is mandatory</u> if the child is to receive this clue to meaning.
	Meaning can be communicated through intonation patterns in natural situations throughout the day:
	
	 • <u>Happiness</u>
	   "You put on your coat all by yourself. Good for you!"
	   "Johnny made a picture for Mommy. Thank you!"
	   "Dada. Did you say Daddy? Hi, Daddy!"
	
	 • <u>Love</u>
	   "I love you so-o-o-o-o much!"
	   "Sleep tight. Mommy will see you in the morning."
	   "Hi, Johnny. Did you wake up?"
	
	 • <u>Anger</u>
	   "That makes Mommy angry."
	   "No. No. Do not run in the street."
	   "Do not dig a hole in the yard. Mommy doesn't like that!"
	
	 • <u>Fatigue</u>
	   "Mommy is so tired."
	   "Let's sit down and rest. I'm tired."
	   "Johnny is sleepy. Do you want to lie down?"

OBJECTIVE: Parent Will Wait For Some Response Such As Cooing Or A Smile.

How the Teacher Helps	What the Parent Does at Home
Sometimes parents get so in the habit of providing language input for their child that they forget to allow him the opportunity to respond. It is important, if we want to set up the ping-pong-like pattern of communication, that the parent waits for some sort of a response, such as a coo or smile. • The teacher can coach the parent to <u>wait</u> after she has given the child an instruction or asked a question. The child's initial responses may only be an eye gaze or a smile, but that response should be reinforced. • Initially, the teacher may need to help the parent recognize these responses. The teacher can point them out during parent-child activities and suggest a response if necessary.	Responses to look for and reinforce at home: • If the child looks toward the <u>object or person Mother is talking about</u>, the parent can go to the object or person and reinforce that gaze by saying something like: "Johnny sees the ball. Here is the ball. Mommy throws the ball to Johnny." • If the child <u>vocalizes or babbles in response to parent's talking</u>, the parent can indicate to the child that she has heard him and reinforce him by saying: "Ga-ga-ga. I hear you. Are you talking to Mommy? Ga-ga-ga. Can you say some more?" • If the child <u>smiles at the parent in response to the parent pointing out something pleasurable</u>, the parent can go to the object and talk about it: "Johnny likes the mobile. See it go around and around?" • If the child <u>smiles at the parent in response to the sound of the parent's voice</u>, the parent can reinforce this smile by talking: "Did you hear Mommy? Mommy is talking to you. I like to talk to my big boy."

OBJECTIVE: **Parent Will Ask The Child For One Or Two Items The Child Has Among His Playthings, Clothing, Food, Etc.**

How the Teacher Helps	What the Parent Does at Home
After the child has had many opportunities to see and hear familiar language associated with routine situations, the parent may challenge the child's listening skills. • The teacher can show the parent how to set up a "closed set" for the child to choose from. For example, when the child is getting dressed, Mother can lay out two clothing items on the bed for the child to choose from. She can then say: "Johnny, get your shoes." "Johnny, get your socks." The child may be able to auditorily recognize the difference in the vowel sounds in those two items, "shoes" and "socks" and choose the correct one. • The teacher can demonstrate for the parent how to choose items that are very different in length or vowel sounds at first so the child will experience success with this task. For example, "shoes versus sweater" is different, whereas "hat versus pants" is too similar in both length and vowel sounds. • The teacher can suggest that the parent do this very naturally by sitting next to the child or by covering her mouth so the child can't lip-read as clearly. The parent must not get in the habit of "testing"the child. That practice would be counter-productive to the atmosphere we want the parent to create.	Parents can do this in natural situations throughout the day. At breakfast: "Get your cup." or "Give Mommy your spoon. At play: "Push the truck." or "Push the car." "Kiss the baby." or "Kiss the teddybear." At lunch: "Eat the banana." or "Eat the sandwich." Outside: "Go get the football." or "Go get your bike." "Put on your coat." or "Put on your mittens." If the child does not demonstrate recognition after one or two presentations auditorily, the parent should avoid frustrating the child, allowing him then to watch and listen as she presents the instruction again.

OBJECTIVE: **Parent Will Use Certain Phrases Such As "Turn The Light On/Off," "Get Your Coat," And Expect The Child To Recognize Them.**

How the Teacher Helps	What the Parent Does at Home
After the child has had many opportunities to see and hear familiar phrases or instructions, the parent may challenge the child's listening skills by asking him to do these things with an auditory-only presentation. • Teacher can discuss with the parent which familiar phrases the child responds to routinely at home. They can make a list of these. • The teacher can suggest that the parent try presenting some of the phrases listed with an auditory-only stimulus. • The teacher can demonstrate for the parent how she can present these with an auditory approach for the child to listen to and then respond. • The teacher will need to remind the parent to get close to the child and be on "ear level" with the child when she initially presents familiar phrases auditorily. When the child knows the topic and has understood the language, the parent can give that language to the child auditorily. Listening is <u>not</u> testing. Hence, in auditory training, the child <u>must know</u> what is being presented through his hearing.	Phrases that would be appropriate to start with are those that are repeated often and those that the child is already familiar with. <u>In the morning</u>: "It's time to get dressed." "Breakfast is ready!" "Brush your teeth." <u>At play</u>: "It's time to clean up." "Put the toys on the shelf." <u>Throughout the day</u>: "Open the door." "Shut the door." "Do you want to go outside?" "Turn the light on/off." "Do you have to go potty?"

OBJECTIVE: **Parent Will *Expect* The Child To Respond To Words, Phrases Or Sentences Within A Restricted Set.**

How the Teacher Helps	What the Parent Does at Home
Again taking familiar information, stories, or rhymes, the parent can challenge the child to listen carefully.	At home, the parent can present these words, songs, phrases, or sentences at natural talking times.

How the Teacher Helps

- The teacher can demonstrate this with teacher-prepared materials that reinforce an in-class experience, i.e., carving a Jack-O-Lantern. The teacher can make a little experience story on cards. She can review the story with the child following the experience. She can then display two to three of the cards (differing in length and intonation patterns) and present the language auditorily. The child is to point to the correct picture.

- The teacher can demonstrate this technique with familiar picture books. She can auditorily give the child instructions, i.e.:
  "Where is the bunny?"
  "Which animal is the doggie?"
  "Please, turn the page."
  "Do you want to open the book?"

- The parent should speak in situations where meaning is clear and wait for a response.

- Comprehension of meaning is necessary before language is meaningful.

What the Parent Does at Home

- The parent can begin to sing a familiar song or say a familiar fingerplay and expect the child to demonstrate recognition by doing the actions or join in the singing.

- The parent can draw some simple picture representing familiar songs or nursery rhymes. (She could also buy some inexpensive nursery rhyme books to cut apart for the pictures and glue them on cards.) She could lay three or four of these pictures out in front of the child. She sings (or says) one of these songs or rhymes with an auditory-only presentation. The child is to choose the correct picture for "Jack and Jill went up the hill to fetch a pail of water," or "Mary had a little lamb."

- The parent can ask questions such as "Do you want cereal?" and accept "Yes" or "No" responses.

- She may rise from her chair preparatory to leaving and ask the child to get his boots. Later she would ask for his "coat," his "cap," etc.

- The parent could expect the child to differentiate between:
  "Throw me a kiss." and "Give Daddy the ball."
  "Use the big spoon." and "Use the wooden spoon."

OBJECTIVE: **Parent Will Expect Child To Comprehend Freely From Unlimited Numbers Of Rhymes, Objects, And Sentences About Experiences.**

How the Teacher Helps	What the Parent Does at Home
Just as all beginning language needs to be experienced-based, so must the beginning auditory learning. • For the child to learn the auditory signals he must understand the meaning of what is being said to him. • Meaning is a clue to language. So is it a clue to what is spoken.	The whole idea that must be implemented at home is that the child may be able to receive information auditorily. • Parent expectation must keep pace with the child's capabilities. • Stick figure drawings of the child's experiences can be drawn following the event. Language captions can be put under each drawing. Each of the "sentence cards" can be read several times to recall the experience. Then the parent can play a game whereby the parent reads one of the language captions and the child selects the correct card. • The task increases in difficulty as the number of experiences increases. The cards serve as a closed set. • Similar games can be played with rhymes forming the closed set.

AREA K:
STRUCTURING
THE VISUAL ENVIRONMENT

Some possible objectives that might be considered at this stage are:

- For the parent to see that she always faces the light, with the light at the child's back. **367**
- For the parent to see that there is sufficient illumination for lipreading. **368**
- For the parent to get to the child's eye level or bring him to hers. **369**
- For the parent to present to the child the full view of her face in order for him to perceive the place-of-articulation. **370**
- For the parent to minimize distractions. **371**
- For the parent to turn off the television when talking to the child. **372**

OBJECTIVE: **Parent Will See That She Always Faces The Light—With The Light At The Child's Back.**

How the Teacher Helps	What the Parent Does at Home

Development of lip-reading ability requires knowledge of environmental factors which can enhance the development of this skill. The parents may need to heighten their awareness of the visual environment of their home.
 	
• Parents need to know about light in relation to optimal conditions for lip-reading.
 	
• The teacher and parent can evaluate the visual environment of the classroom setting or room at the clinic where the child and parent are seen for parent-infant sessions.
 	
   – Is the room arranged so that the child can always have the light at his back?
 	
   – Are there curtains or blinds that can be closed when the child must face the windows?
 	
   – Is there light from windows or lamps that causes a glare?
 	
• The teacher-counselor can position the child in different places throughout the room and ask the parent to evaluate the placement. Where does the light fall: on the child's face? on the speaker's face?
 	
• The teacher can ask the parent to evaluate where she is sitting. Is the parent sitting where the light falls on her face? If not, how can she correct that problem?
	In the kitchen:
	    Look at the place where the hearing-impaired child usually sits. Is the light at his back?
	
	In the living room:
	    Look at the place where the child usually plays games or reads books. Is the light at his back? If not, could the furniture be rearranged to improve this situation?
	
	In the bedroom:
	    Look at the location of the child's bed. When Mother comes in to talk to the child in the morning or read him a book at night, will the light from the windows be on her face? If not, could the room be rearranged to remedy this situation? If not, could Mother pull down a shade in the morning so the child is no looking into the sun when she is trying to talk to him about getting dressed and so forth?
	
	Outside:
	    Mother needs to learn to always be aware of where she is in relation to the sun. When talking to the child, she may need to change places with the hearing-impaired child so the sunshine is on her face and not shining in his.

OBJECTIVE: Parent Will See That There Is Sufficient Illumination For Lipreading.

How the Teacher Helps	What the Parent Does at Home
A home for a young hearing-impaired child should be a well lighted place. • The teacher can demonstrate for the parent by turning on additional sources of light on dark, cloudy days or when the sun suddenly goes behind a cloud. The teacher should be tuned in to these changes so she can demonstrate how the parent can make adjustments in the lighting. • Some families prefer the quiet, subdued feeling of rooms with low illumination, dark wallpaper and draperies. The teacher may need to encourage the family to provide extra, well-placed lighting that can be turned on during those times that the hearing-impaired child is playing and talking in those rooms.	It would be a good idea for the parent of a hearing-impaired child to evaluate her home room-by-room and determine if there is sufficient illumination for lipreading. • How good is the illumination on the child's level? • Does illumination improve if the child is moved to a different part of the room? • Through some modification in natural lighting from the windows, either by opening shades or changing the window treatments, could illumination be improved? • Through the addition of lamps, larger lightbulbs or light fixtures, can the illumination be improved? • Should some rooms be avoided as "talking places" if modifications are impractical?

OBJECTIVE: Parent Will Get To The Child's Eye Level Or Bring Him To Hers.

How the Teacher Helps	What the Parent Does at Home
This objective can be accomplished by some modifications in the way the adult positions herself in relation to her child. • Just as the parent needed to get near the hearing aid for the best amplification, so must she get within good visual range for the best speech (lip) reading. • Proximity to the visual source is necessary for visual perception. • The teacher can demonstrate by always remembering to get to the child's level herself. She can point out to the parent that she has positioned herself thusly to get on the child's eye level. • The teacher can coach the parent during an activity and make suggestions for a change in her position to get on the child's eye level. • The teacher can ask the parent before she begins a parent-child activity where she will position herself to achieve maximum eye level with the child.	At home the parent will practice the techniques of: • kneeling to get on the child's eye level • squatting to get on the child's eye level • sitting on the floor facing the child • picking up the child so he can face her • placing a child safely on a stool or countertop so the child is at the adult's eye level.

OBJECTIVE: **Parent Will Present To The Child The Full View Of Her Face In Order For Him To Perceive The Place-of-Articulation.**

How the Teacher Helps	What the Parent Does at Home
Children need to be able to see place-of-articulation. Much language is visible especially consonants *p, l, m, wh, r, th, t* and *d*. Many phonemes do not have to be taught, but children learn them through observing them. The teacher needs to demonstrate the visibility to the parent. She can ask the parent to evaluate the visual information the child receives when: • The speaker leans over with her head horizontal in relation to the child's line of vision • The speaker bends over the child, i.e., when a mother rests a child's back against her legs to button his coat, for example, and leans over to talk to him, presenting to him her face upside down • The speaker leans over a child lying down and her face is at a variety of angles, one of which could be completely upside down • The speaker turns away before she finishes a sentence • The speaker bends over to pick something up while she is speaking • The speaker scratches her nose, puts her hand over her face or wipes her nose while talking	The parent needs to be aware of her position and activity when talking to her child: • Wait to bend over and pick up that stray sock until she has finished talking to the child. • Finish talking before turning around to get the dishes off the cupboard. • Finish talking before bending over to get the clothes out of the dryer. • Sit directly across the table from the child at dinnertime. • Sit down on the bed next to the child and face him rather than bend over him. • Pin long hair back out of the way so it isn't hanging in front of her mouth when talking.

OBJECTIVE: Parent Will Minimize Distractions.

How the Teacher Helps	What the Parent Does at Home

Lip-reading or speechreading is a difficult task and requires concentration. There are many things that are distracting to a lip-reader and these should be avoided with the young child who is acquiring language.
 	
• Optical competition can deter attention and lip-reading.
 	
• Parent must learn to minimize distractions.
 	
• The teacher can discuss some of the things that are distracting to the lip-reader:
  – gesturing and movement
  – large, dangling earrings or necklaces
  – mustaches and beards
  – long hair that hangs in the face or over the eyes
  – "busy" walls with lots of pictures or wallpaper with large designs behind where the speaker is standing or sitting
  – people or animals that are not involved in the discussion
 	
• The teacher needs to be ever cautious that she is not visually "competing" for the child's visual attention when the parent and child are engaged in an activity. The teacher may need to position herself behind the child or at a distance away from the dyad (the two) so she doesn't present herself as a distraction.
	• Evaluate the personal behavior. Could modifications be made at least during times with the child? i.e., hold hands still, sit quietly, etc.
	
	• Evaluate the visual environment of the places where the child usually sits, plays, works. Look from his point of view. Is the background behind the speaker fairly neutral? If not, are simple modifications possible to improve the visual environment?
	
	• Remove dangling earrings and large necklaces when talking with the child.
	
	• Take the child to another room or another part of the room to remove him from the visual distraction of other people.

OBJECTIVE: Parent Will Turn Off The Television When Talking To The Child.

How the Teacher Helps	What the Parent Does at Home
Television writers and producers spend their days thinking of ways to get and maintain the visual and auditory attention of their viewers. They use many techniques, from lively movement, to loud music, and even to commercials that are louder than the programs they accompany. The young hearing-impaired child who is trying to learn language and listening skills should not have to compete with this powerful auditory and visual stimulus. • The teacher should talk to the parent about turning off the television when speaking. • The teacher should remind the parent that the hearing aid(s) are not discriminatory. They amplify everything, including the television, even when it is in the corner of the adjoining room.	• Evaluate television use at home. • Is the television always on, just for "companionship?" Get in the habit of turning it off when not in use. • Can television viewing habits be changed? For example, some families have a television on during meals in the kitchen or dining room. This makes mealtime conversation and information sharing difficult for everyone, and impossible for the hearing-impaired child. Can the kitchen television be removed or turned off during meals?

AREA L: PARENT'S SPEECH PATTERNS

Some possible objectives that might be considered at this stage are:

- For the parent to speak clearly. **375**
- For the parent not to exaggerate nor slur her speech. **376**
- For the parent's overall rate of speech to the child to be slower than with an older child or adult. **377**
- For the parent to make longer pauses between meaningful units of speech. **378**
- For the parent to stress the content words. **379**
- For the parent to use prosodic features prominently. **380**
- For the parent to mark emotional and attitudinal aspects of her utterance by stress, intensity and other intonational devices. **381**
- For the parent to use proper intonational terminals to mark questions, statements and commands. **382**

OBJECTIVE: Parent Will Speak Clearly.

How the Teacher Helps	What the Parent Does at Home
Many techniques that have been described have emphasized presenting the hearing-impaired child with optimum conditions for seeing and hearing speech. Many recommendations have been made for the environment and positioning the child in the environment.	If the parent is made aware of the things that promote clear speech, she can evaluate herself and other family members at home.

How the Teacher Helps

Many techniques that have been described have emphasized presenting the hearing-impaired child with optimum conditions for seeing and hearing speech. Many recommendations have been made for the environment and positioning the child in the environment.

- The above objective deals with the speaker personally.

- Clarity of speech is of vital importance in lip-reading. Since children can learn place-of-articulation from looking at the speaker's mouth, parent must speak clearly and articulate well.

  The teacher can evaluate the speech of the parent. Are there any habits that interfere with clear speech?
  - Does she talk while chewing gum?
  - Does she talk with a cigarette in her mouth?
  - Does she talk while eating?
  - Does her hair frequently cover her mouth?

- If the teacher notices any of these things in the mother, she can discuss these in general as things necessary to promote clear speech.

- The teacher can coach the parent during an activity and suggest that Mother may want to get rid of her gum while talking to her child.

What the Parent Does at Home

If the parent is made aware of the things that promote clear speech, she can evaluate herself and other family members at home.

- The parent can do some mirror practice. She can talk to herself and see if she can observe movements.

- Parents can talk to each other through a glass door. They can evaluate each other.

- The parent can talk without voice in front of a mirror and see if she can lipread herself.

- The parents can turn TV down low and see if she can lipread/speechread a speaker such as a newscaster. How does he speak to make his message clear? Does he do anything distracting that makes it difficult to lipread/speechread him?

OBJECTIVE: Parent Will Not Exaggerate Nor Slur Her Speech.

How the Teacher Helps	What the Parent Does at Home
In an effort to provide the clearest signal possible to the hearing-impaired child the parent will not exaggerate or slur her speech. • The teacher can talk to the parent about the importance of maintaining the natural rhythm and intonation of language. • The teacher can demonstrate how this natural flow is disrupted when the speaker exaggerates her speech; i.e., "Open the door," has it's own rhythm and flow. However, if the speaker exaggerates and says, "O-pen the do-o-o-r," this flow is distorted and the speaker removes that auditory clue the child can use to identify the message. • The teacher can also demonstrate how slurred or rapid speech can alter the natural flow and rhythm of familiar phrases. • The teacher might use a stop watch to note the time envelope of intervener and parent saying the same sentences. (The second hand of a watch can be used if no stop watch is available).	The parent needs to practice at home speaking as clearly as possible without exaggerating nor slurring her speech. • Think about the way routine phrases and sentences sound naturally: their unique rhythm, intonation and emphasis. • Are speakers in the child's life distorting that natural flow? • Practice talking into a mirror helps eliminate exaggeration. • Parent can note the amount of time other family members take to say the same sentence.

OBJECTIVE: Parent's Overall Rate Of Speech To The Child Will Be Slower Than With An Older Child Or Adult.

How the Teacher Helps	What the Parent Does at Home
Speaking a little more slowly to a young child is a technique used by "Super Mothers" the world over. The pauses between meaning units are longer and the words per minute are fewer than in adult to adult or adult to older child. • The teacher can evaluate the parent's rate of speaking with the child. (Can use stop watch here also.) • The teacher can coach the parent during parent-child activities. She might say: "You might want to slow down your talking just a little bit. It's easier for young children to understand when people talk to them a little more slowly." The teacher can demonstrate an appropriate rate of talking. • The teacher needs to monitor to make sure that when the parent slows down her rate of speech that she doesn't begin to exaggerate her speech. • An "assignment" for the week could be for the parent to listen to herself talking and make sure that she is talking at an appropriate rate for the child. She could time herself and other family members.	The mother can evaluate her rate of speaking at home. • Is she speaking at a rate appropriate for her child? • Are there times of the day when she's in a hurry that she needs to be more careful of her rate of speech? • Can she enlist the help of other family members in monitoring one another's rates of speech?

OBJECTIVE: Parent Will Make Longer Pauses Between Meaningful Units Of Speech.

How the Teacher Helps	What the Parent Does at Home
Another technique to provide a clear message to the hearing-impaired listener is that of phrasing the message into thought concepts and pausing briefly between these meaningful units.	Sample sentences that may occur at home.
• The teacher can demonstrate this technique in her own talk with the child.	• Look both ways before you cross the street.
	(Look both ways)**(before)**(you cross the street.)
• The teacher could provide some familiar, common sentences that might be spoken to the child and talk with the parent about how they might be phrased into meaningful units. Put the banana on the table. (Put the banana) ** (on the table.)	• It's time to come in for supper. (It's time to come in)**(for supper.) • Put the box on the table. (Put the box)**(on the table.)
The teacher can illustrate with print how a sentence is perceived without meaningful planning, with each word running into the next:	• Take the dishes out of the dishwasher. (Take the dishes)**(out of the dishwasher.)
Johnnyputthebananaonthetable.	
• The teacher can also illustrate how the meaning of the sentence gets lost when the sentence is chopped up into words rather than <u>thoughts</u>, as in: (Put the)**(banana on)**(the table.)	

OBJECTIVE: Parent Will Stress The Content Words.

How the Teacher Helps	What the Parent Does at Home
In early days of language learning, the child often keys in on one or two words that he knows to decode the meaning of a sentence. Stressing these meaningful or "content" words will aid the child in decoding that message. • Parent should stress the content words, with some getting more emphasis than others. Are you <u>hungry</u>? Let's go <u>bye-bye</u>. The <u>teddy bear</u> is on the <u>big</u> chair. • The teacher can demonstrate for the parent. The teacher can instruct the child to, "Put the banana on the table." The teacher can ask the parent which words in that sentence she thinks the child knows or understands. The parent undoubtedly will pick one or two, i.e., "banana" and "table." The teacher can further demonstrate for the parent how to gently stress those content words to help the child. Put the <u>banana</u> on the <u>table</u>.	At home, if a child misinterprets part of a message, the parent can stress the misunderstood word or words to clarify the message. • Misunderstood words can be taken out of the context of the sentence for extra emphasis and then put back in for a final complete model. "Put the banana on the <u>table</u>." "the <u>table</u>" "Put the banana on the <u>table</u>." "Put your backpack in the <u>room</u>." "the <u>room</u>" "Put your backpack in the <u>room</u>."

OBJECTIVE: Parent Will Use Prosodic Features Prominently.

How the Teacher Helps	What the Parent Does at Home

The prosodic features of our language mark the emotional and attitudinal features of speech and aid in its comprehension. These features should be used prominently in the speech directed to the hearing-impaired child.
 	
● The evidence is that prosodic features are instrumental in early language acquisition.
 	
● Parents of young children use prosodic features prominently.
 	
● The teacher can remind the parent of the prosodic features:
   pitch
   stress
   duration
   intensity
 	
● The teacher can review with the parent how these features affect the meaning of a message.
	Parent will use pitch:
	   – to indicate a question
	   – to indicate a statement
	   – to indicate that she is finished with her turn
	   – to indicate a command or directive
	
	Parent will use stress:
	   – to emphasize important words
	   – to emphasize the thoughts that are important to her
	
	Parent will use duration:
	   – when calling someone's name
	   – to indicate excitement or an exclamation
	
	Parent will use intensity:
	   – to indicate her emotional state

OBJECTIVE: Parent Will Mark Emotional And Attitudinal Aspects Of Her Utterance By Stress, Intensity And Other Intonation Devices.

How the Teacher Helps	What the Parent Does at Home
The hearing-impaired child needs to hear attitudes and emotions expressed honestly and marked appropriately with intonation. • The teacher can caution the parent against giving mixed messages to the child in which the words don't fit the intonation. For example, at the grocery store, Mother says in a rather casual tone, "Don't do that," instead of in the firm, authoritative tone that would convey its true meaning. • The prosodic features of speech are the primary means by which a speaker expresses meaning. • Speakers organize speech into units, and mark them with prosody, i.e., sentence as declarative, interrogative and exclamatory; phrases with pauses, etc.	The parent needs to mark those thoughts and feelings that are important to her and important for her to communicate to her child by using stress and intensity. I love you so-o-o-o-o-o much. That makes me so-o-o-o-o-o angry. DON'T do that AGAIN!! Come in the house NOW! You are driving me cra-a-a-azy! GO to your ROOM! Are YOU ready to go? Will you PLEASE help me? I need all the BLUE beads. After you eat lunch, (pause) we'll go for a walk.

OBJECTIVE: **Parent Will Use Proper Intonational Terminals To Mark Questions, Statements, And Commands.**

How the Teacher Helps	What the Parent Does at Home
Hearing-impaired children need to have appropriate experiences with different sentence types. There is much valuable information carried in the different intonational contours. • Prosodic features of intonation are very early language skills for a child. If his language has few intonation terminals the intervener needs to go back to see what mother is doing in her talking <u>to</u> and with her child. • Intervener may tape record mother talking to her child telling a story or just interacting. Did the mother use a variety of sentence types? Were they marked with appropriate intonational contours? • Another way the teacher can assess the parent's language to the child is to take a "language sample" on the parent and then evaluate it for the number of different types of sentences the parent has used. If the parent uses a disproportionate number of questions or statements or commands, the teacher can point this out to the parent. • The assignment for the week would be for the parent to try to include more questions, for example, in her natural language situations with her child or to include a rising intonational contour when appropriate when asking questions. (continued)	Parent should be aware of utilizing statements, questions and exclamations in daily activities. • Input has intonation terminals. Parent should be alert to perceiving this in child's utterances. This helps the parent decipher the child's speech. <u>When Playing:</u> • How parents utilize statements: "Johnny is pushing the truck." "The truck is going up the hill." "The truck is full of dirt." • How parents utilize questions: "Do you want more dirt in the truck?" "Is the truck full?" "Is the dirt pile high enough?" • How parents utilize exclamations: "Wow! Look at that dirt pile!" "Look out! The truck is tipping over " "Oops! The dirt is all over your shoes!" <u>When Dressing</u> • How parents utilize statements: "Johnny is putting on his shirt." "I washed your favorite jeans." "Your shirt is in the top drawer." • "How parents utilize questions: "What do you want to wear?" "Do you like that shirt?" "Is that shirt warm enough?" (continued)

OBJECTIVE: Parent Will Use Proper Intonational Terminals To Mark Questions, Statements, And Commands. (cont'd)

How the Teacher Helps	What the Parent Does at Home
• If the parent's language sample points out that she is using a good variety of sentence types, then she should be encouraged to keep up the good work.	• How parents utilize exclamations: "Look out! You're tearing your shirt!"

Recommended Readings
for Parents

Beck, Joan. (1983). *Best Beginnings. Giving Your Child A Head Start In Life.* New York: Putnam.

Braga, J. and Laurie. (1976). *Children and Adults.* Englewood Cliffs, NJ: Prentice-Hall, Inc.

Brazelton, T. Berry. (1969). *Infants and Mothers, Differences in Development.* New York: Dell Publishing Company.

Brazelton, T. Berry. (1974). *Toddlers and Parents.* New York: Delacorte Press.

Brazelton, T. Berry. (1987). *What Every Baby Knows.* Reading, MA: Addison Wesley.

Burtt, Kent and Kalkstein, Karen. (1981). *Smart Toys for Babies.* New York: Harper Books.

Bush, Richard. (1980). *A Parent's Guide to Child Therapy.* New York: Delacorte Press.

Butler, Dorothy. (1982). *Babies Need Books: How to Share the Joy of Reading with Your Child.* New York: Penguin Books.

Callahan, Sidney and Cornelia. (1974). *Parenting: Principles and Politics of Parenthood.* New York: Penguin Books.

Caplan, Frank, Ed. (1977). *The First Twelve Months of Life.* New York: Grosset and Dunlap.

Caplan, Frank and Theresa. (1977). *The Second Twelve Months of Life.* New York: Grossett and Dunlap.

Chase, R.A., Rubin, R.R., Eds. (1979). *The First Wondrous Year.* New York: Johnson and Johnson Child Development Publications, Collier Books.

Church, Joseph. (1973) *Understanding Your Child from Birth to Three: A Guide to Your Child's Psychological Development.* New York: Random House.

Fallows, Deborah. (1985). *A Mother's Work.* New York: Houghton Mifflin.

Frailberg, Selma. (1959). *The Magic Years.* New York: Scribner and Sons.

Friedland, R. and Kort, C. (1981). *The Mother's Book.* New York: Houghton-Mifflin.

Glickman, Beatrice, Marden & Springer. *Who Cares for the Baby?* New York: Schocken Books (Random House).

Jones, Sandy. (1976). *Good Things for Babies.* New York: Houghton Mifflin.

Maynard, Fredelle. (1985). *The Child Care Crisis.* New York: Viking Books.

Pulaski, Mary Ann Spencer. (1978). *Your Baby's Mind and How It Grows.* New York: Harper and Row.

Robertson, James and Joyce. (1982) *A Baby in the Family.* New York: Penguin Books.

Spock, B. (1976). *Baby and Child Care.* New York: Pocketbooks.

Stallibrass, Alison. (1977). *The Self-Respecting Child.* New York: Pelican Books.

White, Burton L. (1980). *A Parent's Guide to the First Three Years.* Englewood Cliffs, NJ: Prentice-Hall, Inc.

White, Burton L. (1987). *Educating the Infant and Toddler.* Lexington, MA: Lexington Books.